Guide to Patient Evaluation

THIRD EDITION

HISTORY TAKING, PHYSICAL EXAMINATION AND THE PROBLEM-ORIENTED METHOD

By

JACQUES L. SHERMAN, JR., M.D., F.A.C.P.
Professor of Medicine
School of Medicine, Health Sciences Center
State University of New York at Stony Brook
Associate Chief of Staff for Education
Veterans Administration Hospital
Northport, New York

and

SYLVIA KLEIMAN FIELDS, R.N., Ed.D.
Associate Professor of Nursing
School of Nursing, Health Sciences Center
State University of New York at Stony Brook

MEDICAL EXAMINATION PUBLISHING Co., INC.
969 STEWART AVENUE   •   GARDEN CITY, N.Y. 11530

INTRODUCTION TO THE THIRD EDITION

The preparation of a third edition, just four years after the completion of the original text, has given us the opportunity to use many constructive suggestions. Some have come from our own use of the earlier editions in teaching and some have been provided by students, other faculty members, and colleagues. Many valuable ideas and critiques have been collected by our publisher who has received reviews from numerous educators throughout this country and Canada. They have helped to identify areas which were neglected, over-complex, or not optimally organized.

Modifications made in the second edition have been retained. These include the addition of a chapter on Examination of the Adolescent, contributed by Dr. Rita Wieczorek of the Columbia University School of Nursing; the Supplemental Exercises; the expanded section on Ocular Fundoscopy; and the more precise nomenclature of heart sounds.

Since the objective of this text remains the description of a sound, *basic* examination, we have minimized the amount of additional material, for expansion can be done almost without limit. The major addition in this edition is a complete chapter on Assessment of the Elderly. Our dental colleagues have contributed a much-needed expansion of the examination of the mouth, and material clarifying examination for lymph nodes has been added.

The nurse author has collaborated with a group of selected nurse educators on the development of programs in which patient assessment is an integral component of the undergraduate curriculum. This collaboration has provided the impetus for modification and rewording of some elements of history-taking. These changes should insure that the greatest users of this text, nursing students and practitioners, can readily apply this process to the nursing role in both traditional, secondary and tertiary care settings, as well as in primary care delivery sites. We believe this expansion, particularly related to the patterns of daily living, will be of value to other health professionals as well.

As we noted in the second edition, although color plates would be a great improvement, our determination to keep the cost of the book as low as possible prohibits their use.

We continue to emphasize that the student must turn to other texts for details of anatomy, physiology, psychology, and pathophysiology to develop competence, based on knowledge and understanding, in patient evaluation. Excellent skills can come only with continuous study and practice.

J.L.S., Jr.
S.K.F.

FOREWORD TO THE THIRD EDITION

I am pleased to once again write the foreword to a new edition of Sherman and Fields' Guide to Patient Evaluation. Since the second edition, the need for such a text has gained in significance. Increasingly, nursing education has been turning its attention toward inclusion of physical assessment at all levels: undergraduate, graduate, and lately, in its continuing education efforts. Approaches to the teaching of this skill are sorely needed as adjunctive tools for faculty, students, and in-service directors as they grapple with identification and integration of the added knowledge base required to develop competency in this skill.

In the present text, two significant additions have been included, involving examination of the mouth, along with the requisites for gerontological assessment. Both areas have sometimes been overlooked in teaching materials which purport to be concerned with total patient evaluation. These additions can only serve to give the guide even wider applicability.

Once again, I highly recommend Sherman and Fields to all engaged in nursing education, regardless of location, as a suitable and eminently usable adjunctive learning tool.

Ellen T. Fahy, R.N., Ed.D.
Dean and Professor
School of Nursing
State University of New York at Stony Brook

DEDICATION
THIS BOOK IS DEDICATED TO
OUR TEACHERS AND OUR STUDENTS.

CONTRIBUTORS

MILTON AGULNEK, M.D., F.A.A.P.

CAROLE BLAIR, R.N., M.A.

ORA JAMES BOUEY, R.N., M.A.

STEPHEN BRODSKY, M.D.

ARTHUR FRIEDLANDER, D.D.S.

VIRGINIA M. GLOVER, R.N., Ph.D.

STEVEN GOLDMAN, M.D.

LEON MANN, M.D., F.A.C.O.G.

LENORA McCLEAN, R.N., Ed.D.

DOROTHY POPKIN, R.N., M.S.

BERNARD POTTER, M.D.

HELEN PURELLO, R.N., M.S.

ROSE RICHMOND, R.N., M.A.

BARBARA-JANE SINNI, R.N., B.S.

RITA WIECZOREK, R.N., Ed.D.

INTRODUCTION TO THE FIRST EDITION

This textbook grew out of the authors' recognition of the need for a guide for teaching the elements of a history and physical examination for the Nurse Clinician, the Nurse Practitioner, the Physician Assistant and other intermediate health care professionals. The standard textbooks of Physical Diagnosis are designed for medical students whose three- or four-year curriculum will be more extensive in the fields of anatomy, physiology and pathology. The medical student is required to collect a somewhat larger data base and to expand the techniques of physical diagnosis as he spends several years of study and practice in clinical medicine.

Recognizing these differences, the authors have designed this text specifically for the non-medical student. The material included here will enable the student to learn to elicit a sound medical history and to perform a comprehensive physical examination which is equivalent to that done by a competent clinical clerk (see Appendix I).This thesis has been proven many times over in our experience.

The text is based upon the physician author's design of courses for Registered Nurses and Physician's Associates at the Northport Veterans Hospital and the Health Sciences Center, State University of New York at Stony Brook. This design has been modified and improved upon with the assistance of Dr. Stephen Brodsky through the presentation of six courses of instruction. The co-author and her colleagues, who were academically and clinically prepared through this program, have also modified the basic design in developing a successful curriculum in which patient evaluation has become an integral component of the baccalaureate program in nursing at Stony Brook.

This is not a "do-it-yourself" textbook; it has been designed and organized to be used in conjunction with a classroom instructor or with a preceptor. While some techniques are described in detail, it is not expected that the student can learn to perform an adequate examination without assistance and supervision.

Although pertinent points of anatomy and physiology are presented to enable the student to understand the principles underlying a satisfactory physical examination, it is suggested that the reader review standard textbooks of anatomy and physiology. The more the student knows about these subjects and the more information he has about psychic and somatic disease, the better will be his performance.

To this end we have included a few descriptions and illustrations of abnormal findings, although the major emphasis of the text is on the principles and techniques of the history and the examination. We expect the student to be able to recognize and to describe deviations from the normal well enough so that they can be identified by a more experienced practitioner. We further expect that the student will understand that the ability to conduct an excellent history-taking and physical examination is a matter of continuous learning and practice.

In this text we have used the metric system throughout, despite the fact that there are many convenient expressions in the "foot-pound" system. The national commitment to the metric system is clear and we encourage students to use it from the beginning.

A word about sex and language may be in order. We have used the pronoun "he" throughout the text to signify the patient and the examiner except in specific situations where examination of the female breast and genitalia are described. The use of the awkward "he/she" pronoun form or the untried "ter" was felt to be unnecessary. The interests of simplicity and linguistic habits in this textbook override our clear recognition of the fact that many examiners and patients are women.

As noted earlier, there are many excellent textbooks on patient evaluation. The student is encouraged to become familiar with some of these and to use them as references. The fact that somewhat different techniques, emphases, sequences, or approaches will be found should not be a source of confusion. The assessment of a patient's problem is not a mathematical science but rather an art — with rules — made up of various practices and skills. The general references given at the end of the text are selected for their value as supplements to this textbook. There are others of equal value which the student may use with profit.

At the end of each chapter which describes specific examination techniques there is a suggested outline for recording normal findings. These are collected in Appendix I which is a model write-up of the full normal physical examination.

Following this, in some chapters, a brief "patient problem" is presented in the form of a problem-oriented note. This illustrates the way in which pertinent data may be selected from the total data base and put together for an analysis of one of the problems which the patient may have. We do not intend to imply, however, that the actions recommended should necessarily be considered directions for practice.

Our goal is to present a patient-based program for the student's guidance. It stresses the concepts expressed by Sir William Osler in an address, reported in 1903 by *Medical News:* "In what may be called the natural method of teaching, the student begins with the patient, continues with the patient, and ends his studies with the patient, using books and lectures as tools, as means to an end . . . . The whole art of medicine is in observation, as the old motto goes, but to educate the eye to see, the ear to hear and the finger to feel takes time, and to make a beginning, to start a man on the right path, is all that we can do."

We should like to express our acknowledgments to the many persons who assisted us in the preparation of this book. The list is long and includes colleagues, students, secretaries, artists, photographers, models, patients, and friends. To each of these we are deeply grateful. We should also like to express our gratitude to Dr. Harry Fritts, Jr., Chairman, Department of Medicine, for his review and critique of the manuscript, and to Dr. Ellen T. Fahy, Dean of the School of Nursing, for her motivating spirit and continual support. Our special thanks are offered to our families, whose contributions of patience, encouragement and understanding have been essential. We are greatly indebted to Mrs. Harriette Sherman, who, with the force of righteousness as her sword and the Oxford English Dictionary as her shield, attempted to defend the integrity of the English language throughout.

September 20, 1973

J.L.S., Jr.
S.K.F.

FOREWORD TO THE FIRST EDITION

Historians of twentieth-century medicine will easily be overwhelmed by the breakthroughs and technological wonders wrought by the fruitful marriage in our era of medicine and experimental science. They may easily overlook some of our more human and equally difficult accomplishments in the organization and delivery of health care. One of these most surely is the emergence of the team concept and the sharing of clinical functions, formerly the sole province of the physician, by a variety of other health professionals.

To respond adequately to the social mandate to make health care available on an equitable basis for all, we must begin to make genuine progress toward the optimal use of all health manpower. In that endeavor, medicine and all the other health professions will undergo a redefinition of their roles and functions within new models of health care teams. The social utility of team care which will emerge may well come to rival our brightest technological triumphs.

If this is to happen, we must encourage the sharing of a common language among all who engage in clinical care of patients, enabling them to communicate with each other, as well as to exchange and share certain functions which the needs of patients may dictate. The ancient arts and techniques of history taking and physical examination constitute the most basic common language. A first step in building an effective health team is fuller sharing of the responsibilities for collecting clinical data about the patient. Educators and practitioners now appreciate that future team members should be taught together if they are later to share some of their functions and to understand their own contributions more clearly. One of the most feasible and effective methods of interdisciplinary education is to teach the elements of pathophysiology and the detection of abnormal states by history and physical findings. Students in all the health professions can easily share this knowledge, which enhances the capacity of each to contribute to the assessment of the totality of the patient's needs.

Sherman and Fields' book is, therefore, a timely effort, consciously intended to introduce the essentials of history taking and physical examination to those who work most closely with the physician — physician's assistants and nurse-practitioners. It is based on the authors' experiences in teaching this subject and in making use of its principles in an experimental model of team care in operation at the Northport Veterans Administration Hospital.

The book, as the authors point out, is not a replication of standard texts of physical diagnosis. The number of these abounds, and scarce justification can be found for producing yet another. Rather, the authors have aimed at a special category of new health professionals and their special requirements for these skills as members of a co-ordinated team. The same material will be valuable for the pharmacist, the dentist, and other health professionals as they too become less isolated from the mainstreams of medical and health care.

Sherman and Fields' manual will facilitate cooperation among health professionals by introducing nurses, physician's assistants, and others to the acquisition of a common set of terms, techniques, and criteria. The collection of clinical data about the patient by the time-tested methods of history taking and physical examination will be improved thereby. This book meets an urgent present need and it will surely be followed by others.

Edmund D. Pellegrino, M.D., F.A.C.P.
Vice-President for Health Sciences
Director, Health Sciences Center, and
Professor of Medicine
Health Sciences Center
State University of New York at Stony Brook

September 20, 1973

GUIDE TO PATIENT EVALUATION

Third Edition

CONTENTS

CHAPTER 1

PROBLEM ORIENTATION

INTRODUCTION

The concept and method for implementation of problem-oriented medical records (POMR)* were developed several years ago by Dr. Lawrence Weed to bring a logical system into the recording of information, opinions, and plans related to a patient's problems. The organization of the POMR is based upon the scientific method and is designed for problem solving and for preserving the logic used in arriving at solutions. Its primary purpose is to provide a method for communication among those responsible for providing health care.

Although this textbook is concerned with the techniques of history-taking and the physical examination, it is valuable to understand the context in which the history and physical are used in the records of the health care process.

The POMR serves well, in our opinion, as a framework into which the initial history and physical can be inserted. An understanding of the process of problem orientation can also clarify the reasons for checking and repeating elements of the history and/or the physical examination. The recording method also serves to maintain the integrity of initial plans and as a method for evaluation of management and of educational programs.

This brief outline of the POMR serves as only an introduction to the concept; the technique of development of the POMR is described only superficially, and many important features are not included. Nonetheless, the student may gain an idea of the way in which such a system may help to organize his thinking in the process of patient evaluation. The system has undergone modification since Weed first introduced the concept, and various agencies and institutions have adapted the system to their individualized needs. A major advantage of the POMR is its flexibility and adaptability.

The problem-oriented medical record is a tool to aid in the management of the patient's problems - not "nursing" or "medical" problems - and it organizes these problems for assessment, management, and evaluation. All of this also leads to another advantage of the system - it is ideal for teaching. Schools of Medicine, Nursing,

---

* - Often referred to as Problem Oriented Record (POR), or (POS) Problem Oriented System.

and Allied Health Professions have readily identified these additional benefits and encourage its implementation in locations where
students are having clinical learning experiences.

The concept of the POMR is simple; data must be presented in a
form that makes sense for problem solving. The POMR identifies
all of the patient's problems and provides a uniform system of recording, so that anyone who deals with the patient can use the record. It reflects the plans for management of the whole patient and
his problems - holistic patient care.

No diagnostic or therapeutic regimen is sufficient unless complete
and properly expedited. No method of communication is of value
if the information is inaccurate, incomplete, or illegible. A problem oriented record openly displays thoroughness or sloppiness in
record-keeping or in patient care. It can help in management of a
single problem or of the whole patient, but it cannot perform this
management.

METHOD

The system includes four basic components for a POMR:

1. Data Base: The record of the patient's history, physical
   examination, and laboratory reports.

2. Problem List: A list of the patient's identified problems
   which require a separate plan for management.

3. Plans: A written plan for each major problem identified,
   including the writer's own assessment of the factors involved and processes occurring, with recommended further
   studies, treatment, and patient education.

4. Action Phase: The records of implementation of plans and
   of the patient's progress. These include orders (diagnostic
   and therapeutic), consultations, records of additional information from history, or further physical examination,
   and records of the monitoring of the patient's response to
   treatment.

All of these actions generate and record new data which modify the
data base and lead to continued re-evaluation of the Problem List,
etc.

These components are represented in the following flow diagram
which reflects the "closed loop" nature of the system:

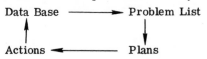

Although this formulation is somewhat different from Weed's description, it represents a system of chart recording which follows the pattern of logical thinking by the clinician in problem solving - the object of Weed's system.

THE DATA BASE: This information is initially collected in the usual way and recorded in standard format for the Medical History and the Physical Examination. The Data Base also contains important historical data from previous medical records, any immediately available laboratory values, and observations such as the color of urine, character of vomitus, etc. Additional data obtained during the patient's course are recorded in problem-oriented progress notes.

The Data Base should be well defined so that any practitioner will gather the same basic information. A complete Data Base should contain:

1. The chief complaint or reason for contact
2. History of present illness(es) or patient's perception of current health status if there is no illness present
3. Past health history
4. A logically arranged review of systems
5. Family health history
6. Personal/social history
7. Patient profile
8. Complete physical examination, and
9. Results of initial laboratory tests

Each of these elements of the Data Base will be described in the chapters to follow.

The initial collection of the Data Base should be as thorough as the patient's comfort and physical condition will allow. Uniformity and thoroughness of Data Base will enable easier assessment of the patient's problems, course of treatment, and need for education.

THE PROBLEM LIST: No better description can be given to the Problem List than Dr. Weed's: it is a "table of contents" and an "index" to the patient's problems. The precision and skill with which the patient will be managed may often depend upon the precision and skill with which the patient's problems are defined.

A "problem" is defined as any significant deviation that has influenced, is now influencing, or may influence the patient's state of health or his ability to function normally. It may be of medical, of psychiatric, or of social significance. This is not a very precise definition, and titles will not always be the same in the hands of different clinicians, but that is a minor deficiency compared to the benefits to be derived from such an index.

The Problem List will contain two types of problems: "active" and "inactive" (or, "resolved"). An active problem is any major or significant problem which is presently affecting the patient, e.g., diabetes, schizophrenia, blindness, unemployment, rectal bleeding. An inactive (or resolved) problem is any past problem of major significance which is NOT presently affecting the patient, e.g., an appendectomy, history of pneumonia, a fracture which healed without sequelae. The words "major" and "significant" are critical, for if every hangnail, childhood disease, and upper respiratory infection are recorded, the Problem List could become pages long and thereby lose its effectiveness.

It is apparent from the above that problems are not necessarily diagnoses. In fact, the initial entry on a Problem List is quite often a sign, a symptom, or a syndrome, but is not a diagnostic possibility or "rule out." The problem entered is the most specific that is possible at the time - one defines the problem in terms of exactly what he knows about it - no more and no less. The following list illustrates various classes of problems:

1. A proven diagnosis - e.g., emphysema
2. A physiologic entity - e.g., congestive heart failure
3. A syndrome - e.g., hyperventilation
4. A sign - e.g., hepatomegaly
5. A symptom - e.g., chest pain
6. An abnormal lab value - e.g., elevated alkaline phosphatase
7. An allergy, including drug sensitivities (this should always be an active problem) - e.g., anaphylaxis to penicillin
8. An operation - e.g., subtotal gastrectomy
9. A risk factor - e.g., 2 packs per day smoker
10. A psychological problem - e.g., depression
11. A social problem - e.g., unemployment

The practitioner enters problems at his level of understanding. For example, patient Z gives a history of myocardial infarction in 1969 and angina since 1970. Practitioner A may list two separate problems: #1 - Myocardial Infarction, 1969; #2 - Angina Pectoris, 1970. Practitioner B may list one problem: #1 - Arteriosclerotic Heart Disease, 1969. Both are correct; the latter merely indicates an understanding that the infarction and the angina are part of the same disease entity. However simple or complex, the Problem List must contain only factual data, not speculations.

Since both the patient and his disease are subject to change, the Problem List must also be dynamic and expected to change as well. As more information is gathered, some of the problems listed initially may turn out to be parts of a single problem, and the Problem List will reflect this modification. Changes indicate that thinking is going on, not necessarily that the clinician has made errors. For example, when several problems turn out to be separate manifestations of a single problem, the Problem List is modified. If problems

Arthritis and Pericarditis are later recognized as being due to
Lupus, then the two entries are eliminated as separate problems,
and a new problem, Lupus, is entered on the Problem List.

As problems are clarified, altered or further delineated, the original Problem List is modified accordingly. This modification is
accomplished not by erasure, but by inserting an arrow, followed
by the new diagnosis or by noting "dropped," "resolved," or "inactive." All of these changes should be dated and initialed.

Although the techniques used for modifying the Problem List vary
from place to place, one principle is constant - keep the Problem
List up to date.

Minor episodes may arise in the course of a patient's illness which
the practitioner may hesitate to define immediately as a significant
problem on the Problem List. This should be recorded in a progress note and titled "Temporary Problem." If it is subsequently
decided that the problem is significant, it is then entered on the
Problem List. If not, a note on the progress sheet should indicate
that it is a transient episode of little significance. An example
might be a brief episode of "constipation probably due to inability
to use the bedpan."

A hypothetical Problem List which might appear on the face sheet of
a hospital record will demonstrate its value as an index to the record (see sample of hospital record face sheet on the following
page).

At a glance it can be seen that on June 28th the practitioner dealt
with the initial medical problems of cough, fever, hyperglycemia
and the social problem of unemployment. Three days after admission, problems 1 and 2 were judged to be the single problem of
pneumonia which was then considered resolved 8 days after admission. Problem 3 presented as the laboratory finding of hyperglycemia, and on the 16th hospital day was refined to the problem of
diabetes mellitus.

From this "table of contents" a reviewer cannot tell on what basis
problems 1 and 2 were made into the single problem of pneumonia,
or why it took 3 days to make that judgment - but he knows that a
progress note entitled Pneumonia should have been written on
7/1/73 which should explain the situation. That progress note should
have all of the pertinent data, the practitioner's reasoning, and a
plan for therapy and patient education on the problem of pneumonia.
The reviewer should not need to look through the laboratory slips,
the x-ray slips, nurses' notes, etc. in order to find the story.

Problem Number	Approx. Date of Onset	Date Problem Recorded	Active Problems	Inactive/ Resolved Problems	Date Resolved
1	6/24/73	6/28/73 7/1/73	Cough Pneu- monia		7/6/73
2	6/24/73	6/28/73 7/1/73	Fever Pneu- monia		7/6/73
3	Unknown	6/28/73 7/14/73	Hyper- glycemia Diabetes mellitus		
4		6/28/73		Subtotal gastrec- tomy	8/ 1963
5	4/30/73	6/28/73	Unem- ployed		
6		6/28/73		Appen- dectomy	1938

DOE, John M
SS# 123-45-6789
D.O.B. 1/12/1920
Admitted 6/28/1973

University Hospital, HSC, Stony Brook, N.Y.

Similarly, the reviewer might with to know why the problem of hyperglycemia took over two weeks to resolve. He might be interested to find out about the impact of unemployment or the subtotal
gastrectomy on the patient's current status.

From this brief view of the problem list it may be evident that problem
orientation of the medical record can serve as a useful teaching tool
and as a method for audit of the patient care process. Whether this
method will improve patient care itself is a matter for resolution in
the future.

THE INITIAL PLAN: In a problem oriented medical record, significant problems will be discussed in terms of a plan designed to resolve that problem. Prior to determination of the plan, a summary
of pertinent data is noted and an assessment of the situation established, which should reflect the practitioner's thinking about the

problem. The format which is used later for progress notes, includes the number and problem title and follows the "SOAP"
outline:

S - Subjective - pertinent complaints, observations and past
history elicited from the patient, his family, or his previous records related to a specific problem.

O - Objective - current physical findings and laboratory data
collected by practitioner.

A - Assessment - analysis and synthesis of the data; interpretation and evaluation of the problem, the data, possible
implications, and the prognosis. This is the place for
opinions, guesses, and "rule-outs."

P - Plan - diagnostic studies, therapeutic regimen, and patient
education.

The plan is organized into these three sections - diagnostic, therapeutic, and patient education - in which the clinician will outline
his program of further management. Under patient education, a
statement is made as to what the patient has been told about his
disease, i.e., possible course, and what he should know and understand about his medications and therapy and self-care for his own
benefit in the future. It may indicate collaboration with other health
personnel or the patient's family.

It is important to note here that a plan is generally formulated for
each active problem on the problem list, with the corresponding
number of the problem on the list. If no actions are considered
necessary, this should be specified.

After an initial plan has been written, subsequent modifications of
the plan are incorporated into the progress notes.

ACTION PHASE: As stated earlier, these are records of the actions
taken for resolution of the patient's problems.

Orders should be organized and titled. The first set of orders should
be titled "General" and include such items as medication for pain,
position (e.g., ambulatory), vital signs, etc. All other orders
should appear under separate headings corresponding to a problem
on the Problem List. This organization helps the practitioner to
group orders related to one problem and assists other health personnel in their understanding of the program for the patient.

Progress notes are always dated and include the number and problem title for each note, as well as information about the specific
problem. The information then follows the SOAP outline.

Properly titled and organized progress notes will enable any practitioner to read all data regarding a single problem by locating
those numbered and titled entries, without having to search through
information pertaining to other problems. Communications are
thus simplified and are more clearly defined than the traditional
entries in which several problems may be cited in a single
paragraph.

All data, however, do not have to be recorded in narrative form.
As part of the progress record, data essential to the patient's problems which require frequent monitoring may be recorded on a flow
sheet. Flow sheets similar to the graphic chart used to record
vital signs can be designed for individual situations, e.g., diabetes,
post partum, renal dialysis, hypertension, etc. The flow sheet
may include space for a variety of entries, such as medications ad-
ministered, significant lab test results, vital signs, intake and output, all correlated and coordinated for the evaluation of treatment
regimens for individual patients and their problems. If flow sheets
are used for complicated problems, an entry under "objective" in
the progress note may simply state, "see flow sheet."

There is a place in the progress note for general information, e.g.,
"constipation has been relieved" or "patient's morale is greatly improved" - items which may not relate to a major problem. Such
entries are perfectly acceptable and should appear under the heading
"General."

Individual institutions may elect to maintain separate consultation
sheets; however, these notes should preferably be in the same format as for Progress Notes (SOAP).

EVALUATION

The POMR has been in use on a limited scale for only a few years,
but its advantages are so great that year by year more schools,
clinics, offices, and hospitals are adopting the system. It has
proven to be an excellent teaching device; it allows for better audit
of the patient's record; it tends to emphasize data rather than memory; and, of very great importance, it serves as a superb tool for
communication among members of a health care delivery team.

At the end of each of several chapters of this textbook, a sample
problem oriented progress note is included to illustrate the method.
Note that only items considered pertinent to the problem under discussion are included. This selection of data is a matter of judgment,
subject to review, to discussion, and to differences of opinion, all of
which are of use to the patient and to the teaching process.

SUPPLEMENTAL EXERCISES

1. Select a common disease entity from a standard textbook of Medicine or Surgery and rewrite the pertinent items into problem oriented (SOAP) format.

2. Review the chart of a patient written in standard form. Attempt to reorganize it into a Problem Oriented Record. Make a Problem List. See if you can identify the plans and specifically describe the recommended actions. Write the "orders" according to the "problem" they appear to accompany. Abstract the physicians' progress notes and the nurses' notes as well as any other professional inclusions and put them together on one progress form according to historical sequence rather than by practitioner. Use the SOAP form. Develop a flow sheet for all the observations and essential clinical data accumulated. Alter the problem list as indicated. Write a discharge summary according to SOAP format for each problem.

   Compare your two records. Can you evaluate the effectiveness of plans and actions for audit in both records? Ask a colleague to audit for you.

REFERENCES

1. Weed, L.L.: Medical Records, Medical Education and Patient Care: The Problem-Oriented Record as a Basic Tool. Case Western Reserve University Press, Cleveland, 1969.

2. Hurst, J.W. and Walker, H.K.: The Problem Oriented System. Medcom Press, New York, 1972.

3. National League for Nursing. Problem Oriented Systems of Patient Care. New York: NLN, Papers presented at the 1973-74 Workshop Department of Home Health Agencies and Community Health Services. Pub. No. 21-1522, 1974.

4. Wooley, F.R. et al.: Problem Oriented Nursing. Springer Publishing Co., New York, 1974.

5. Sherman, J.L. Jr. and Fields, S.K.: Series on Health Asessment Techniques: Problem Oriented Medical Record, Multimedia Program. Westinghouse Learning Corporation, New York, 1974.

6. Walter, J.B., Pardee, G.P., and Molbo, D.M.: Dynamics of Problem-Oriented Approaches: Patient Care and Documentation. J.B. Lippincott Co., Philadelphia, 1976.

7. Bentz, P.M. and Niland, M.B.: A Problem-Oriented Approach to Planning Nursing Care. Nursing Clin. North America 9: 235, 1974.

CHAPTER 2

THE PROCESS OF INTERVIEWING

INTRODUCTION

The development of a complete and accurate data base is essential
for conducting a successful health assessment of an individual. It
is from this base that one begins to identify specific health problems, as well as the appropriate treatment plan. Much of the desired completeness and accuracy of the first portion of the data
base - the health history - is dependent upon the examiner's ability
to set up an effective communication system with the patient. The
interview is the first step in this process.

Successful interviewing requires that several specific objectives be
kept firmly in mind and that these objectives be reached as rapidly
as possible:

1. to establish between the patient and the practitioner a working relationship which is necessary for proper diagnosis and
   treatment

2. to obtain accurate information about the patient's medical
   and emotional state of health; and

3. to give the patient an understanding of his illness and to support him through the period of treatment and follow-up

The patient interview and the taking of the initial health history come
first in evaluation because they are the most important tools in establishing the patient's problems and diagnoses. Well over half the
problems presented in the general health clinics are psychogenic in
origin and may be diagnosed by establishing adequate rapport and obtaining a careful medical history.

DYNAMIC INTERVIEWING

When people are faced with health problems, they experience a wide
range of reactions. In addition to the impact of the diagnosis itself,
these reactions are determined in part by age, sex, personality, and
cultural, social, and economic circumstances. These facets of the
patient's life need to be considered when conducting a health assessment, for understanding them provides the key to an accurate interpretation of both the verbal and nonverbal communications of the
patient.

The patient who seeks medical assistance frequently experiences fear and anxiety, because the impact of the health problem on his present and future is uncertain. Even if these fears or emotional responses are not founded in reality, it is still necessary for the examiner to know to what extent they exist in the mind of the patient, so that distortions or misconceptions can be corrected or eliminated. Even though it may differ from that of the clinician, the patient's perception of reality must always be respected.

It is essential that the clinician be in tune with the feelings of the patient from the earliest moments of the professional contact, so that he may encourage the expression of these feelings and follow up with appropriate and consistent support throughout the entire period of health care. The health professional must have a strong grasp of the principles of human behavior and an appreciation of the psychosocial forces that affect the patient's life.

First, and foremost, the practitioner must develop his sense of caring. There is, perhaps, no better general advice on this subject in the world's literature than the essay entitled "The Care of the Patient" by Francis Peabody. The concluding sentence reads, "One of the essential qualities of the clinician is interest in humanity, for the secret of the care of the patient is in caring for the patient." This article should be read in its entirety by all involved in patient care.

Through his teachers and through experience, the practitioner will develop certain verbal skills and techniques. In addition, however, he must cultivate the ability to respond to an individual with warmth, concern, and support. Occasionally, a patient is embarrassed or has difficulty in expressing certain thoughts or ideas. Quick recognition of this problem may enable the interviewer to assist the patient. Simple verbal acknowledgement of the patient's difficulty is frequently supportive and may retain or strengthen rapport.

GENERAL TECHNIQUES

Although each professional functions in accordance with his own unique characteristics and patterns of behavior, effective communication channels can best be established with the patient when certain principles and techniques are understood. These general guidelines must always be modified to suit the specific situation, but they do apply in most practitioner-patient relationships.

PRIVACY: The place selected for the initial interview and subsequent contacts should always assure the maximum possible privacy for the patient. Unnecessary interruptions or noise should be avoided and every effort expended to focus on the patient and his concerns.

IDENTIFICATION: The position of the interviewer in the health care delivery team should be made clear to the patient at the outset. The

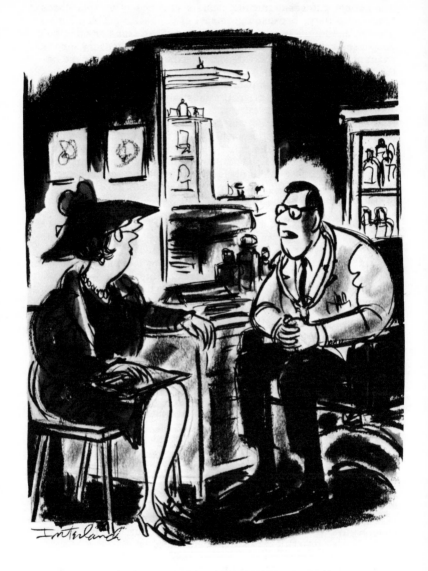

"Frankly, Mrs. Powers, 'like hell' isn't much of a symptom."

patient has initiated the interview by seeking help, and he is entitled
to know with whom he is dealing. If the interviewer is a student, it
is often useful to have him introduced by name to the patient by a
more senior member of the team; but, in all cases, it is important
to present the interviewer to the patient for what he is - student,
nurse practitioner, physician's assistant, or physician.

LISTENING TO THE PATIENT: This sounds simple, obvious, and
unnecessary to say, but is, in fact, none of these. Imagine for a
moment the following exchange:

> Interviewer: Now, Mr. Blank, tell me just what happens when
> you walk for several blocks during the cold weather. Do you
> get chest pains in that situation?
>
> Patient: Yes.
>
> Interviewer: Now, Mr. Blank, tell me about the type of chest
> pain which develops. Is it a sharp pain, or is it heavy, with
> some shortness of breath?
>
> Patient: Er--would you repeat that, please?

Note that the patient has 100% of the desired information, but it is
the interviewer who has been talking for 90% of the time. This
method of interviewing - direct questioning - which requires a yes
or no answer - is more useful after the general story has been told
by the patient.

LISTENING WITHOUT BIAS: It is extremely important to listen to
all of the patient's history before coming to a judgment. Premature
conclusions, or "snap diagnoses," triggered by some aspect of the
story, may turn off the clinician's thoughtful perceptions of what the
patient is saying or cause the examiner to cut off the patient's flow
of information. Dangerous prejudgment must be forcefully and deliberately resisted.

LISTENING TO EVERYTHING: Listen to what the patient is saying,
even though it does not come in the order in which you want the information or in which you will record it. The next chapters will
outline the preferred form for reporting a history. Make very brief
notes as the patient is talking, but make no attempt to fit the patient's story into your format. Later, when you wish to verify a
point or a time relationship, clarification will be given freely by the
patient who is pleased that you have listened. There are few things
so frustrating and annoying to the patient as having an examiner ask
a question which shows that he wasn't listening when the patient explained that particular point. The clear implication of not listening
is lack of interest.

As much as possible, it is the interviewer's task to get the patient talking and, as long as he is providing pertinent information, to keep him talking. Listen carefully, for these are the most important medical sounds you will ever hear - the sound of the patient trying as best as he can to tell you just what is wrong with him.

"Open-ended" dialogue is designed to get the maximum number of words per minute from the patient and a minimum from the examiner. The examiner's role is to keep the story going, to keep it from wandering too far afield, and to obtain necessary details. One can assist in keeping the story moving by short periods of silence or by use of cues such as "Yes?" or "Tell me more", or repeating the patient's last words. Before turning off the patient's story in order to get in some of your own words, remember that you have no information and the patient has all the information regarding his problems, so listen carefully before deciding that no further useful information is forthcoming.

CONSENSUAL VALIDATION: Each person uses familiar language to convey his needs, describe his complaints, and identify his problems. As patients tell their story to the interviewer, it is important that there is a mutual understanding of what is being said. Under stressful circumstances, the interviewer may sometimes accept what is being said by the patient but attribute meaning to an expression that the patient did not intend. For example, if a patient says he is "bothered by stiff joints," the interviewer should not record that the patient is "bothered by arthritis" until that diagnosis is made. So that the interviewer reports what the patient says and only what the patient says, it is helpful to summarize what the patient has said periodically during the interview and ask for the patient's agreement. For example: "Now as I understand it, you said you have had stiff and swollen joints in your legs and feet for eight days. Is that correct?" Then the patient has the opportunity to validate these data as being correct or in error.

NON-VERBAL COMMUNICATION: The student must continually remind himself of the great importance of non-verbal forms of communication in the establishment of rapport and in transmitting information. These non-verbal methods are a part of our normal communication and will be used naturally by both the examiner and the patient. Discipline over the use of certain words and phrases is often readily learned by the interviewer, but failure to learn control over non-verbal situations or actions can effectively prevent the establishment of rapport or the obtaining of information. For example, dirty fingernails may "turn off" a patient within moments of the introduction, as may an inappropriate smile when the patient expresses fear of cancer over an insignificant skin blemish.

Proper understanding of non-verbal signs can be used positively to encourage the patient to continue a story, to assure him of your interest, to shift to another subject, to comfort him, to relieve some of his anxieties, etc. Watching the patient's use of non-verbal signs may assist in obtaining information, both at this point and later on during the physical examination.

THE "THIRD EAR": There is another aspect of receiving communications which is commonly referred to as "listening with the third ear." This means that the interviewer pays close attention not only to the words, per se, but also the way in which they are expressed. Changes in the quality of the voice, such as its tone and loudness, may be clues to the importance of what is being said. Facial expressions, body movements, hand positions, and nervous mannerisms are non-verbal signs which modify the words being spoken. In addition, the "third ear" listens to what is not said. Important omissions, vagueness, evasiveness, and sudden changes in the subject are all methods for avoiding expression of thoughts which are sensitive or disturbing to the patient.

APHORISMS

There are a few other guidelines which are important in the medical interview process. These may be briefly stated:

1. Never express surprise or judgment at the patient's statements. You are a data collector and a health professional, not a judge.

2. Always express interest and concern for the patient's problems. The patient's problems are the basis for your profession.

3. Remember that there is no adequate way to measure pain other than the taking of a careful history by requesting specific descriptions from the patient.

4. Try to like your patient. He will recognize your sincerity and become a more willing partner. Diagnosis and treatment will be made easier and more effective.

5. Don't believe everything you hear. Patients forget; they may deliberately suppress information (often because of fear), they may unconsciously repress information, and they may falsify (often for purposes of compensation or insurance payments).

6. Try to avoid too many "why" questions, for they are often challenges to the patient's competence. The question "Why did you stop taking medication?" can lead to confrontation and hostility, whereas more neutral and open-ended expressions such as, "Tell me about your reasons for not using the medication," may maintain rapport and obtain information.

7. Do not express judgment about the previous course of treatment given the patient by other practitioners. It is a safe assumption that neither you nor the patient has adequate information to make such judgments hastily.

8. Be <u>certain</u> that words used by you and the patient mean the <u>same</u> things. <u>You</u> know that all tumors are not cancers - does the patient? Use medical jargon carefully to avoid misunderstanding and be sure that the patient understands your language and questions clearly, or his answers may be inaccurate.

9. Be as quantitative as possible. "Once upon a time . . ." is a pleasant way to start a fairy tale but is inadequate for a medical history. "At 2:00 p.m. yesterday, about 1/2 hour after eating a large meal, Mr. X arose from the table and vomited about two quarts of partly digested food mixed with bright red blood . . ." may not be a pleasant way to start a story, but it is quantitative and informative.

10. Keep in mind the patient's reason for seeking professional help. If he came for treatment for a cold, don't forget this complaint as you get involved in other aspects of the patient's problems.

11. Remember that during the medical interview you will also be completing the first portion of the physical examination on the patient: observing general state of alertness, body build, skin tone, eye lesions, hair problems, muscle tics or tremors, voice quality, etc., etc., etc.

Remember that you are the health professional, and therefore, the guide in this relationship between you and the patient. Together you can achieve the goals desired of the medical interview - the establishment of a good working relationship and accurate information regarding the patient's physical and emotional health.

There are several fine texts on interviewing, a few of which are suggested at the end of this chapter. Needless to say, it is impossible to learn interviewing skills by reading this brief chapter. It is most advantageous to read several resources and practice with fellow students. The video camera is an excellent tool for recording the interview and then for reviewing the effectiveness of the examiner's skills. Whenever possible, an experienced interviewer should be available to critique performance and offer advice.

REFERENCES

1. Peabody, F.: The Care of the Patient. JAMA 88:877, 1927.

2. Reik, T.: Listening With the Third Ear. Farrar, Strauss and Co., Inc., New York, 1948.

3. Engel, G.L. and Morgan, W.L.: Interviewing the Patient. W.B. Saunders Co., Philadelphia, 1973.

4. Benjamin, A.: The Helping Interview. 2nd Ed., Houghton-Miflin Co., Boston, 1974.

5. Bernstein, L. and Dana, R.H.: Interviewing: A Guide for the Health Professional, 2nd Ed., Appleton-Century-Crofts, New York, 1974.

6. Froelich, R.E. and Bishop, F.M.: Clinical Interviewing Skills. 3rd Ed., C.V. Mosby., St. Louis, 1977.

7. Garret, A.: Interviewing: Its Principles and Methods. 2nd Ed., Family Service Association of America, 1972.

CHAPTER 3

THE HEALTH HISTORY - PART I

INTRODUCTION

A health history is the first element of the data base because it is the single most important element in establishing the patient's problems. A comprehensive history should give the examiner a picture of the person's current and past health problems and information about the individual as a whole in his environment.

The content of the health history should not vary if it is to be complete and comprehensive, but the format for recording the history differs somewhat from author to author. The one presented in this text is a model which has been satisfactory for our use and for our students.

This history consists of the following elements: Chief Complaint, Present Illness, Past History, Review of Systems, Family History, Personal/Social History, and Patient Profile.

Each of the above elements has a specific goal, or set of goals, which must be clear to the practitioner, so that when he has achieved his purpose with one element, he will know that it is time to shift and to explore the next. Briefly stated, these objectives are as follows:

Chief Complaint (CC): to establish the major specific reason for the individual's seeking professional health attention.

Present Illness (PI): to obtain all details related to the Chief Complaint

Past History (PH): to give the examiner a picture of the patient's previous illnesses and injuries.

Review of Systems (ROS): to bring to light any health problems related to the PI or the PH which were not mentioned earlier.

Family History (FH): to identify the presence of genetic traits or disease which have familial tendencies; to learn if the patient has had prolonged contact with a communicable disease in a family member; and to assess the patient's ability to cope with stress induced by disease or death in his family.

Personal/Social History (P/SH): to develop an understanding of the patient as an individual and as a member of a family and of a community.

Patient Profile (PP): to summarize in the examiner's mind the totality of the individual within the context of his medical, psychological, and socio-economic background.

In actually taking a history, the practitioner should let the patient report any information in any order, as long as it seems pertinent to the complete history. Do not force the patient to conform strictly to this outline, but rather keep him talking. However, the practitioner can, and should, report the history using the above format by rearranging the elements given to him by the patient.

CHIEF COMPLAINT (CC)

This represents the specific reason for the patient's visit to the office or admission to the hospital. Since the CC may be thought of as the title, and the PI as the story of the patient's major problem, the two are often intermixed as the history is being evolved. It is important to determine, as much as is possible, the major problem facing the patient at the moment, and its duration.

Often, there may be no problem or complaint. The individual may want a routine annual check-up or may require a pre-employment examination. This is simply listed as the Reason for Contact.

The CC should be briefly recorded, using the patient's own words (in quotation marks) where possible. An attempt should be made to have the patient identify the major problem, even if there seem to be several closely related complaints. These other problems will be recorded elsewhere. It may not be possible for the patient or the examiner to isolate one chief complaint, in which case the CC will contain several entries.

The examiner should begin the history-taking with an open-ended, neutral question or statement, as free as possible of confrontation, judgment, or misinterpretation. "How may I help you?", "Tell me about what is bothering you." "What problem led you to seek help?" and "What is your trouble?" are relatively good ways to start. The question, "What is your sickness?" implies that the patient is, in fact, sick. "What brought you to the hospital?" may readily be answered by "The ambulance!" or "My wife!", and the interview could begin with an unnecessary humorous note or with some hostility, which may adversely affect the relationship.

There is no single question which is guaranteed to get the interview started without a possible negative reaction on the part of an already hostile patient, but the neutral questions suggested above are frequently successful openings.

The following are samples of desirable recordings of chief complaints because they are brief, specific, and to the point, and, in effect, serve as titles for the story (PI) to follow:

CC: "Terrible chest pain," 2-3 hours' duration.
CC: "I think I've got the clap," 2 days' duration.
CC: Cough, fever, insomnia of 4 days' duration.
CC: Coma, unknown duration.
CC: None. Routine annual examination.

Do not translate the patient's story into a diagnosis! If the chief complaint was of passing black stools, record it as such, not as "gastrointestinal bleeding." "Chest pain" is not to be translated as "Angina Pectoris," "substernal pain," "heart attack," or any other term.

A chief complaint with multiple entries often confuses the examiner, the reviewer, and the consultant. Thus: CC: "High blood pressure, chest pain, numbness of fingers, palpitation, nausea, cough, and vomiting of several days' duration" presents a series of problems which may or may not be related. The examiner may be unable to focus in on just what bothered the patient most or what made him concerned enough to seek help now. Were all these problems "of several days' duration," including the high blood pressure?

PRESENT ILLNESS (PI)

If there is no problem or chief complaint, as for the person who comes for a routine examination, this section may be retitled "Current Health Status," and will record the patient's perception of his state of health.

A clear history of the Present Illness will be a narrative, beginning with the earliest onset of the complaint and describing its progression to the present. It is quite important to obtain information about the reason for the patient's seeking help now.

In a history of arthritis, for example, it might well be found that the acute attacks which began five years ago, recurred once four years ago, then twice in the next year, and have become almost monthly in frequency in this current year. Such a story, presented to the appropriate consultant, would suggest the characteristic progression of gouty arthritis.

How does a student learn which questions to ask without knowing, for example, that acute attacks of gouty arthritis generally become progressively more severe and occur with increasing frequency? This comes by dissecting the story into its critical parts:

The details of onset
The complete interval history
The current status
The reason for seeking advice now

An expert would achieve the results more quickly but he must obtain the same critical bits of information as the novice - onset, interval history, current condition, and reason for being in the office
today.

Thus, a CC: "Cough and fever 3 days' duration" should prompt the
examiner to find out why the patient came today, not 2 days ago or
yesterday. Did the cough become worse? Did the fever become
worse? Did the cough change? A CC of "Arthritis of 5 years' duration" must be explained, in the PI, in terms of how it began five
years ago, what went on over the five-year period, and what it is
like now. The story should end with a statement of the reason for
the patient's visit to see the examiner today. Many valuable diagnostic clues will be uncovered by obtaining the history of a complaint, from its onset, through the interval period, and up to the
present moment. Additionally, a fair amount of insight into the patient's personality and motivation may be uncovered by digging into
details of the story. In the example cited of "CC: Cough and fever
3 days' duration," the clinician might uncover, as a reason for coming today, the fact that the patient's cough was no worse, but that he
became afraid that he had tuberculosis or cancer.

It must be remembered that patients seek help because of changes
in their clinical status; because of behavioral changes (increase in
anxiety, loss of tolerance to pain, etc.); and because of social pressures (increased stress at home or at work, etc.). Any one or all
of these may play a part in the patient's decision to seek help today.

There are some basic bits of information about various problems
which are important to obtain and the student must develop a pattern
of history-taking which will elicit these vital facts. No one could, or
should, memorize a series of routine questions but should learn what
basic information must be obtained.

Knowledge of pathophysiology will enable the student to develop a
background of knowledge of syndromes or clustering of symptoms
characteristic of specific problems. For example, when the patient's chief complaint is "difficulty in urinating" it becomes important to branch from that complaint to the commonly found associated
symptoms of blood in the urine, dribbling, burning, incontinence,
etc.

An excellent example of a pattern to be followed is in dissection of
the story of pain - an extremely common complaint. The critical
features of pain are:

Type
Location
Severity
Duration
Influencing factors
Associated symptoms

A report incorporating each of these characteristics will be more complete and informative. For example, here is such a history recorded in highly condensed form: "Crushing, heavy (Type), substernal pain radiating to left shoulder and arm (Location), which causes patient to stop all activity (Severity), occurring for past three months at about 7-10 day intervals, each attack being only 1-2 minutes in duration (Duration). This often occurs about an hour after meals, especially while walking. Brought on by severe job tension, cold weather, large meal, climbing two flights of steps. Relieved by stopping activity (Influencing factors). Associated with sweating of few minutes duration and fear of impending death. Does not recall if he is short of breath during attacks (Associated symptoms)."

This, of course, is the typical pain of angina pectoris due to coronary heart disease.

Note that these are entries for each of the six critical features of pain. The type of information desired for each of these features of pain will not vary no matter what pain syndrome is being investigated. A few details regarding each of these features may assist in obtaining all the necessary diagnostic information.

TYPE: The character of pain is of great importance and it is useful to have the patient's description. Let him choose the words as long as you understand just what the pain is like. "Like a headache" is not adequate, since there are many types of pain associated with headache; but "Like being stabbed with an ice-pick" is highly specific. In the PI recorded above, the patient used the term "heavy," to describe his pain, and this is clear enough for the clinician to distinguish the type of pain from "sharp," "knife-like," throbbing," or "sticking."

LOCATION: Try to ascertain just where the pain is perceived. The patient may need to be helped to locate pain by indicating to him the importance of such localization. "Head pain" is an inadequate description of pain located deep behind both eyes, or in other locations such as over the left occiput, over the left eyebrow, at the top of the head, at the right mastoid process, at the angle of the jaw, across both temples, etc. Each of these is, indeed, head pain, but each is possibly due to a different disease process in a different structure. Often the patient may add non-verbal means of description by pointing with a finger-tip, or by spreading an outstretched hand over an area. A clenched fist pressed against the mid-sternum may be used to describe both location and type of pain.

Location should also be defined in terms of the patient's perception of whether the pain is superficial or deep, and whether or not it radiates to some other anatomic site. For example, radiation to the left shoulder and arm, or into the neck, is often associated with pain of coronary heart disease; radiation from the low back down the posterior thigh and calf frequently is found with sciatic nerve pain; radiation to the tip of the right scapula from the abdomen may help in identifying gallbladder disease.

SEVERITY: This feature is generally best described by having the patient tell you how the pain affects his normal activity. Adjectives are too frequently and too loosely used. Thus, an attack of "terrible" pain during which the patient goes on with playing cards, walking, or other usual activities may not be regarded by the clinician as being truly severe, despite the patient's words. Pain, on the other hand, which causes the patient to stop in mid-stride, or half-way up a flight of stairs, to fall to the ground, to double-up, or to lose consciousness, is clearly understood by the examiner. It is always preferable to record the effect of the pain on the patient's activity of daily living, than to quote adjectives.

DURATION: This should include the duration and timing of a single attack as well as the frequency of attacks, since the onset of the problem.

INFLUENCING FACTORS: These include a wide range of factors which seem to the patient to precipitate the pain or to make it worse, or which relieve the pain partially or totally. Factors such as exercise, excitement, meals, medication, smoking, standing, bending over, cold or hot environment, fatigue, time of day or season of the year, may all be pertinent in tracking down the possible cause of pain or its relief.

ASSOCIATED SYMPTOMS: This category will include symptoms in body regions not directly involved by the primary pain. Thus, in the example of angina pectoris given above, sweating and fear of impending death were considered to be associated with the chest pain. If the patient had noted nausea as an accompaniment of the angina, it would properly be included here.

The student must memorize these six critical features of pain, and with these guide-posts and experience, he can obtain an accurate history which will often enable a reviewer to make a diagnosis, suspect a particular disorder, or, at the least, to focus attention on a specific organ system.

This outline, designed for eliciting a history of pain, may not be able to be followed exactly for other symptoms, but should give the examiner a general pattern of questioning to follow. Complaints like blurring of vision, chronic cough, constipation, palpitations, nausea or fever, will require somewhat different guide-posts, but questions about type (or character) of the symptom, severity, duration, influencing factors, and associated symptoms are all as pertinent for these symptoms as they are for pain.

PAST HISTORY (PH)

Having obtained enough information about the CC and the PI, the examiner then directs the interview toward other medical and surgical problems. This is ordinarily an easy shift to make.

A convenient organization of this element of the history is: medical, surgical, injuries, allergies, immunizations, and current medications. As before, in obtaining a CC and PI, the patient is encouraged to "tell me about all other illnesses and operations you have had." This is an open-ended invitation for the patient to detail what he thinks important. If, later in the interview other important facts turn up, the examiner may have obtained information about the patient's memory, or perhaps about his reluctance or fears in revealing information earlier. If such a delay occurs, the examiner should use this situation to reinforce the rapport and confidence developing between practitioner and patient, but must never confront or chastise the patient over such a lapse, no matter what the reason.

Entries here are previously established diagnoses with dates of occurrence, severity, and complications, if any. Try to establish the fact that the diagnosis reported by the patient was provided by a physician and not simply assumed to be a diagnosis by the patient. Thus, with a report of "a heart attack in 1972," the examiner should inquire as to how the diagnosis was established, the length of hospitalization and convalescence, and the name of the physician-of-record. A reply such as, "Oh, I had some chest pain and the doctor said that it might have been a heart attack," is improperly classified as indicating a true coronary occlusion. Such a story should be entered in the Review of Systems where symptoms are recorded.

By such evaluations the examiner makes the PH a listing of known and established medical facts. Relationships between these facts and the PI may or may not exist, but until they are clearly recorded, it is impossible to evaluate such relationships adequately. Since the entries are established diagnoses, questioning can be brief, and need not go into much detail beyond confirming the fact that the patient is reporting the diagnosis accurately.

Translation into brief medical terminology is desirable here, so that if the patient describes pain in the right lower quadrant, vomiting and removal of an inflamed appendix three years ago, the entry may simply be: "Appendectomy - 1975."

MEDICAL: Included here are diagnosed and medically important illnesses. Remember that symptoms and complaints which are un-diagnosed belong in the section on Review of Systems. Entries should be as brief as possible, e.g., "Pneumonia, right - 1966"; "Cholecystitis - 1969, no attacks since, no stones." Some illnesses may require more details to give an adequate picture, e.g., "Hy-pertension discovered in 1969 on routine check-up. BP said to be moderate requiring no treatment. More severe by 1971 when medi-cation (type not known) was begun. Patient discontinued Rx in 1972 and has taken none since."

Listing of usual infectious childhood diseases such as measles, mumps, chicken-pox, etc. may be of importance in the evaluation of an adolescent patient or pregnant woman (has she had rubella?), but is unlikely to shed much light on the overall medical status of an 80-year-old widower suffering from depression. This remains a matter of judgment.

To assist the patient in recalling such diseases, it is often useful to ask about any illnesses which confined the patient to bed for several weeks or which required hospitalization.

SURGICAL: This is principally a listing of operations, e.g.,

Appendectomy - 1950, Mountainside Hospital, N.Y. Partial Hysterectomy - 1972 for prolonged bleeding due to fibroids. No malignancy reported. Westview Hospital, N.J.

In more complicated situations, include as much information as is necessary to indicate exactly what the disorder was and the results, e.g., "Kidney stone passed 1969. Second stone 1970 removed by surgery. Third stone removed surgically late 1970 led to work-up for parathyroid disease and parathyroidectomy in 1971. No stones since."

INJURIES: The history of old or recent accidents may shed as much light upon the patient's balance and stability as upon the possible consequences of the injury. In obtaining the history of a fall, it is important to ascertain why the patient fell as well as learning what injuries occurred. Learning the reason for a fall may reveal the first clues to such diverse disorders as night-blindness, epilepsy, stroke, vertigo, or syncope. Obviously, a history of repeated falls or accidents must be carefully reviewed with the patient to find a reason, if possible, for his being accident-prone. Damage to the brain, heart, lungs, liver, spleen, kidneys, bladder, and other or-gans may follow blunt injury whether or not there were fractures, so the interviewer must not discard the story of such trauma simply be-cause the patient is sure that "no bones were broken."

ALLERGIES: The patient should be asked about commonly known allergic disorders such as hay fever or asthma and also about any unusual reactions to food, drugs, or contact agents such as fabrics. It is particularly important to prompt the patient to describe the reaction if he reports an allergy to a drug, since a patient will often confuse a known side-reaction of a drug with an allergy to the drug. True drug allergy must be carefully recorded in this section of the history and also brought forward to the summary of abnormalities and the active problem list, if the POMR is used.

IMMUNIZATIONS: This is of particular importance in examination of infants and children for whom a record should be made of immunizations to diphtheria, pertussis, tetanus, poliomyelitis, measles, and vaccination against smallpox. Information on smallpox vaccination and tetanus booster is usually adequate for adult patients.

CURRENT MEDICATIONS: A complete list of the medications being taken by the patient may be invaluable to an understanding of his past or present illnesses. Although some of this information may have been recorded in the PI, all medications should be listed here including name, dose, schedule, duration, and reason for the treatment. If circumstances are appropriate, ask the patient to bring in, on his next visit, all such medications for your review, particularly if there seem to be many. It is not unheard of to have the patient return with a large bag containing a dozen or more vials and bottles including two or three sedatives and several stimulants as well as several other similar medications prescribed by different physicians. This will often provide useful information about the patient's physical and emotional health. Additionally, since many of the modern potent drugs are capable of producing illnesses themselves ("Diseases of Medical Progress" as Dr. R.H. Moser has called them), the list may offer significant diagnostic clues.

REFERENCES

1. Engel, G.L. and Morgan, W.L.: Interviewing the Patient. W.B. Saunders Co., Philadelphia, 1973.

2. Froelich, R.E. and Bishop, F.M.: Clinical Interviewing Skills, 3rd edition. C.V. Mosby Co., St. Louis, 1977.

3. Small, I.: Introduction to the Clinical History, 2nd edition. Medical Examination Publishing Co., Inc., New York, 1971.

4. Mechner, F.: Taking a Patient's History. Am. J. Nurs. 74: 293, February 1974.

5. Baer, Ellen D., McGowan, Madeline N., and McGivern, Diane O.: How to Take a Health History. Am J. Nurs. 77:1190, July 1977.

6.   Mahoney, E.A., et al.: How to Collect and Record a Health History, J.B. Lippincott, Philadelphia, 1976.

See also pertinent chapters in General References cited at the back of this text, on page 356.

CHAPTER 4

THE HEALTH HISTORY - PART II

INTRODUCTION

In obtaining the Chief Complaint (CC), Present Illness (PI) and Past History (PH), it is desirable to use open-ended questions and/or prompting to assist the patient in telling you his medical story. The remaining sections of the complete medical history will require more direct guidance on the part of the examiner. It may also be more difficult to obtain patient cooperation from this point on, since the lines of questioning may seem to be leading further away from the patient's CC, which is his main concern. Therefore, a brief explanation is in order to assure the patient that you have not forgotten the prime reason for his having come to the office or hospital. Both the practitioner and the patient need to be aware of the reasons for obtaining further history, i.e., the details of the medical, social, familial, and economic background on which the current problems are based. Accurate evaluation is usually not the product of inspiration, but more often depends upon carefully putting together all of the information about the person himself, not just a disease.

REVIEW OF SYSTEMS

This portion of the history reviews all current and pertinent past symptoms in order to be sure that no important clues have been overlooked by either patient or practitioner. Often, the history of the PI will be a complete review of the system related to the CC, so additional questioning on that system is often unnecessary. For example, if the CC was "cough of 6 weeks' duration," the examiner should have obtained at least as much information in the PI as is suggested for the review of Respiratory System in the listing which follows. Do not make the patient repeat this story here, but add only any information on the system not obtained in the PI.

The listing of items of data to be obtained in the ROS is, to some degree, arbitrary. There is no practical limit to the questions which might be asked, but those suggested were selected as ones related to the more common problems found in adult practice. The suggested order is also arbitrary and is roughly in anatomical order, so that the reviewer can proceed with his questioning in some sort of systematic way.

Questioning will, of course, vary with circumstances. The items pertinent only to adults will not be asked of the parent of the infant or child.

Although medical terminology is listed here, the questioning must be in words commonly used and clearly understood by the patient. Failure of the patient to understand will lead to responses which are inaccurate and misleading. Each of the items is briefly asked about and, if denied, may be so recorded. If positive responses are elicited, additional information is obtained. Thus, for example, a "yes" answer to the question, "Have you ever been told that you had high blood pressure?" should be pursued with either an open-ended statement such as, "Tell me more about it," or with a series of more direct questions. The examiner should know, no matter which interview technique is used, additional details such as when hypertension was first found, how discovered, how high pressures were, how or if it was investigated, how persistent or transient it was, what treatment was suggested or given, whether it was followed regularly, what the most recent pressures were, etc.

In reporting the ROS, remember that this is a part of the history, so that the patient's responses are recorded, not physical findings. These will come later. A useful technique for this review is to start with general questions for a system, e.g., "Have you had any problems with your lungs or your breathing?" Specific questions can be asked later to cover items not mentioned by the patient.

General: Overall state of health, fatigue, unexplained weight changes, exercise tolerance, fevers, night sweats, frequent infections, ability to carry out activities of daily living

Integument: Eruptions, rashes, pruritis, pigmentation, unusual hair growth or loss, disorders or deformities of nails

Head: Headache, trauma

Eyes: Visual problems, pain, lid edema, use of glasses, date of last examination, tests for glaucoma, scotomata, excessive tearing

Ears: Hearing, tinnitus, discharge

Nose: Smell, nasal obstruction, epistaxis, sinusitis

Mouth, Teeth, and Gums: Dental problems, fit of dentures (if present), last visit to dentist, soreness of tongue, bleeding or swelling of gums

Throat and Neck: Frequent sore throat, hoarseness, tonsilitis, neck stiffness or pain

Breast: Discharge, bleeding, lumps

Respiratory: Wheezing, cough, hemoptysis, sputum production, shortness of breath at rest or on exertion,
orthopnea, paroxysmal nocturnal dyspnea, last
chest x-ray

Cardiovascular: Chest pain, palpitations, heart murmur, peripheral edema, hypertension, claudication, varicose veins, thrombophlebitis, Raynaud's phenomenon,

Gastrointestinal: Dysphagia, appetite, food intolerance, jaundice, abdominal pain, indigestion, bleeding,
nausea or vomiting, bowel habits, laxatives,
blood or mucus in stools, tarry stools, acholic
stools, use of antacids

Genitourinary: Dysuria, frequency, urgency, hesitancy, incontinence, nocturia, force of stream, bleeding,
stones, venereal disease, discharge, hernia,
prostatitis

Gynecological: Menarche, catamenia, menorrhagia, metrorrha-
gia, date of last menstrual period, type of con-
traception (if used), dyspareunia, post-coital
bleeding, vaginal discharge, pruritis, infertility,
date and result of last Pap smear

Obstetrical: Pregnancies, full-term deliveries, abortions,
living children, complications of pregnancies

Musculoskeletal: Weakness, neck, back or joint stiffness, pain
or swelling, radicular pain, muscle cramps,
deformity

Neuropsychiatric:
1. General: syncope, seizures, vertigo, tremors, paralysis/paresis, dizziness, memory,
insomnia, nightmares
2. Sensory: paresthesia, hyperesthesia,
hypesthesia
3. Affect: appropriateness to situation, anxiety,
nervousness, depression.

Lymphatic and Hematologic: Lymph node swellings, excessive
bleeding or bruising, anemia, blood transfusions

Endocrine: Intolerance to weather changes, thyroid disorder,
sugar in blood or urine, polydipsia, polyphagia,
polyuria, excessive sweating, change in voice

FAMILY HISTORY (FH)

As stated earlier, the family history can shed light on the potential existence of hereditary diseases in the patient, on the patient's reactions to illness and death in the family, and the possible exposure to communicable disease.

In most situations, brief questioning about first-order relatives (parents, siblings, children) is adequate. Questions should be asked about disorders which tend to run in families, such as heart disease, hypertension, diabetes, cancer, bleeding disorders, sickle-cell anemia, allergies, and mental disorders.

Unless there are other family members with disorders similar to those of the patient, further exploration is usually not necessary. If a full history is deemed necessary, it may well be deferred to a subsequent visit, since this may require as much as an hour and the construction of a genogram or a table (Fig. 4.1).

PERSONAL AND SOCIAL HISTORY (P/S H)

Information on the "patient as a whole" in his socio-economic environment is needed in the process of evaluation. Sir William Osler's dictum, that it is as important to know what kind of patient has a disease as to know what kind of disease the patient has, is as pertinent as ever in our complex, stressful world.

Questioning the patient at this point in the interview is generally easier, since good rapport may have been developed. The patient may not construe this questioning as "prying" if he has confidence in the practitioner's interest in him and his problems. However, rapport is not automatic and if the clinician is aware of some hostility on the part of the patient, the questioning about personal and private matters must be done carefully, sensitively, and minimally.

The format developed here is not a universally accepted standard but, in one way or another, information of this type should be generated and recorded for a full picture of the patient.

As with other elements of the history, the amount of detail sought by the clinician must depend upon clues and leads which develop during the patient-practitioner contact. Thus, if the examiner senses that he is dealing with someone who seems to be psychologically sound and whose problem appears to be a straightforward organic one, the personal and social history can be brief.

On the other hand, patients who seem tense or anxious and who present with obvious psychic or psychosomatic disorders deserve more detailed interviewing about personal and social aspects of their life.

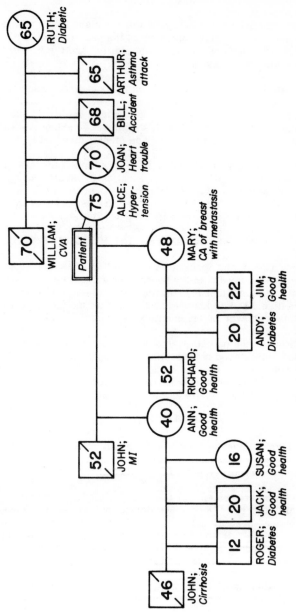

FIG. 4.1: Example of a genogram

Such a distinction may be difficult to make and the clinician may err in his judgment, but he must use it to perform a proper history. Experience is obviously a necessity in this task.

ACTIVITIES OF DAILY LIVING: A considerable amount of pertinent information can be developed by asking the patient an open-ended question, such as, "Tell me about the way in which you spend an average day." You will want to hear specific details about the patient's typical diet, his sleep pattern, his work and recreation, and his use of tobacco, alcohol, and drugs of any type. If sufficient detail is not given, prompting or direct questioning may help to obtain specific information.

DIET: The examiner should know about the type and approximate quantity of food and fluid intake over an average 24-hour period as well as the frequency of meals and snacking.

SLEEP: Information about the average number of hours of sleep, the frequency of waking during sleep, and recent alterations in sleep patterns will help to clarify the patient's physical and mental status.

OCCUPATION: Record the details of a typical work day and the general history of work patterns. An individual who, for example, has held fifteen to twenty different jobs in as many years may be giving you useful information about an unstable person who is chronically ill or chronically dissatisfied. The type of job or hobby may provide a clue to environmental hazards, such as coal dust for a miner, asbestos dust for a construction worker, or exposure to toxic solvents by a chemical factory worker or even by an office worker, whose hobby may turn out to be cleaning and repairing old guns with carbon tetrachloride.

Knowledge of the patient's occupation will also be useful in the clinician's judgment about the patient's ability to continue working or the convalescent time which might be required upon discharge, if the patient is hospitalized.

If the patient is unemployed or retired, he will generally discuss his financial problems and may readily go on to express hostility or resentment toward society or individuals, if these feelings are present.

Patterns of recreation will often provide insight into a person's personality and social environment.

HABITS: The pattern of use of tobacco, alcohol, and over-the-counter drugs should be explored in quantitative terms. Cigarette smoking at present or in the past should be estimated in packs per day and "pack-years." Since the terms "social drinker" or "a few drinks" are nonspecific, the actual weekly intake of beer (number of bottles, cans, or glasses) should be ascertained. Similarly, for hard liquor, some estimate of specific amounts is needed in terms of drinks per day, fifths of liquor per week, or other measurement of intake.

The regular use of over-the-counter drugs provides an important clue to symptoms which may not have been uncovered earlier, and, again, the clinician's task is to try to quantitate the types and amounts of the use of such drugs.

Obviously, a patient's admission that he is using narcotics, "uppers," "downers," or other dangerous substances will provide the examiner with a significant lead, requiring investigation into the patient's reasons for starting or continuing use of these agents. It is important to re-emphasize the point, made earlier, that the examiner's personal bias or prejudice about drugs must not be expressed, nor should it interfere with the conduct of the interview.

GEOGRAPHIC EXPOSURE: Items of importance are birthplace and travel or residence in tropical or sub-tropical areas which have a high incidence of certain unusual diseases. Inquiry into military service in this context is necessary, for even people who have "lived their entire life" on the Eastern Seaboard may neglect to mention a tour of military service in Korea, Okinawa, or Vietnam.

MARITAL AND SEXUAL HISTORY: The interaction between sexual problems and psychic or somatic disease is well-enough known to most patients, so that too much resistance may not follow questioning. In addition, the health care professional should be alert to potential problems. For example, certain anti-hypertensive agents may lead to male impotence. Uncovering and correcting such a problem may be of tremendous help to the patient and may provide relief of much tension.

Despite the openness and frankness on sexual matters of our society, many people are still reluctant to discuss their own problems. Prompting and professional interest may help to overcome this reluctance. The discussion is preferably opened by relatively open-ended questions such as, "Do you have any concerns about your sexual life?", or "Are you having any problems with sexual activity?".

INTERPERSONAL RELATIONSHIPS: While it is important to identify sources of hostility and/or conflict in the patient, detailed questioning about all contacts is not desirable or necessary. The clinician should have picked up clues from earlier portions of the history which may be pursued, or he may simply ask the patient about any difficulty in "getting along" with family members, friends, or coworkers. Ask, "Are there any problems at home or work that you'd like to discuss with me?"

INTRAPERSONAL EVALUATION: The patient may be asked to give a brief view of himself, his life style, his way of coping with stressful situations, his own strengths and weaknesses, his usual mood, and his current concerns.

Coming at the end of the interview an open-ended request for such information is often well-received and may be productive of a picture of the patient's self-image.

PATIENT PROFILE (PP)

This is your evaluation of the "patient as a whole." All the data will have been collected and recorded prior to this evaluation, so the PP will not provide additional information from the patient.

Review, briefly, the patient's socio-economic status, his current family structure (with whom does patient live?), and his income in terms of meeting basic needs for food, shelter, and clothing. Give your opinion of his adjustment to his situation (e.g., "This 45-year-old ex-Marine is employed full-time and lives at home with his wife and children. His wife works to help support the family. He seems well adjusted but is afraid of spending too much time in the hospital because of concern about losing his job.") Ignoring this evaluation may occasionally lead to missing the real problem. An illustrative actual case is the story of an elderly man who had repeated admissions to a hospital for "intractable congestive heart failure." Properly managed on each admission, he was placed on a low-salt diet, appropriate medications, and adequate rest with good results, and then was discharged. A careful history, finally taken on about his fourth admission, revealed the facts that he lived alone in a fourth-floor walk-up apartment and that his income was inadequate to purchase the more expensive low-sodium foods prescribed for him. When the PP was properly written about this poor, quiet, shy old man who had to walk eight flights of steps daily to buy his food, the "medical" problem of intractable heart failure was supplemented by a socioeconomic problem of poverty, loneliness, and overexertion which fortunately, was readily correctable by the proper agencies. Knowledge about both types of problems allowed for adequate total treatment of the patient.

The student should review the purposes of each of the elements of the complete health history (page 32), and should then examine the model of a normal history (Appendix I) to summarize for himself the concept and methods of the health history.

SUPPLEMENTAL EXERCISES

1. Construct your own, or a patient's, family genogram. Look up and use standard symbols.

2. There are about 30 drugs in common use which may cause impotence (of which about 30% are anti-hypertensive agents). Collect a list of drugs with this potential side effect.

3. In an "open-ended" interview, if a patient begins to wander far from the medical history, what clues should you look for to see if this behavior is due to a memory defect? Learn to distinguish between loss of long-term and short-term memory and also learn the significance of each type of loss.

CHAPTER 5

THE PHYSICAL EXAMINATION

INTRODUCTION

The basic premise in performing a physical examination is that the examiner, by use of all of his senses, can detect variations from the normal state which will become the second part of the data base on a particular patient. It is apparent from this premise that the examiner must know the range of normal findings for each of the modalities of the physical examination. This knowledge is based upon a sound foundation in anatomy and physiology and is developed with practice under the guidance of an experienced preceptor. There are, of course, some abnormalities which are obvious to any untrained individual, but most abnormalities which will be of importance in the establishment of a sound data base are not obvious without learning, training, experience, and practice - and more practice.

The student must learn how to inspect and observe - not just to see. He must learn to feel accurately and sensitively and he must learn to use techniques of percussion and auscultation which are outside the realm of everyday experience. The chapters which follow will assist the student in developing the needed skills and in establishing a systematic pattern of examination so that he will not miss important findings or forget to examine certain areas.

The examination described is a sound, basic routine evaluation which will identify almost all significant abnormalities. It must be recognized, however, that it does not represent a complete examination. There are hundreds of observations, signs, and tests which are not described in this text. For example, in Dorland's Medical Dictionary, under the term "Sign" there are 695 entries, almost all of which relate to the physical examination! The cardiologist can add a number of special examinations, the neurologist can continue the neurological examination for ten or more minutes beyond what is described, and, in turn, every specialist can add to this base. Thus, in the real world, there is no such thing as a "complete physical examination."

The student or practitioner who can perform the described examination well and thoroughly need have no concern on this score, for this examination is an excellent screening examination which will identify the presence of almost all important findings.

As in history-taking, when one finds an abnormality, further and more detailed examination is indicated. For example, it is not ordinarily necessary to listen over each square centimeter of the lung during routine auscultation. But if rales are heard in a particular area, it then becomes mandatory to cover that entire area - centimeter by centimeter - to determine the exact extent of that abnormality.

The history has provided the practitioner with clues relating to certain areas deserving special attention. As he performs the examination, the clinician will frequently find things not mentioned by the patient during the history-taking. Significant skin lesions, scars, deformities, rales, muscle weakness, heart murmurs, etc., may require a continuation of questioning. As mentioned earlier, history-taking is a continuous process extending throughout the physical examination, at the discussion after the examination, and at each subsequent visit.

Interviewing and teaching are continued during the examination to obtain additional information and, often, also serve to place the patient at ease. The examiner should explain what he is doing and what the patient may expect. Surprises should be avoided. Where patient cooperation is required, clarity and patience will most often be rewarded by better examination and the development of confidence. Maintenance of eye contact with the patient will assist greatly in development of good rapport and may often provide clues to assist in evaluation of the degree of pain induced by any movement or pressure during the examination.

Of utmost importance, is the professional demeanor of the examiner. Careless behavior, lack of preparation, inappropriate jokes, impatience, lack of proper draping, and other evidences of lack of consideration for the patient may all inhibit a proper relationship and a thorough examination.

The clinician must always guard, very carefully, his verbal and non-verbal behavior when he finds something unexpected. Inappropriate reactions will often frighten the patient or may "turn him off" as a partner in the necessary interchange between patient and clinician.

At the completion of the physical examination, after the patient is dressed and the examiner and patient are together for a summing up, it is useful for the clinician to ask the patient, "Is there anything else that you'd like to discuss with me?" By this time the patient should have more confidence in the examiner and may give additional, and often important, information which he withheld earlier.

ORGANIZATION

As much as is practical, the physical examination will be described by general body regions such as the head and neck, the thorax and its contents, the abdomen, etc. Thus, the examination of the peripheral vascular system, for instance, will not be described in any single chapter, but rather will be incorporated into the examination of the neck, the abdomen, and the extremities.

While there are some exceptions to this format (e.g. skin, neurological system) the teaching of examination by body region will more nearly match the technique of the actual physical examination.

TECHNIQUES

GENERAL: The four classical techniques of the physical examination are inspection, palpation, percussion, and auscultation. These will be described separately and should, in general, be performed one at a time in sequence.

With certain major exceptions, the right and left sides of the body are nearly symmetrical. The heart extends into the left hemithorax much more than into the right. The liver lies in the right upper portion of the abdomen, the stomach and spleen in the left upper, and on both sides these organs are covered by the thoracic cage. Thus, the examiner will find normal asymmetry in his examination of both the thorax and upper abdomen. In the remainder of the body, symmetry is to be expected, and abnormalities may be identified by comparing one side of the patient with the other. There are slight deviations from side to side which fall within the normal range, so the observer must not expect perfect symmetry but must learn by experience when deviation is to be considered abnormal - and therefore significant.

An important part of the physical examination is the evaluation of function of the part or organ as well as examination for anatomical change. For instance, in the examination of the head and neck, the facial muscles are tested for strength and symmetry of motion, the eyes for motion and vision, the ear for hearing, the jaw for motion, the tongue for motion, the pharynx for swallowing, etc.

SOUND PRODUCTION: Since interpretation of sounds will be extremely important in the examination, a few basic points should be reviewed at this time.

All sound is produced by vibration of an object or substance. Strings in vibration produce the sounds of the guitar or violin, reeds vibrate in the clarinet, the player's lips in the trumpet, the head of a drum, and an air column in a pipe-organ.

Physiologically, we shall evaluate the vibrations of the larynx in voice production, vibrations of the thorax and abdomen as we percuss them, vibration of air, mucus, and fluid in the lungs; valve closure in the heart; and abnormal vibrations in the heart and blood vessels by auscultation.

While it is not necessary to describe pitch in absolute numbers, it may be of interest to know that middle C on the piano is tuned to 262 cycles per second (cps), the tuning fork recommended for diagnostic kit has a pure tone of 128 cps, and the normal human voice ranges from about 80 to 2,000 cps.

Heart sounds are of relatively low pitch, 30 - 70 cps, while some murmurs reach 600 cps. In the abdomen, normal peristaltic sounds are generally below 1000 cps, while peaks of over 2000 cps may be produced in intestinal obstruction.

The important qualities of sound for the clinician are pitch and loudness. Pitch is related to the number of vibrations (frequency) per unit of time, recorded as cycles per second (cps). The fewer vibrations per second, the lower will be the pitch of the sound.

Striking a firm, hollow object (such as a drum) will produce a low-pitched, booming sound which will have a long duration since the drum-head vibrates freely. On the other hand, a soft, solid object (such as the thigh), which does not vibrate freely, produces a very short, high-pitched sound.

Loudness of the sound (intensity) is related to the force which produces the sound, and the ability of the object to vibrate. Thus, in the example above, striking the thigh gently will not produce a very loud sound. Striking it more forcefully will produce a louder sound, but the pitch will not change.

SOUND TRANSMISSION: In order to hear a sound, the vibrations produced at the source must be transmitted through various media to the air and thence to the ear drum. Thus, closure of the heart valves will vibrate those valves and the heart itself; this vibration will be transmitted to the chest wall to the stethoscope, through the air column in the stethoscope to the ear drum.

Factors which influence the transmission of sound are of great importance in understanding physiological and pathological phenomena. In general, sound vibrations are best transmitted through firm solids (e.g., metal, wood), less well through fluid, and poorest through air.

For example, when one applies a stethoscope to a patient's chest and asks the patient to speak, the vibrations are transmitted from the larynx, through the trachea, the bronchi, the air-filled lung, the chest wall and thence, through the stethoscope to the examiner's ear. However, if there should be a consolidation of the underlying lung (as with advanced pneumonia), the voice sound will be transmitted much better than normally. This finding (see p. 154, bronchophony) will indicate to the observer that the underlying lung is more solid than normal - a definite pathological finding.

These principles must be kept in mind during the examination by percussion and auscultation to properly interpret the findings by these techniques.

SEQUENCE OF EXAMINATION: There is no single, perfect, "right" way to do a physical examination and various patterns are used by different practitioners. (See Chapter 19 for a recommended sequence.) No matter what the exact sequence may be, however, no physical examination is adequate which neglects to examine each area and region by all of the necessary techniques. It should be an absolute rule, however, that inspection of the part to be examined should always come first.

PHYSICAL EXAMINATION

INSPECTION: Most of what we have learned in life has come through our sense of sight and a great deal of the data on which a diagnosis will be based will come from inspection. It is a psychological truth, however, that we perceive more of what we look for than what we look at. Skill in inspection will come in learning what to look for and how to observe carefully.

The master detective, Sherlock Holmes, used to astound Dr. Watson with his deductions based on observation. In one of the stories, Holmes, in explaining the principle involved, asked Watson how many steps there were on the stairway leading to their flat. When the doctor admitted that he did not know, Holmes pointed out that while Watson had seen those steps for years, he had never observed them. We all see all there is to see, but the trained eye observes, and that is the essence of inspection in physical examination.

Adequate lighting and proper exposure of the area being observed are essential. Instruments such as a penlight, otoscope, ophthalmoscope, nasal speculum, and vaginal speculum are aids in the inspection process.

PALPATION: Because the sense of touch is highly developed, with training and experience it can become an important diagnostic tool. The hand can distinguish many variations between hard and soft (e.g., a nodule within a thyroid gland), rough and smooth (e.g., a fine papular skin rash from a macular rash), stillness and vibration (e.g., absent fremitus from diminished fremitus), and heat and cold (e.g., increased temperature surrounding an early inflammation from normally warm skin). In general, the fingertips are most sensitive to touch, the palm and ulnar surfaces of the hand to vibrations (fremitus), and the ulnar and dorsal surfaces of the hand to temperature. Sensitivity to touch can be dulled by heavy pressure on the fingertips and by continued pressure. Thus, as a rule, light palpation is preferred for most examinations. It is often necessary to

increase pressure to make certain distinctions, and better dis-
crimination will result from pushing down several times rather
than holding the fingertips in place for a long period.

Deep palpation is necessary to accomplish a thorough examination
of the abdominal contents and heavy pressure may be achieved by
pushing the fingertips of one hand with the fingers of the other hand.
A preferred technique for deep palpation is to place the fingers of
one hand over the area to be palpated, and then to place the fingers
of the other hand immediately in front of the first set of fingers and
to push deeply with both hands (Fig. 5.1).

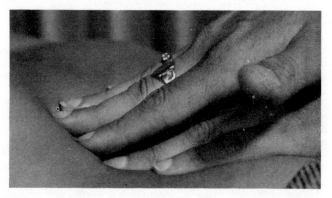

FIG. 5.1: Position of fingertips for deep palpation. Note the
overlapping.

Bimanual techniques also include using both hands to entrap an organ or mass between the fingertips or to fix an organ in place with
one hand while palpating with the other.

Another useful technique of palpation is ballottement. The term
comes from the French verb meaning to toss or bounce a ball. This
consists of a bouncing or tapping motion of the fingertips. Performed very lightly, ballottement of the eyeball through the closed
lid may sometimes give a better sense of eyeball tension than will
simple gentle pressure.

Light ballottement is also useful in the initial palpation of the abdomen where the fingertips are rapidly bounced along the abdominal
wall from the lower to upper portion. A sense of resistance which
may be missed by firmer palpation can often be appreciated in this
way.

PERCUSSION: This is the act of striking a portion of the body to
evaluate the condition of underlying structures. Blunt percussion

will produce tenderness in an underlying inflamed tissue or organ. Thus, striking a blow over the kidney may produce pain if there is renal infection (see Fig. 15.3, p. 233) and tapping over an infected sinus will often induce pain. A special form of blunt percussion over a tendon is used to stretch the muscle and produce a reflex used in the neurological examination.

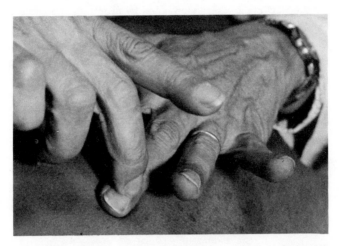

FIG. 5.2: Percussion. Only the pleximeter finger is flat on the chest wall. The distal phalanx is struck by the tip of the third finger of the other hand.

The other purpose of percussion is to identify and demarcate underlying structures by vibrating an area of the body surface. This is ordinarily performed by placing the middle finger of the left hand (for right-handed examiners) flat and holding it firmly against the area to be percussed. This is called the pleximeter finger. The percussion blow is struck by the tip of the middle finger of the right hand (Fig. 5.2). Obviously, the fingernail must be trimmed short; otherwise the examiner will use the pad of his finger, producing a poorer sound. The target for the percussing fingertip is the area immediately distal to the last joint of the pleximeter finger.

Those who have played percussion instruments will know without further instruction that in order to produce a sharp, crisp note, the blow of the percussing finger must be brisk and short; otherwise the vibrations produced will be damped and muffled. The wrist should be used to produce the striking force and the blow should be so controlled that the percussing finger bounces off the pleximeter rather than poking it.

In addition to listening to the sound produced by percussion, the examiner should concentrate on the vibrations felt by the pleximeter finger. Both the sense of touch and the sense of hearing will assist the examiner in detecting changes in vibration as the pleximeter finger is moved from one area to another.

This technique cannot be learned by reading the above description alone. After obtaining assistance from a preceptor, the student should practice this technique until it is easily performed. One can produce the important percussion notes by practicing on one's own body, if no other cooperative one is at hand.

The vibrations produced by percussion depend upon the nature of the tissue underneath the pleximeter. Verbal descriptions of the various notes are nearly useless so definitions are best given in terms of examples. Normal percussion notes over the thorax and abdomen are resonance, dullness, and tympany:

Resonance: the low-pitched sound produced by percussion over normal lung (i.e., right anterior thorax above the level of the breast)

Dullness: A higher-pitched sound produced over more solid tissue (i.e., over the heart or liver)

Tympany: An even lower-pitched sound produced by percussion over an air-filled organ (i.e., most of the abdomen)

Two abnormal percussion sounds are flatness and hyperresonance:

Flatness:*   An extreme degree of dullness sometimes referred to as "absolute dullness." This is higher pitched than dullness and may be simulated by percussion of a totally non-aerated tissue such as the thigh.

Hyperresonance: An even lower-pitched sound than resonance, produced over abnormally air-filled lung, such as in severe emphysema or pneumothorax

It is not necessary to produce a loud percussion sound. On the contrary, the best diagnostic information is obtained by quiet percussion since, by striking lightly, the examiner vibrates only a small area and can pick up smaller lesions or variations from the normal.

---

* - Some authors describe the normal percussion sound over the mid-portion of the heart or liver as "flat." It is our preference to reserve this term for an abnormal note such as that produced over a large pleural effusion.

One final point - percussion will not produce vibrations of deep
structures. Therefore, any organ or mass more than four or five
centimeters deep will not be detectable by this technique, and structures smaller than four or five centimeters cannot ordinarily be
detected.

AUSCULTATION: The most important factor in being able to do
diagnostic auscultation is an adequate stethoscope that fits. This
is the one piece of equipment which must be fitted for you and which
you must own, carry, and use. When you come to the examination
of the ear and use the otoscope, you will appreciate the fact that
there is great variation in the diameter and angle of individual external auditory canals. There may be variation also between one's
own left and right canals. It then will be obvious to you that no one
stethoscope can possibly fit all ears.

The ear-plugs must be of the right size; the metal ear pieces must
be properly angled for each of your canals; the tension spring must
hold the ear pieces tightly enough to block out most extraneous
noises but not so tightly that your ears are uncomfortable; the tubing should be of 1/8 inch internal diameter, of fairly thick outer
diameter, about twelve to fifteen inches long; there must be no leaks
anywhere in the tubing or connections; the instrument should have
both bell and diaphragm chestpieces. Anything less than this may
be adequate for taking blood pressures, but nothing less than this
will do for clinical auscultation. The time spent with a box of extra
ear plugs, a pair of pliers, an otoscope, and an instructor will be
one of the most important investments you will make in learning
auscultation.

However, one must also keep in mind Dr. J.V. Warren's reminder
not to forget the most important part of the system - "that between
the earpieces."

The diaphragm of the chestpiece amplifies sounds and transmits
higher-pitched sounds better than lower frequency sounds. When
using the diaphragm, press it firmly against the chest wall to get
maximum benefit from its ability to amplify sounds. The bell fil-
ters out high-pitched sounds and is therefore useful in listening for
low-pitched sounds. The bell should be placed lightly on the skin,
just enough to make good contact. If pressed tightly, the bell will
stretch skin across its orifice and, in effect, will become a diaphragm chestpiece. Both diaphragm and bell are used in the routine
examination of the heart, whereas the diaphragm is generally adequate for examination of lungs, since most of the chest sounds are
of higher pitch. There are areas in thin persons and children where
the diaphragm will not lie flat, such as at the lung apices above the
clavicles or between ribs where the bell may be needed.

EQUIPMENT: As has been suggested, a properly designed, carefully adjusted stethoscope is the one piece of equipment which the examiner must own. All other instruments can be borrowed or are available at diagnostic stations.

If the student intends to pursue physical assessment as an integral part of his career, there are a few other items which should be purchased. At a minumum these include a:

> penlight
> reflex hammer
> C-128 tuning fork (128 cps)
> tape measure (180-200 cm.)
> transparent ruler (15 cm.)
> blood-pressure set (with adult and pediatric cuff)
> otoscope-ophthalmoscope set
> carrying bag for the above items

VITAL SIGNS AND MEASUREMENTS: It should be obvious to all that no physical examination is complete without certain vital signs and measurements. Yet, all too often these elements are absent or taken casually. Routine blood pressures - even in only one arm - are rarely recorded in certain offices and clinics, particularly in some of the specialty areas. Many patients will depart from a hospital stay without a single body weight ever having been recorded.

The practitioner must incorporate these simple but vital examinations into his practice. The measurements, made routinely, should include, at a minimum, height, weight, pulse, temperature, respiration, and several blood pressures. While there are, of course, circumstances in which height and weight cannot be measured immediately, these must not be forgotten and must be recorded at the first opportunity. All of these measurements serve as a part of an adequate data base and may give important clues during the follow-up period.

Blood pressure should be taken in both arms and in at least two positions. A useful routine is to take pressures after the patient has been supine for a few minutes. Record pressure in one arm, move the cuff to the other, record pressure, then with cuff still on the arm , ask patient to sit up and repeat pressure. Pressures should not normally vary from one arm to the other by more than 10 mm Hg, and on sitting up (or standing), there should be no more than a 10 mm lowering of either systolic or diastolic pressure. Variations in either situation of more than 10 mm warrant rechecking at some time prior to completion of the full physical examination.

Conditions such as orthostatic hypotension, paroxysmal hypertension, coarctation of the aorta, among others, may be first suspected by careful measurement of blood pressure and repeated recordings at each visit.

As an aid in patient evaluation, other measurements can assist in determining variation from normal standards and in evaluating change. The student and practitioner are encouraged to use the metric system which will soon become the national standard. A 15-centimeter transparent pocket ruler and a 180-200 centimeter tape measure are essential ingredients of the diagnostic kit and should be used often. In addition to recording height, weight, and blood pressures in the infant, head circumference and crown-rump height are also routinely measured.

To these, one should add measurement of significant asymmetry of any part of the body, the size of masses, the size of organs (such as the liver), the degree of swelling of an extremity with thrombo-phlebitis, etc. The simple act of carrying a ruler and tape measure at all times will assist in making such measurements a matter of routine practice.

RECORDING

The development of skill in reporting is important to provide a record of the findings at a particular time. Communication of these findings is necessary for others who may examine the patient and to the examiner himself when he repeats parts of the examination at a later hour or date. Remember that the focus is upon what the examiner sees, feels, hears, or measures, not subjective information which he has read in the patient's chart or learned from the history.

Examples will be given in each chapter to assist in learning this skill. In general, the term "normal" is used sparingly. Rather, the report should describe what has been done and found. For instance, a report, "Pharynx normal," communicates little information as to what was examined, and is therefore an inadequate report. A report: "Pharynx - mucosa pink, no lesions, tonsils absent, uvula rises in mid-line on phonation, gag reflex present bilaterally," is specific, useful for communication, and serves as a basis for a comparison at a repeated examination.

Vital signs and measurements are best recorded in traditional tabular form:

Ht: 163 cm. (5'4"); Wt: 61.4 Kg. (135 lbs); Temp: 37°C.
    (98.6^{O}F.) oral
Pulse: 80 reg.; Resp: 16 reg.
BP: RA 135/80; LA 130/80 supine
              LA 130/80 upright

CHAPTER 6

GENERAL SURVEY

INTRODUCTION

In a typical visit, the patient will have walked into the office and the examiner will have introduced himself, shaken hands, and directed the patient to a chair. By this time, the physical examination, starting with inspection, will have been unobtrusively under way for several minutes, and the astute observer will have collected dozens of bits of information. He will be aware of the patient's sex, race, apparent age, state of grooming, and gait. He will know whether the patient's palms are dry or sweaty and will have observed the presence or absence of skin pallor, flushing, cyanosis, or jaundice. Facial tics, jerky, uncoordinated limb motions, obesity or asthenia, speech impediments or foreign accent, facial asymmetry, stare, and many other abnormalities will have been noted.

Not all of these findings - positive or negative - will be recorded as part of the general survey, but all will find their way into the patient's record, and all will have given the clinician some leads into the history-taking and the physical examination.

THE PATIENT AS A WHOLE

"Mrs. A is an alert, ambulatory, well-developed, moderately obese 47-year-old white woman appearing of about stated age who is in mild respiratory distress. No speech defects."

This is a typical introduction to the physical examination. There are no rigid rules for such an introductory statement, but the features described in that paragraph should provide the reader with an image of the patient, so that details of the physical examination about to be presented can be put into a general context.

Most of these observations are not related to a single body system, but reflect constitutional factors which give a picture of an individual's general state. The recommended elements of this introduction are mental status, body development, nutritional state, sex and race, chronological versus apparent age, presenting appearance, and speech.

Remember that these introductory statements are intended only to sum up the gross total appearance of the patient and do not need to be detailed descriptions. For instance, Mrs. A's "mild respiratory distress," noted in the sample introduction, will be described fully in the report of the physical examination of the thorax and lungs.

MENTAL STATUS: This brief general statement of the patient's mental condition should describe the patient as alert or dull, oriented or confused, and may include a statement about the level of education or intelligence.

BODY DEVELOPMENT: Any patient whose height and body build fall within the wide range of acceptable normals may be simply characterized as "well-developed." Gigantism is a pathological variation, usually due to hypersecretion of growth hormone prior to maturation, in which height and weight are well beyond the normal range. This is usually associated with retarded sexual development. Where the anterior pituitary hypersecretion occurs after full body growth has been completed, the condition is called acromegaly. Here, there is enlargement of the nose, jaw, hands, and feet, producing the characteristic appearance seen in Fig. 6.1.

The opposite of gigantism is dwarfism. The ateliotic dwarf or midget is simply an abnormally small adult with normal body proportions. Another type of dwarf is the achondroplastic dwarf in whom the head and body are frequently normal size but the extremities are very small and short.

There are other congenital and metabolic disorders which produce abnormalities of body size, shape, and proportion. Any such abnormalities should be reported here.

NUTRITIONAL STATE: This may be reported in terms of malnourishment, the normal state, and obesity. A record will be made of actual height and weight so that the evaluation of overweight or underweight will not depend totally upon the examiner's concepts of the ideal. Height and weight charts should be available to the examiner for subsequent discussion with the patient who falls outside the normal range. In infants and children such data should be recorded on standardized growth charts.

SEX AND RACE: The patient's sex will, of course, be obvious to a reviewer, but it is useful to state it here to assist in presenting a picture of the patient, as a whole. Since there are disease entities which are predominantly found in persons of a particular racial origin, this factor must also be recorded.

STATED AGE VERSUS APPARENT AGE: There is often a difference, to the examiner's eye, between these ages. While this is admittedly a matter of subjective judgment, it is important to record such an apparent difference. Frequently, the person harboring a chronic disorder may appear definitely older than his actual age, and the

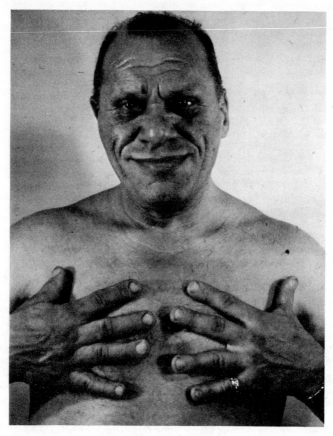

FIG. 6.1: Acromegaly

notation of such a clue may assist in uncovering such a disease, if it exists. Pathological extremes such as <u>progeria</u> or <u>precocious puberty</u> are rarely seen.

PRESENTING APPEARANCE: This may be a specific observation such as, "in acute respiratory distress," or "writhing in pain." More general subjective observations such as "appearing chronically ill," "in no acute distress," or "seeming to be in excellent health" also assist in providing the desired overall survey of the patient.

There are other general abnormalities which may well fit into this introductory report. One of these is his position, often referred to as <u>station</u>. The examiner's interest here is not in simple poor

posture due to habitual stooping or slumping, nor in skeletal deformities, which will be examined carefully later on. Rather, the
abnormalities of station are those related to physiologic disturbances
such as the position taken by the patient in severe respiratory distress. Here, he will lean forward, bracing his arms so that he can
use the accessory muscles of respiration (see Fig. 11.7, p. 144).
In left-sided congestive heart failure with severe pulmonary edema,
the patient will sit or stand nearly upright and will not lie supine
comfortably. He may lean to one side to splint a fractured rib or
have his knees drawn up to relieve abdominal pain. Station refers
to any feature of the patient's position and where pertinent, should
be specified if it helps to give a picture of the whole patient.

Abnormalities of speech may be recorded here or in the neurological
examination. Speech is a highly complex act which involves mental
processes, the cerebellum, several cranial nerves, the mouth, palate, tongue, larynx, and the respiratory system. As with many
other problems, the exact mechanism for speech defects may not be
known at the completion of the history and physical examination, but
a careful, complete description of the defect will have important diagnostic value.

As stated earlier, many observations will be made at the very outset of the interview. In general, however, it is a useful procedure
to describe abnormal findings in the system or region in which they
are located, and to reserve this general survey for a brief, orient-
ing, introductory picture of the "patient-as-a-whole."

SUPPLEMENTAL EXERCISES

1. Obtain a height-weight table for adults. Note the way in which
    data were collected. If the table is in feet and pounds, add
    scales for height in centimeters and weight in kilograms for
    easy reference.

2. What abnormalities might be observed on the initial observation
    of a patient with advanced Parkinson's disease?

CHAPTER 7

THE INTEGUMENTARY SYSTEM AND MASSES

INTRODUCTION

Since the skin is the individual's showpiece to the world, it becomes a medium through which the personality is frequently expressed. Tattooing, use of make-up, wigs and hairpieces, and other cosmetic aids are also considered when the practitioner is making a psychological assessment, since their use may reflect the individual's self-image, as well as his cultural identity.

Examination of the skin, hair, and nails begins with general inspection during the interview early in the process of health evaluation, and continues throughout the physical examination of each organ or body system. The condition will ordinarily be described along with other elements of a particular region. Thus, absence of genital hair will appear as a part of the inspection of the genitalia, and a skin rash limited to the abdomen will be described in the report on that region. However, if there is a condition which involves all or nearly all of the body, it is useful to describe it in this general section. Examples of widespread abnormalities which belong here are: total absence of hair, absence of skin pigment (albinism), jaundice, or a generalized rash.

TOPOGRAPHICAL ANATOMY

Fig. 7.1 may be of value in identifying the different layers of the skin and its appendages, but its inclusion here is primarily to help the examiner establish a framework for further study, particularly of invading lesions.

PHYSIOLOGY

The skin is an organ which serves many functions in addition to protection of underlying vital organs, such as controlling temperature, elimination of wastes, and providing a system for sensory stimulation.

The normal skin and its appendages, the hair and nails, vary according to sex, age, race, endocrine influence, and genetic messages. They are also especially affected by factors of climate and nutrition and reflect the internal as well as external environment of the body, so that many disease processes alter their function and appearance. The general color and a number of pigmentary alterations are examples of inherited characteristics.

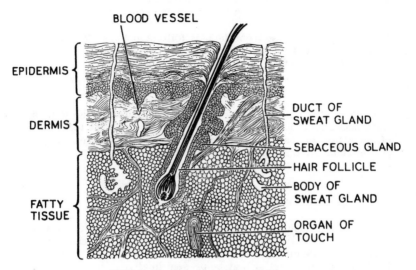

BLOOD VESSEL

EPIDERMIS

DERMIS

FATTY
TISSUE

DUCT OF
SWEAT GLAND

SEBACEOUS GLAND

HAIR FOLLICLE

BODY OF
SWEAT GLAND

ORGAN OF
TOUCH

FIG. 7.1: Cross section of skin.

It is important to remember, however, that a variety of alterations
in character and consistency may be quite normal in certain
individuals.

The child's skin is normally thick, elastic, and well lubricated; but
as the years advance, there are changes which result in thinning,
less elasticity, drying, and wrinkling. Also, the skin long exposed
to sunlight is coarser, dryer, and rougher.

The amount of hair growing over the skin varies from individual to
individual and is also a genetic and endocrine determined trait.
Thus, males develop hair on the face and chest in addition to the
axilla and pubis at puberty. The rapid rate of hair loss from the
male head after age twenty-five is certainly a well-accepted fact of
normal development. Of course, in today's American society where
the male wig is widely worn, baldness may not be readily seen, and
history becomes the source of information, rather than simple inspection. (We hope it is unnecessary to mention that inspection of
the skin on the head will require removal of any appliance worn by
males or females.)

In Fig. 7.1, the sweat glands can be seen to arise from the subcutaneous tissue; they are distributed generally over the skin, particularly on the palms, soles, and forehead. These glands aid in regu-
lation of the body temperature and will begin to secrete in the normal,
healthy, resting individual when the temperature reaches approximately

$30^{o}C$ ($86^{o}F$.). In addition, they also respond to emotional stress, and evidence of hyperactivity is frequently demonstrated by axillary perspiration and moisture on the palms and soles of the feet.

Sebaceous glands arise from the hair follicle and are a frequent source of infection and cyst formation, especially over the scalp, neck, back, and genital area.

TECHNIQUE OF EXAMINATION

For the most part, the methods used in examination of the skin and its appendages require no special instruments, only the techniques of inspection and palpation, a good light, and a transparent flexible pocket ruler for measurement of any lesions found.

EXAMINATION

GENERAL PHENOMENA:

The examiner should note the color in general and identify such deviations as pallor, flushing, cyanosis, or jaundice. Each of these may involve one or more small areas of the body (e.g., cyanosis of the lips and nail-beds) or may be present in all.

When the practitioner notices any areas of increased or decreased pigmentation, further history from the patient should be elicited regarding their duration. There are some changes in pigmentation which are temporary or which are of no real significance. Chloasma gravidarum, for example, consists of brown patches on the forehead and cheeks of the pregnant women, known as the "mask of pregnancy." This increase of pigmentation usually disappears spontaneously after childbirth.

Table 7.1 identifies some of the color and pigmentation alterations which may be observed and which require recording.

Texture: The texture or turgor of the skin should then be assessed by grasping a small section between the examiner's fingers (see Table 7.2). It may feel thin, inelastic, and dry, due to lack of moisture within the skin itself, or thick and mushy if the skin is overhydrated. When the water content of the skin is excessive, edema is present and is characterized by pitting upon pressure (see Fig. 15.1, p. 221).

A special type of thickening called myxedema, often seen over the tibia, may be present in hypothyroidism; it has the sensation of mushiness, but does not pit. More extensive hardness of the skin is seen in systemic sclerosis where the changes tend to be symmetrical, involving the face, extremities, and anterior chest. Thickening and hardening of thin and fragile skin may be due to disease and should always be described as accurately as possible.

TABLE 7.1		
COLOR CHANGES OF SKIN		
COLOR CHANGE	BASIS	EXAMPLES
Erythema-reddish tint	Increased amounts of blood flow or RBC	Fever, sunburn, poly-cythemia vera
Cyanosis-bluish tint	Increased amounts of deoxygenated blood	Pneumonia, congenital heart disease with right-to-left shunt
Pallor-whitish tint	Decrease in hemo-globin content	Anemia, shock
Greenish-yellow	Increased bilirubin in skin or sclera	Jaundice due to blood pigments in hemolysis or biliary tract obstruction
Orange-yellow	Increased amounts of carotenoid in skin but not sclera	Ingestion of excess amounts of food with carotene, occasionally in pregnancy
Gray	Deposition of metal-lic salts such as silver, gold, and bismuth	Prolonged ingestion of such salts
Increased or decreased pig-mentation	Absence or excess of melanin	Exposure to sunlight, Addison's disease, albinism, vitiligo
Localized pig-mentation superficially	Injection of carbon-containing particles	Tattoo

Temperature: In general, increased warmth of the skin is due to increased blood flow as a result of the body's response to inflamma-tion and also in an attempt to lower the body temperature. Increased coolness is frequently due to reduction of blood flow to the integument in an attempt to preserve body heat or to supply vital organs, as in shock.

Local coolness usually exists in extremities due to decreased blood flow and/or as a result of peripheral vascular disease.

TABLE 7.2		
CHANGES IN SKIN TEXTURE		
TEXTURE AND TURGOR	BASIS	EXAMPLES
Excessive moisture	Autonomic nervous system stimulation	Perspiration
Dryness	Endocrine imbalance, dehydration	Hypothyroidism, post menopausal fluid loss
Wrinkling	Loss of skin elasticity	Rapid weight loss, aging
Velvety smoothness	Endocrine imbalance	Hyperthyroidism
Puffiness and indentation on pressure	Fluid and electrolyte imbalance	Edema
Thickening without dryness	Endocrine imbalance	Myxedema

LOCAL PHENOMENA:

Skin

SKIN LESIONS: The skin is subject to so many types of lesions that the principal task of most nonexperienced observers is to describe lesions accurately. They should be described according to distribution and location, size, contour, and consistency. The following charts have been prepared to assist in the recognition and recording of lesions. It is important to understand that eruptions consist of one or more primary lesions (see Table 7.3) which can be either discrete or confluent, and with or without secondary lesions (see Table 7.4). Certain lesions affect only exposed areas (e.g., poison ivy), while others prefer typical locations such as the trunk and neck in pityriasis rosea or the root of a nerve in herpes zoster. An important test of the practitioner's examination ability requires that he differentiate among lesions which are commonly found, those which are pre-malignant, and malignant neoplasms which require immediate attention.

TABLE 7.3			
PRIMARY SKIN LESIONS*			
TYPES	DESCRIPTION	SIZE	EXAMPLES
Macule	A flat circumscribed area of color change without elevation of its surface	1 mm to several cm	Freckles, flat pigmented moles, vitiligo, café-au-lait spots
Papule	Circumscribed solid elevation of the skin	less than 1 cm	Acne, lichen planus
Nodule	Solid mass extending deeper into dermis than does a papule	1 to 2 cm	Erythema nodosum, pigmented nevi
Tumor	Solid mass, larger than nodule	over 2 cm	Epithelioma, dermatofibroma
Cyst	Encapsulated fluid-filled mass in dermis or subcutaneous layer	over 1 cm	Epidermoid cyst
Wheal	A relatively flat localized collection of edema fluid	1 mm to several cm	Mosquito bites, urticaria (hives)
Vesicle	Circumscribed elevations containing serous fluids or blood	less than 1 cm	Herpes simplex, herpes zoster, chickenpox, smallpox
Bulla	Larger fluid-filled vesicle	over 1 cm	Pemphigus, 2nd° burn
Pustule	A vesicle or bulla filled with pus (larger collections of pus are called furuncles, abscesses, or carbuncles)	1 mm to 1 cm	Acne vulgaris, impetigo

* - Some determatologists include plaques as primary lesions, while some do not. In any event, a plaque may be defined as a flat, elevated lesion, more than 1 cm in size. Some plaques appear to be made up of clusters of papules which have coalesced into a single lesion.

TABLE 7.4		
SECONDARY SKIN LESIONS		
TYPE	DESCRIPTION	EXAMPLES
Crust	The dried exudate of serous oozing, purulent infection, or blood	Eczema, vesicular or pustular eruptions, impetigo
Scale	Flakes of skin	Psoriasis, pityriasis rosea
Excoriation	Scratch marks	Pruritus, needle marks
Fissure	A crack in the skin, usually through the epidermis	Eczema, chapping
Ulcer	A circumscribed loss of epidermis which may extend deeply into the corium and subcutaneous tissue	Chancre, malignant growth, stasis ulcer as with severe varicose veins
Scar	Replacement of destroyed tissue by fibrous tissue or excess collagen	Postoperative scar, keloid
Striae	Long, slightly depressed lines, appearing like scars but without disruption of the skin, often shiny and colorless when due to stretching of subcutaneous tissue, or reddish-purple when due to excess adrenal steroids	Pregnancy, marked obesity, Lupus erythematosus, Cushing's disease

Pigmented nevi or moles are usually raised dark brown or black
lesions varying in diameter from the size of a nodule to a tumor
and may or may not contain hairs. Although commonly found and
usually benign, they may occasionally develop into malignant mela-
nomas (Fig. 7.2). It is important to ascertain historical data relative to the duration of their existence and change in characteristics.
If there is evidence of rapid enlargement, change in color, consistency, crusting, or bleeding, it may signify malignant degeneration,
and warrant biopsy or excision.

Vascular Lesions: The examiner should note the presence of unduly
dilated superficial veins, telangiectasia, or spider angiomas. Some
of these are caused by interference with normal blood flow and are
usually significant in determining diagnosis, depending on location.
Some are more related to severe pathology than others. Telangiectasia are localized, fine red lines due to dilated blood vessels that
may be venules, capillaries, or arterioles. They frequently appear
on the alae nasae of almost every adult but may occur at any age,
in both sexes, and anywhere on the skin or mucous membranes.
Their presence is rarely of diagnostic value. Spider angiomas
(vascular spiders) are cutaneous lesions frequently found in areas
drained by the superior vena cava. They have a central red pulsating
arteriole representing the body from which small fine vessels radi-
ate like the legs of a spider over a reddened area one to ten millimeters in diameter (Fig. 7.3). When the central arteriole is compressed, the branches become blanched, and upon release, fill
again from the center. Although they may occur in normal individuals, and during pregnancy, they are most frequently found in
chronic liver disease.

Bleeding Lesions: The term purpura, strictly used, means a disorder
characterized by hemorrhage into the skin. There are two purpuric
lesions which are important to differentiate because of their different causes.

The presence of individual tiny red or red-brown capillary hemorrhages known as petechiae, no more than 0.5 millimeters in diameter, located within the skin papillae, may be indicative of capillary
fragility due to vitamin deficiency, blood dyscrasias, or severe infections. Larger hemorrhages under the skin referred to as ecchymoses, or bruises, varying in size from several millimeters to
several centimeters, may be due to trauma or blood dyscrasias.

Hair

There are many normal variations in hair distribution but only a few
abnormalities are of importance. These are unexpected general or
local hair loss (Fig. 7.4), distinct change in the character of the
hair, and excessive hair growth in women. Any of these findings
should be the subject of a careful history to be sure that a change

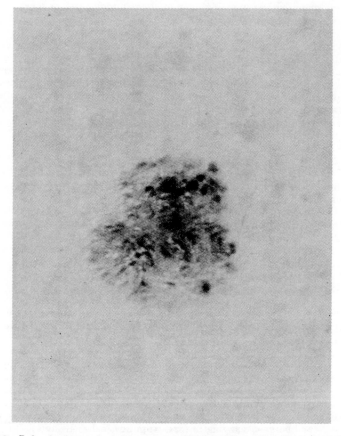

FIG. 7.2: Malignant melanoma, enlarged X 3. Note the irregular margins, and particularly the variation in pigment in different parts of the lesion.

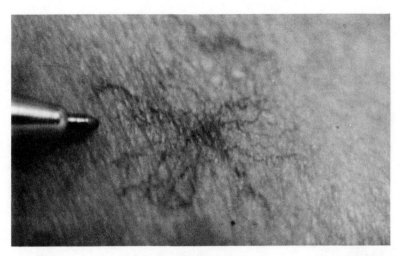

FIG. 7.3: Spider angioma

has occurred. Baldness is certainly not unusual in middle-aged or
elderly men, but is worthy of questioning and reporting in a man
under 25 years of age or in a middle-aged woman. Disappearance of
body hair from a region where it is ordinarily present (see Fig.
15.14 p. 234) is to be reported.

A change from normal hair texture to rapidly thinning, fine, silky
hair is often associated with hyperthyroidism, while in hypothyroidism the hair becomes dry and brittle and may begin to disappear
from the lateral portions of the eyebrows.

In women who have excessive hair, the areas which should be carefully examined are the face and chest. The presence of coarse hair
forming a beard or an excess of hair across the anterior chest are
suggestive signs of hirsutism due to an endocrine tumor, while excess hair on the arms, upper lip, or abdomen is more often an abnormality without known cause. Since this disorder may be a serious one from either an endocrine or cosmetic point of view, the
presence of excess hair on a woman should always be a matter of
report.

Nails

The nail bed can be seen through the transparent nail and it may be
one of the first places that cyanosis will be seen. The appearance of
badly mutilated, bitten nails may alert the examiner to consider the
presence of an emotional or personality disorder.

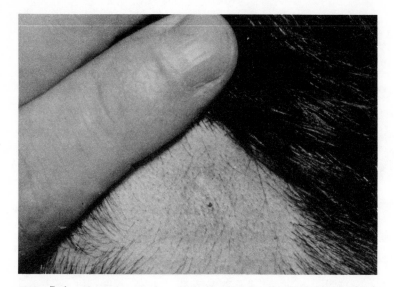

FIG. 7.4: Alopecia areata. Note the localized area of loss of hair without scaling of the scalp and with normal hair elsewhere.

Nails grow outward at a regular rate which is ordinarily interrupted only by disorders such as a major operation or serious infection. As the nail continues to grow, a deep horizontal line across each nail will become visible. These are called De Beau lines, and the time of occurrence of the illness which caused them can be roughly calculated by remembering that outward growth is about at the rate of one millimeter every ten days.

A most important lesion to identify is clubbing. This is an abnormality which involves both the nail and the terminal phalanx but which is evident earliest in the nail. The normal nail meets the skin fold (called the eponychium) where the cuticle develops, at an angle (Fig. 7.5). As clubbing develops, the proximal portion of the nail is elevated, eliminating this angle. Light palpation of the base of the nail will identify a softening of the nail bed. As clubbing becomes more severe, it also becomes much more obvious. The nail becomes curved ("watch-glass" deformity) and the terminal phalanx becomes widened and rounded ("drumstick" deformity). Clubbing is generally a sign of chronic oxygen lack often seen with certain congenital heart diseases, chronic pulmonary disease, arteriovenous shunts and, rarely, with other disorders. It may also be a normal, familial trait.

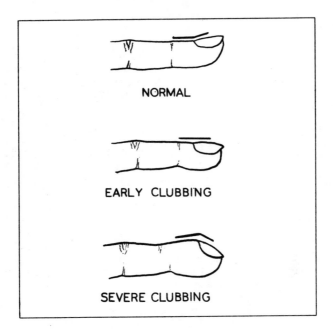

NORMAL

EARLY CLUBBING

SEVERE CLUBBING

FIG. 7.5: Clubbing of nail. Note the normal angle between the eponychium and the nail. This is true even with curved nails. The loss of angle seen in early clubbing is replaced by a reversed angle as the proximal nail bed elevates.

The nail should also be inspected for chronic infection and for "splinter" hemorrhages which are thin, brownish, flame-shaped lines in the nail bed. These most often are a result of tiny emboli associated with subacute bacterial endocarditis, which occur throughout the body but are not visible under the skin.

EXAMINATION OF MASSES

Any swelling or tumor larger than two centimeters in diameter is generally referred to as a mass. Its significance, of course, depends upon the nature of the mass. While the observer may not be able to identify its nature, he must be able to examine it critically and to describe the mass so accurately that a skilled reviewer may be able to identify it from the description alone. There are several fundamental attributes of all masses which must always be described. These are location, shape and size, consistency, mobility, and tenderness. Additional features which should be described, if present, are pulsations, temperature, and changed color of overlying skin.

Location: Define as exactly as possible the area of the body involved.

Shape and Size: Describe the shape of the mass (e.g., spherical, oval, irregular, nodular) and draw a simple sketch to show the outline of its surface. Measure the greatest length and width and record these in centimeters. Measure depth if possible or give an approximate measurement.

Consistency: Use the most descriptive terms possible. Often used are adjectives, such as stony-hard, hard, firm, rubbery, plastic, soft, and mushy.

Mobility: The movement or fixity of a mass is related to the structures to which the mass is attached and is of considerable diagnostic importance. Note carefully the mobility of any mass in relation to both deeper and overlying tissues.

Pain and Tenderness: Pain refers to a spontaneous uncomfortable sensation, while tenderness means the induction of pain by pressure on or movement of a part. These characteristics should be noted in any description of a mass.

Other Features: If pulsation is present, it is important to determine the reason for this motion. Taking the mass between the fingers may assist in making this distinction. An aneurysm of an artery will pulsate in all directions, while a mass being moved by an underlying artery will pulsate only upward. The temperature and color of the skin may be changed by the mass and, if so, should be noted. Occasionally, the actual color of the mass may be identified through the skin.

While the characteristics listed above are used for the description of masses, they are useful also in the description of enlarged organs such as the thyroid, liver, spleen, testes, etc.

LYMPH NODES

A special type of mass is the enlarged lymph node. Under normal circumstances lymph nodes are not palpable as they are small (1 - 5 mm. in diameter), soft, mobile, and underneath the skin. While there are many lymph nodes throughout the body, there are only three regions where enlargement is frequently found - the neck, the axilla, and the inguinal area.

Palpable nodes often occur in clusters, although solitary nodes are occasionally seen. The most common cause of enlargement is infection somewhere in the body region from which lymphatic channels drain toward the nodes (Table 7.5). Metastases from neoplasms are often trapped in the nodes, leading to enlargement, and there are

TABLE 7.5		
LYMPH NODE ENLARGEMENT		
SITES	BODY REGION DRAINED	EXAMPLES
Submaxillary	Mouth, pharynx	Abscessed teeth, carcinoma of mouth, tongue, etc.
Anterior cervical	Mouth, pharynx	Tonsilitis, pharyngitis
Posterior cervical	Scalp	Severe dandruff, lice
Supraclavicular:		
Right side	Right lung	Tuberculosis, sarcoidosis
Left side	Left lung, upper abdomen	Sarcoidosis, carcinoma of stomach
Axilla	Breast, chest wall	Mastitis, carcinoma of breast
Inguinal-femoral	Lower extremities, pelvic area, genitalia	Athlete's foot, skin infections
All or many	----	Hodgkin's disease, lymphoma

systemic disorders which sometimes lead to generalized lymphadenopathy including infectious mononucleosis, rubella, rubeola, as well as neoplastic lesions of the lymphoid tissue itself such as Hodgkin's disease, lymphomas and leukemias.

There is a general tendency for nodes which are draining infections to be of moderate size, firm, separate and tender. Nodes involved by metastatic disease are often stony hard and are, as a rule, not tender. With involvement of the nodes by lymphatic neoplasm; the nodes are firm or rubbery and have a distinct tendency to be matted together as though bound by fibrous tissue. These are not absolute rules, by any means, since there can be a great variation in characteristics.

Palpation for nodes in each of the common locations will be described in the examination of each region later in the text. It should be noted, however, that sites other than these common ones may show lymph node enlargement. These include the areas immediately anterior to and posterior to the ear lobes, the epitrochlear area just above the median condyle of the humerus, and the popliteal space.

Whenever and wherever lymph nodes are visible or palpable, all of the characteristics described for masses in the previous section must be included in the examination and report. In addition, since lymph nodes tend to appear in clusters, it is important to determine if they feel like separate masses (like grapes on a stem) or if they seem to be matted and bound together in lumps.

It is preferable to report lymph node enlargement (lymphadenopathy) in the specific locations where detected. Even for generalized lymphadenopathy, description region by region provides more accurate information.

RECORDING

> Skin: pink in color, good turgor, warm to touch, no excoriations or lesions.
> Hair: normal distribution and consistency.
> Nails: no deformities, nail beds pink, no clubbing.

PATIENT PROBLEM

Mr. T.J.R. is a 17-year-old white adolescent with a chief complaint of "skin lumps" of two years' duration.

Problem: Skin Masses (Fig. 7.6)

Subj: History of development of non-tender lumps on the back over the past 2 years, most of them within the past 6 months. No family history. Pt. is concerned that this may be venereal disease.

Obj: Skin - pink color, freckled, good turgor, warm. There are about 10-12 light brown macules over the back averaging 2.5 cm. in diameter without inflammation or excoriation. Masses - There are hundreds of scattered lesions of the skin varying in size from papules to tumors over 4 cm. in diameter. These are distributed principally over the back, neck, and posterior surface of the arms, with a few on the thorax and abdomen. None on face or genitalia. They lie in the skin not fixed to subcutaneous tissues and are firm and generally non-tender.

Assessment: Coming on after puberty, associated with freckles and large brown macules (café-au-lait spots), these fit the description of neurofibromas. Not a venereal type of lesion.

Plan: Diagnostic: Refer to dermatologist.
Therapeutic: None.

Patient Education: Patient told that these are probably not venereal, malignant, or contagious, but that examination by a specialist is mandatory. Discussion of patient's sexual activity cleared up several misconceptions.

_____
                                 Signature

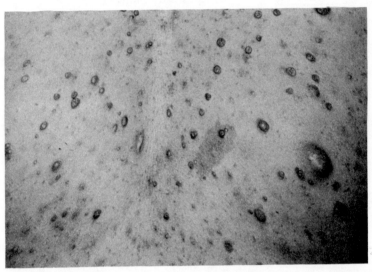

FIG. 7.6: Neurofibromas of the back. Note the multiple nodules of varying sizes. A café-au-lait spot can be seen just to the right of the center of the photograph.

SUPPLEMENTAL EXERCISE

1.   Look through a color atlas of skin lesions several times to familiarize yourself with the appearance of many skin lesions.
     Try to describe in your own words the appearance, as well as you can, from the pictures.

REFERENCES

1.   Levene, G.M. and Calnan, C.D.: Color Atlas of Dermatology. Year Book Medical Publishers, Inc., Chicago, 1974.

2. Sauer, G.C.: Manual of Skin Diseases, 3rd edition. J.B. Lippincott Co., Philadelphia, 1973.

3. Roach, L.B.: Assessing Skin Changes: The Subtle and the Obvious. Nursing '74 3:64, March 1974.

4. Roberts, S.: Skin Assessment for Color and Temperature. AJN 75:610, April 1975.

5. Kimmig, J., et al.: Frieboes/Schoenfeld Color Atlas of Dermatology. W.B. Saunders Co., Philadelphia, 1966.

CHAPTER 8

THE HEAD, FACE AND NECK

INTRODUCTION

This chapter will describe the examination of the head, including the face and the neck, leaving for other chapters the examination of the eyes, ears, nose, and mouth. Evaluation of the head and neck is principally accomplished by inspection and palpation, supplemented by percussion and auscultation to a limited degree.

TOPOGRAPHICAL ANATOMY

As seen from front or back, the head, face, and neck are nearly perfectly symmetrical on the right and left sides. Slight normal differences should be readily discernible to the observer. Viewed from the side, the short cervical portion of the spine is seen to have an anterior concavity (see Fig. 15.2, p. 222).

The sternomastoid muscles which extend from the sternum (and the medial portion of the clavicles) to the mastoid processes divide the neck into anterior and posterior cervical triangles. The carotid artery (see Fig. 8.4) courses upward from the thorax, passes under the sternomastoid muscle and extends to a point just anterior to the angle of the jaw.

The upper portion of the thyroid cartilage - the "Adam's Apple" - is found in the midline of the neck, and the thyroid gland is attached to its lower portion and to the trachea (Fig. 8.1). Below the thyroid cartilage the trachea extends down the midline into the thorax. Because it angles posteriorly, the trachea lies several centimeters behind the sternal plate as it enters the thorax.

PHYSIOLOGY

Because of its musculature and structure, the face is normally quite mobile, producing familiar facial expressions which are indicative of an individual's physical and emotional state.

The head moves on the cervical spine which should be flexible enough to allow the closed jaw to touch the chest in flexion and to reach the plane of the ears in hyperextension. In rotation, the jaw reaches laterally over the right and left shoulders without difficulty, and in lateral flexion the head tilts approximately 45° to either side (per JRS, RPT, DOM).

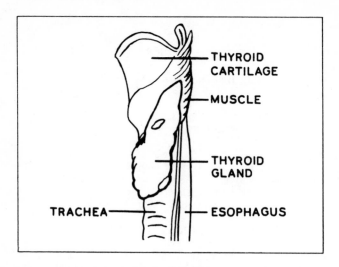

FIG. 8.1: Lateral view showing the position of the thyroid gland low on the thyroid cartilage and upper trachea.

EXAMINATION

HEAD: The normal shape and size of the head vary considerably from individual to individual. Although there are no measurement guides for head size of the adult as there are for infants and children, the observer will have little difficulty in judging an abnormal variation simply because of a lifetime of experience.

Brief palpation of the scalp and underlying skull is ordinarily adequate to identify the presence of underlying tenderness and the character of the hair. Of course, if there is a history of persistent itching of the scalp, localized pain, or a history of old or recent head trauma, both inspection and palpation will be much more detailed.

Percussion is not performed routinely. If, however, the patient has given a history suggestive of sinusitis or of persistent headache localized to a particular region, percussion should be done. Here, blunt percussion with the finger tip or a knuckle may elicit tenderness signifying some underlying pathology.

Auscultation is not performed routinely in the examination. Infrequently, patients may complain of a distinct humming somewhere in the cranium and in such circumstances, auscultation of the skull should be performed, preferably with the bell of the stethoscope. The presence of a bruit may indicate an underlying vascular brain lesion. Bruit literally means "noise" and the term generally refers to a vascular sound produced over an artery or aneurysm. The term "murmur" (see p. 188) is commonly reserved for a specific abnormal cardiac sound either heard over the heart or transmitted along the larger arteries to some distant location.

THE FACE: In addition to the general skin lesions described in Chapter 7, a few items are of special interest in the facial area. Pallor, which may be seen elsewhere, is particularly prominent in the face, and cyanosis is readily seen in the mucous membrane of the lips. Flushing, due to fever and blushing, is also best seen in the face.

Hypothyroidism, in addition to producing a coarse, thickened facial skin, often modifies the patient's countenance to a dull, sleepy expression (Fig. 8.2). This is in contrast to the excited staring or startled expression often associated with hyperthyroid states. Another characteristic organic change of expression is the "mask-like" facies of the patient with Parkinson's disease.

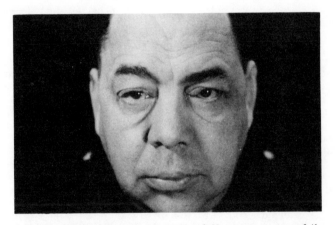

FIG. 8.2: Myxedema facies. Note the dull appearance and the edema of the eyelids.

The facial muscles should be carefully observed for significant asymmetry. Bell's palsy, a paralysis of the 7th (facial) cranial nerve, leads to smoothing out of the forehead and cheek, sagging of the lower eyelid, and drooping of the corner of the mouth on the involved side. Small degrees of paralysis may be present without much asymmetry when the face is at rest, so routinely the patient should be asked to shut his eyes, clench his jaw, and show his teeth. The presence of unilateral facial weakness will become obvious when only one side of the mouth can be raised or one eyelid does not fully close. (This technique of testing for weakness of

muscles by having the patient put them into action is a general one
and should be used whenever muscle groups are being examined.)
Similar findings, although of lesser extent, may be seen in the facial
muscles after a stroke involving the nucleus of the 7th cranial nerve.

Palpation of the face is generally reserved for the investigation of
painful areas or swellings. Enlargement of one or both parotid
glands, which occurs in mumps, is a common cause of swelling of
the cheeks in children and young adults. The enlarged gland is pal-
pably firm and tender.

The face should be touched lightly in several places on both sides to
be sure that the patient has no areas of anesthesia or significant differences in touch sensation from one side to the other.

THE NECK: A complete examination of the neck must include inspection and palpation of the skin, cervical spine, muscles, blood
vessels, thyroid area, and trachea. Masses in or under the skin
should be searched for and carefully reported.

Skin: As elsewhere in the body, the skin is inspected and palpated
for changes in color and texture, for scars, and for the presence of
lesions.

Cervical Spine and Muscles: The curve of the cervical spine is inspected to see if it is exaggerated or absent. Active range of motion
(ROM) is tested by having the patient move his head in flexion and
hyperextension, in rotation, and in lateral flexion, as described
earlier. Limitation of motion may be due to arthritis of the spine or
to muscular stiffness or weakness. Evaluation of muscle strength is
performed by having the patient attempt movements of the head
against moderate resistance by the examiner's hand.

Blood Vessels: Veins of the neck ordinarily are not full except when
the patient is recumbent and they do not pulsate. Engorgement of
veins in the Fowler's or the upright position is evidence of increased
venous pressure due to obstruction or to right heart failure (Fig. 8.3).
Pulsation of veins (be sure that this is not simply due to pulsation of
the carotid artery) may be evidence of cardiac disease and should be
reported.

The carotid arteries should be palpated for forcefulness and for
equality. Because some individuals have a particularly sensitive
carotid sinus reflex, palpation should be done lightly to avoid production of bradycardia or, in rare instances, syncope.

If carotid pulses are unequal, weak, or absent, auscultation should
be done to check for a bruit (Fig. 8.4). Also, if certain cardiac
murmurs are found, it is advisable to listen over the carotid arteries to see if the murmur is transmitted upward into the carotid

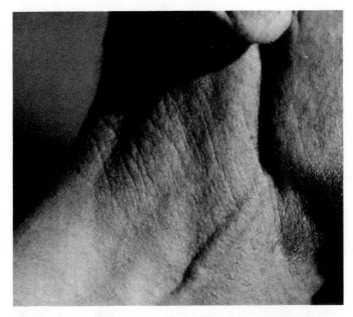

FIG. 8.3: Dilation of neck veins with patient sitting up.

arteries. Detection of an absent carotid pulse, with or without a bruit, is evidence of partial or complete carotid artery occlusion - a most important finding.

Thyroid Gland: As is evident in Fig. 8.1, the gland lies at the lower pole of the thyroid cartilage and the upper trachea. Gross enlargement (goiter) may be seen on inspection (Fig. 8.5). Palpation is performed to evaluate a visibly enlarged gland for its consistency and for the presence of nodules, and palpation is routinely done to detect lesser enlargements. While there are several techniques for palpation of the thyroid gland, they all follow the principles of adequate exposure, comparison of one side of the gland to the other, and the use of motion of the gland through the fingers.

A satisfactory technique is to press gently on one side of the gland, displacing the larynx and trachea laterally (Fig. 8.6). The opposite side is then well exposed and is palpated lightly. Then, keeping the fingers lightly in place, ask the patient to swallow. This motion will move the gland past the finger tips and will help to identify nodules, if present. The gland may be examined with the examiner standing behind or in front of the patient. Both techniques should be learned.

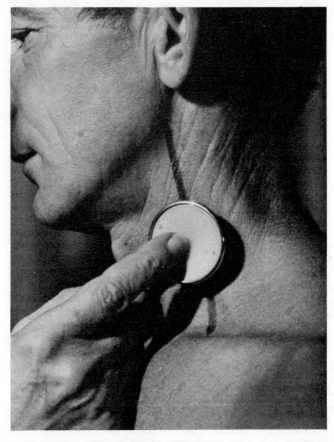

FIG. 8.4: Auscultation for carotid bruit. The line marks the course of the artery in the neck.

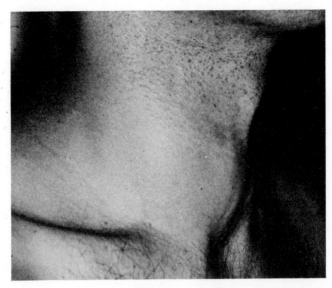

FIG. 8.5: Enlargement of the thyroid gland. Note the position of the thyroid gland in relation to the prominence of the thyroid cartilage. Compare with diagram in Fig. 8.1.

The normal thyroid gland is so soft that its lobes are hardly palpable. Thus, detection of tissue in the proper location which moves on swallowing is possible evidence of thyroid enlargement and should be reported. If one or both lobes of the gland are enlarged, auscultation over the enlarged area may detect a bruit which is due to the great increase in blood flow to an overactive gland.

Trachea: This is inspected and palpated primarily to determine if it lies properly in the mid-line and several centimeters behind the sternum (Fig. 8.7). The trachea should be directly posterior to the suprasternal notch and far enough posterior to allow a fingertip to be inserted between it and the sternum. Displacement from this normal location must be reported, as it may be due to shift of the lung, or to tumor.

Lymph Nodes: Nodes of the face and neck are grouped in four general areas, each of which should be carefully palpated for lymphadenopathy (Fig. 8.8): under the jaw, in the anterior triangle of the neck, in the posterior triangle, and in the supraclavicular space. Occasionally, nodes may be found anterior or posterior to the ear lobe. If palpable, lymph nodes should be described using the criteria noted in the previous chapter.

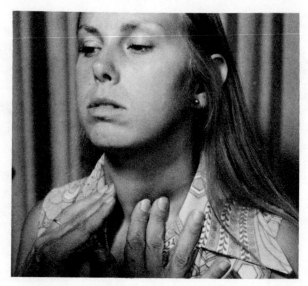

FIG. 8.6: Palpation of the right lobe of the thyroid gland. The examiner is displacing the larynx to the right and palpating with his left fingertips.

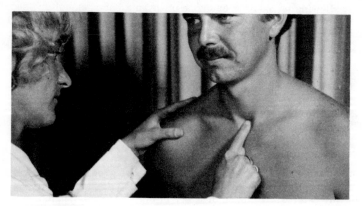

FIG. 8.7: Palpation of the trachea. The trachea is felt directly posterior to the suprasternal notch and several centimeters behind the sternum.

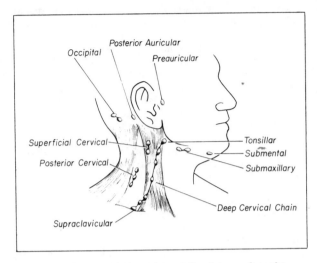

FIG. 8.8: Lymph nodes of the face and neck.

RECORDING

<u>Head</u> - Symmetrical, normocephalic. Normal hair distribution.
<u>Face</u> - No muscle weakness. Appropriate facial expression. Touch intact.
<u>Neck</u> - Full ROM. Veins not distended. Carotid pulsations equal and of good quality. Thyroid not palpable. Trachea midline. No lymphadenopathy.

PATIENT PROBLEM

Mrs. Jean R., a 25-year-old white mother of 3 young boys, presents with a CC "sore throat for 3 weeks."

<u>Problem: Sore Throat</u>

S: Three weeks ago noted cold symptoms; slight cough, sore throat, swollen glands, slight fever, aches and fatigue. Since 2 of her youngsters were ill, she was unable to get rest. One week ago, when symptoms remained, she had CBC and throat culture by personal M.D.; both negative. Has slept poorly, feels tired, depressed, irritable; appetite OK; has lost 2 pounds in 2 weeks. Still has sore throat, thinks she had "palpitation of heart" during argument with husband over boys' behavior. Has difficulty in swallowing, hoarseness, constant achy pain over anterior neck, radiating to both ears.

O: V.S.   T. 37.8°C. (100°F.), P. 130, R. 24, B.P. 120/80

Insp: Pale, thin, well-developed white woman who appears older than stated age. Skin moist, nails bitten and ungroomed, hair thick and normally distributed. Restless.

Palp: Neck: veins not distended. Carotid pulsations strong, rapid and equal. ROM limited. Unable to flex to chin, turn to shoulders, or hyperextend without pain. Thyroid palpable, tender and generally firm to hard. No masses noted. Cervical lymph nodes under jaw are palpable and tender. Nodes in left anterior triangle palpable and tender. No other lymphadenopathy.

A: In view of clinical manifestations of mild hyperthyroidism, negative throat culture with normal white count, thyroiditis is suspected.

P: Dx - CBC, T3, T4, SMA12. Chest x-ray. Consult with MD.
Rx - Complete bed rest, encourage fluids and high vitamin diet as ordered.
Pt. Ed. - Discussed need for period of bed rest with patient and husband. Since no other family member available for assistance, referral made to social service for homemaker. Alternate plans for temporary child care suggested with discussion of possible need for professional help regarding behavior problems.

_____
Signature

SUPPLEMENTAL EXERCISES

1. What is Bell's palsy? Describe the typical physical findings.

2. Palpation for lymph nodes in the supraclavicular fossa is to be done routinely. Of what significance is the finding of a firm or hard node in the left fossa?

REFERENCES

1. Alexander, M.M. and Brown, M.S.: Physical Examination, part 6: The Head, Face and Neck. Nursing '74 4:47, January 1974.

2. Mechner, F.: Patient Assessment, Examination of the Head and Neck. Am. J. Nurs. 75:839, May 1975.

CHAPTER 9

THE EYES

INTRODUCTION

The eyes may readily reveal to the observer many clues to the physical and emotional status of the patient. They may, in their appearance or upon examination, reflect evidence of local or systemic disease processes. Any abnormal findings, or history of pain or loss of vision requires referral to a physician.

TOPOGRAPHICAL ANATOMY

The eye is composed of the eyeball (Fig. 9.1) and accessory structures, including the eyebrows, eyelids, conjunctiva, lacrimal apparatus, and extraocular muscles. These are set into the orbits, the bony sockets of the skull, which provide protection for this entire structure.

The Eyeball

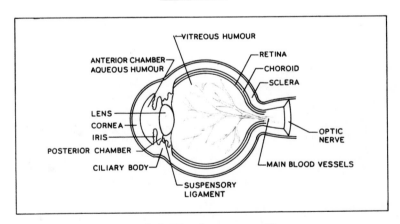

FIG. 9.1: Eye in cross section.

The outer hard coat is the sclera (the white of the eye) to which the eye muscles are attached. The anterior portion of the sclera extends outward in a convex curve and becomes the transparent cornea. The middle coat includes the choroid, a brown membrane just beyond the sclera, the ciliary body, a muscular thickening extended from the choroid, and a suspensory ligament which supports the elastic capsule that encloses the lens of the eye. The ciliary muscle changes the shape of the lens and thus alters the refraction of light rays.

The conjunctiva is a fine transparent membrane divided into two portions, palpebral conjunctiva which lines the inner lid surfaces, and bulbar conjunctiva which covers the eye up to the limbus (junction of cornea and sclera).

Small blood vessels and nerves penetrate the sclera and may be visible as tiny dark dots about a half centimeter outside the limbus These are more prominent in dark complexioned persons.

The iris is a round, pigmented disc, continuous with the ciliary body, containing the pupil.

The innermost coat of the eyeball is the retina, a complex sensory organ. This will be described in association with the examination of the ocular fundus (p. 111).

ACCESSORY STRUCTURES: The accessory structures include the eyebrows and the upper and lower eyelids which normally cover the eye completely when closed. When the eyelids are open and the patient is gazing straight ahead, the lower lid meets the iris, while the upper lid covers a small fraction (two to three millimeters) of the iris. The free edges of the eyelids carry the eyelashes and lubricating glands (Fig. 9.2).

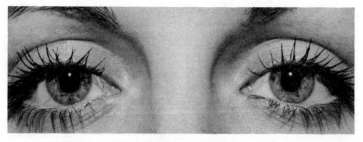

FIG. 9.2: Note the normal palpebral fissures in which both lids are equally separated. The lids are in normal relationship to the iris. The pupils are perfectly round and are equally and moderately dilated.

PHYSIOLOGY

MECHANICS OF VISION: Vision depends upon light rays which enter the eye and, passing through the cornea and pupil, are then focused on the retina by the lens. Muscular activity of the iris regulates the size of the pupil and, therefore, the amount of light which enters the eye. The pupil will constrict in response to bright light and widen when looking from a near object to one in the distance (accommodation). The lens is pulled by the ciliary muscle to change its shape as needed so that the light rays will focus properly on the retina even though the object being viewed moves further away from or nearer to the eye. Any event which interferes with the ability to focus on the retina will result in blurred vision.

In binocular vision the light rays from an object normally strike corresponding points on the two retinas. The two somewhat differing images are interpreted by the brain as a single fused image. In the event that there are two images seen, for whatever reason, diplopia is said to be present.

Color blindness occurs in about eight per cent of the male population. It is due to the absence of certain color receptive cones in the retina. It is an inherited recessive trait and sex-linked; color blindness occurs in less than 0.5 percent of the female population.

TEARING: Blinking, which normally occurs several times per minute, carries lacrimal gland secretions over the eye, bathing it continuously and carrying dust and foreign bodies to the inner or medial angle (canthus) where they can be readily removed. The nasolacrimal duct opening on the lower lid margin at the inner canthus drains away the tears into the nasopharynx.

EXTRAOCULAR MOVEMENTS (EOM): The motions of the eyeball are controlled by six pairs of extraocular muscles which are innervated by cranial nerves III, IV, and VI. Both eyes normally focus on the same point and, at a distance (6 meters or more), the visual axes of the eyes are essentially parallel. The eyes normally operate together, moving simultaneously in the same direction when tracking an object at a distance (conjugate movements), and moving symmetrically inward (nasally), when tracking an object nearing the nose (convergence).

Divergence (strabismus) is an abnormal condition in which both eyes do not fix at the same point either at rest or while in motion (Fig. 9.3).

EXAMINATION

The complete examination of the eye includes inspection of external structures, measurement of visual acuity, determination of visual fields, evaluation of extraocular motion, estimation of intraocular pressure, and exploration of the ocular fundus.

Development of skill in estimation of intraocular pressure and exploration of the ocular fundus will require special instruction and a good deal of intensive practice.

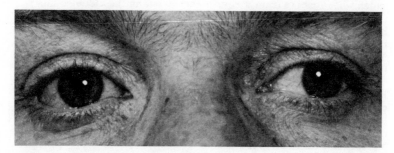

FIG. 9.3: Strabismus or divergence. Note the increased amount of sclera visible in the left nasal angle, and the different positions of the spot of the reflected flash between the right and left eyes. Compare with the symmetrical positions of the light reflections in Fig. 9.2.

INSPECTION OF EXTERNAL STRUCTURES

Eyebrows and Eyelashes: The quantity, distribution, color, and texture of the eyebrow and eyelashes should be determined, keeping in mind the fact that tweezing, make-up, and false eyelashes are the rule rather than the exception for today's woman. The complete absence, however, of eyebrows and lashes may be due to disease, an inherited characteristic, or a manifestation of severe neurotic behavior in which the individual unconsciously removes the hairs.

Eyelash follicles can become infected, producing a painful red sty (hordeolum). A painless cyst-like mass in the eyelid is usually a chalazion - a mass of collected debris due to an obstructed meibomian gland. When infected, it becomes uncomfortable and annoying, so the patient should be referred for treatment.

Eyelids: Very frequent or very infrequent blinking should be noted. Inspect the external surface of the eyelids for any abnormalities in color, lesions, superficial vascularity, or the presence of edema. Because the skin of the eyelid is very thin and loosely attached to underlying tissue, edema can readily occur as a result of a wide variety of systemic and local disturbances. For example, eyelid edema is a common sign in allergic reaction, glomerulonephritis, hypothyroidism, and cavernous sinus obstruction (see Fig. 8.2, p. 85, and Fig. 9.5).

Be certain to observe whether the eyelids close completely, for when this function is impaired, as in Bell's palsy, or in the unconscious patient, corneal drying occurs, leading to ulceration, scarring, and loss of vision unless preventive measures are taken.

The palpebral fissure of each eye should be compared for symmetry (see Fig. 9.2). Ptosis (drooping of the upper lid) may be a congenital condition or early sign of involvement of the third cranial nerve (Fig. 9.4). Observe the position of the lids for eversion (ectropion) and inversion (entropion). Lashes which are misdirected into the eye may cause corneal irritation.

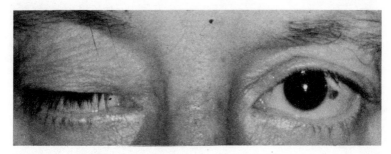

FIG. 9.4: Ptosis of the right eyelid. The spot on the temporal side of the left eye is a sub-conjunctival hemorrhage.

Eyeballs: The globes are inspected to determine if they lie deep in the socket (enophthalmos) or if they project forward (exophthalmos or proptosis). Enophthalmos is often due to dehydration and is frequently associated with an abnormal softness or "mushiness" of the eyeballs to palpation.

Exophthalmos may be suspected if sclera can be seen between the upper lid and the iris. This may be due to actual protrusion of the eyeball, or to stare, in which the patient unconsciously raises the upper lid. Stare can usually be eliminated by asking the patient to gaze into the distance without focusing on any specific object.

True early exophthalmos may be difficult to determine, but if it is suspected, the patient should be referred for accurate measurement. Greater degrees of exophthalmos, which do not allow for full closure of the lids, are dangerous since corneal drying may occur, as mentioned previously. Exophthalmos is also important to recognize because it is usually due to hyperthyroidism or to tumor behind the eyeball. Occasionally, the exophthalmos is unilateral (Fig. 9.5).

PALPATION FOR OCULAR TENSION

Abnormal hardness or softness of the globe is detected by gentle palpation. Softness, as noted above, is often related to dehydration and enophthalmos.

Glaucoma is a serious condition in which there is increased resistance to aqueous humor outflow at the iridocorneal junction resulting in the build-up of intraocular pressure. As the pressure rises,

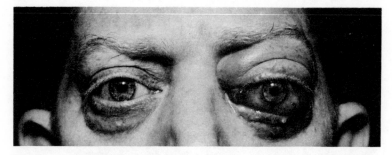

FIG. 9.5: Unilateral exophthalmos. Note the edema of the upper
and lower lids and the severe conjunctivitis of the involved eye.

the retinal artery is compressed, reducing blood flow to the retina.
Permanent progressive atrophy of the retina and optic nerve ensues,
resulting in blindness if treatment is not instituted.

Although adequate examination for glaucoma, which should be done
annually in all individuals over forty, requires a tonometer, screening by simple palpation for eyeball tension should be performed
(Fig. 9.6). The patient is directed to look downward, moving the
cornea down, and the tip of the examiner's middle finger is placed
on the patient's forehead to steady his hand while the index finger is
placed on the upper eyelid. Gentle downward pressure is applied on
the eyeball with the index finger to feel for excessive hardness.

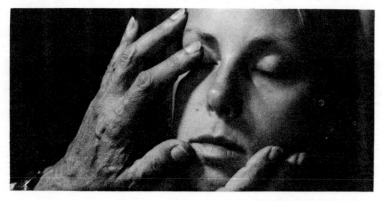

FIG. 9 6: Palpation of the eyeball for ocular tension.

CONJUNCTIVAE

Examine both the palpebral conjunctivae lining the lids and the bulbar conjunctivae covering the sclera. Adequate examination of the lower portions of the membrane can be obtained by pulling the skin below the lower lid downward and having the patient look up. If necessary because of symptoms, or conjunctivitis, the upper portions of the conjunctivae can be visualized by eversion of the upper lid. This may be accomplished by the following procedure:

1. With the patient looking down, grasp the upper lashes and pull downward gently; push down gently on the upper tarsal border with an applicator, finger, or tongue blade, and evert the lid by bringing the lashes to the brow.

2. When inspection is complete, remove the applicator and gently pull the lashes forward and downward as the patient is directed to look up.

Dilation of the small blood vessels (injection) causes the characteristic redness of conjunctivitis (Fig. 9.7; also see Fig. 9.5). A small degree of injection is normally seen at both angles of the eye.

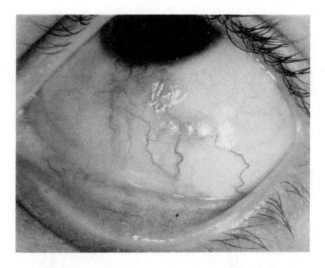

FIG 9.7: Severe conjunctivitis secondary to inflammatory disease of the iris, choroid, and sclera. Note the petechia in the lower lid.

SCLERAE

Observe the sclerae for color change. Normally they are white; however, they may be yellow-tinged with jaundice, or (rarely), if the sclerae are quite thin, they will be blue. Scleral color should always be reported, whether normal or not.

CORNEA AND IRIS

The cornea is an organ which may be the site of opacities (cataract) and abrasions which interfere with its transparency and subsequently affect the individual's visual capacity. The cornea should be inspected from the side with a flashlight for scars, irregularities, and for the presence of foreign bodies (Fig. 9.8). Superficial irregularities create the appearance of a defect in the light reflection on the surface. A common finding in older persons is the deposition of an arc or circle of gray material in the cornea a few millimeters within the limbus. This is arcus senilis (see Fig. 24.1) which may or may not be of clinical significance. Of distinct significance, however, is the presence of a ring of greenish golden pigment just inside the limbus. These are Kayser-Fleisher rings and are associated with a disorder known as Wilson's disease in which there is serious neurological and liver damage.

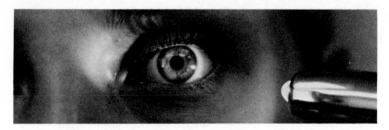

FIG. 9.8: Examination of the cornea by lateral lighting.

PUPILS

Normally, the pupils are of equal size (see Fig. 9.2) and, in a room of average illumination, will not be widely dilated or "pinpoint" in size. The inner margins should be smooth, forming a perfect circle. Significant inequality is always abnormal (Fig. 9.9).

The test for reaction to light is performed by shining a bright light into each pupil and watching for pupillary constriction. The light is brought rapidly into the field of vision from the side to avoid having the patient looking at the light as it approaches. Shine the light into one pupil, and note the response of that pupil (direct reaction). The normal constriction should be prompt, not sluggish or absent. Repeat

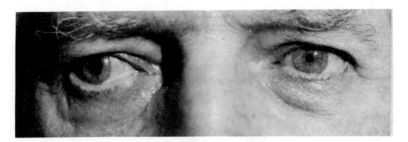

FIG. 9.9: Inequality of pupil size. Note also the strabismus.

this procedure in the same eye, this time watching the other pupil, which should also constrict, although to a lesser degree (consensual reaction). It is important to test for this direct and consensual reaction in both eyes.

Pupils normally also accommodate to near and distant vision by dilating to bring in more light when the individual looks at a distant object. Have the patient look at the examiner's finger, held approximately 15 cm. from the eyes, and watch for some narrowing of the pupils. Then have the patient look past you at any distant object; this accommodation to distance should cause pupillary widening.

VISUAL ACUITY

Distant visual acuity and color vision are best tested with the familiar eye chart (Snellen Chart, American Optical Company, Fig. 9.10). If the patient uses corrective lenses for distant vision, he should wear them for this examination.

Test one eye at a time by having the patient cover the other eye with a card, not his hand, to avoid "peeking." The patient is placed at the test distance just 20 feet (6.1 meters) from the chart and is asked to read lines of smaller and smaller letters until he can no longer read almost all the letters in one line.

The recording system is expressed in relative fraction form. Until the metric system comes into general use, record visual acuity by the common system, in feet. The chart is so constructed (Fig. 9.11) that the number in feet or meters in the right margin represents the theoretical distance from which a person with normal distant vision could have read that line accurately.

Thus, if the patient can read all (or almost all) of the letters in the test line 8, vision in the tested eye is normal, or 20/20. He has read, from a distance of 20 feet, what a normal eye should be able to read at 20 feet.

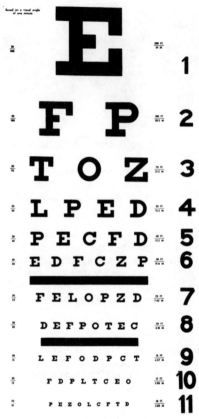

FIG. 9.10: The Snellen Chart. The bar below the letters of line 6 is colored green and that below line 8 is red. Asking the patient to "read the letters over the red line" will quickly identify the patient's color perception, and if he reads the letters correctly, he has 20/20 vision in the tested eye.

If, however, the patient can read the letters of line 6 but not line 7, vision in the tested eye is 20/30, since he has read at 20 feet what the normal can read at the greater distance of 30 feet.

Record vision in each eye separately, viz.: Right eye (O.D) 20/70, left (O.S.) 20/40. If either eye tests below 20/20, the patient should be asked to read the smallest letters he can with both eyes open; [viz.: Both eyes (O.U.) 20/40].

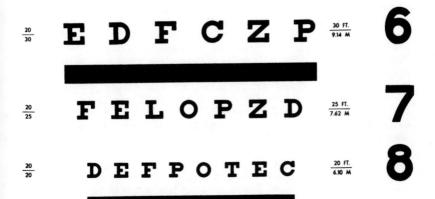

FIG. 9.11: The Snellen Chart, lines 6 through 8. Note distances in feet and meters in the border to your right, and visual acuity for each test line on the left.

If no Snellen (or similar) chart is available, the examiner should try to test distant vision with anything at hand. Large letters in newspaper headlines, textbook titles, labels on equipment boxes, etc., may be used for a crude test. Place the object at any distance at which you can just read the letters clearly and compare the patient's ability to read from the same distance. While such a test cannot measure the patient's distant vision, it can give a clue as to the patient's need for referral for a proper examination.

Since the Snellen Chart tests distant vision, the use of a small commercial pocket card is perhaps convenient, but useless, for this purpose.

Near vision may be tested readily by use of the small print in a newspaper or magazine. Newsprint should be able to be read at 15 to 30 cm. (6-12 inches). If the patient uses reading glasses, they should be worn for this test. Inability to read clearly at less than 30 cm. warrants referral for refraction.

This failure of near vision is called presbyopia, or "far-sightedness." The term myopia means "near-sightedness" and refers, simply, to distant vision below the normal of 20/20.

VISUAL FIELDS

These are superficially tested by comparing the patient's peripheral vision with your own, by noting when both you and the patient can see an object as it enters into the field of vision. Place yourself about 1 meter from the patient and at about the same height, so that your eyes are at the same level. Test one eye at a time by having the patient close one eye (i.e., his left) while the examiner closes the opposite eye (i.e. his right). Instruct the patient to keep his eye on yours so that you are both looking straight forward. Then extend your arms wide apart, placing your hands and raised index finger on a line midway between yourself and the patient (Fig. 9.12). Now move your hands slowly together, asking the patient to notify you as soon as he sees either finger. Wiggling the index finger may assist in being certain that both of you actually see the target. The procedure is then repeated to test the horizontal fields of vision by moving a finger from above and from below the head (Fig. 9.13). This technique is known as gross confrontation and any significant reduction of the patient's fields must be confirmed by a specialist.

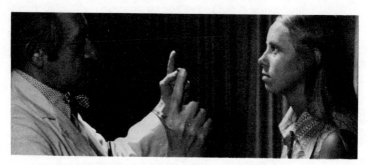

FIG. 9.12: Testing of horizontal fields of vision by gross confrontation. The fingertips must be midway between the examiner and the patient.

EXTRAOCULAR MOVEMENTS (EOM)

The positions of the eyeballs are examined both at rest and in motion. Simple inspection may detect strabismus (see Fig. 9.3) but a better test is examination of the corneal light reflection (or reflex). Stand about one meter in front of the patient, and direct the beam of a small flashlight or penlight into the patient's eyes. The corneal light reflection should be seen in almost the same location in each of the patient's eyes (see Fig. 9.2). If the patient's visual axes are not parallel, the corneal light reflex will not be symmetrical and will indicate strabismus (see Figs. 9.3, 9.5, 9.9). If this condition is of recent origin, the patient may have complained of diplopia. In longstanding divergence, the patient will have learned to suppress the vision in one of his eyes.

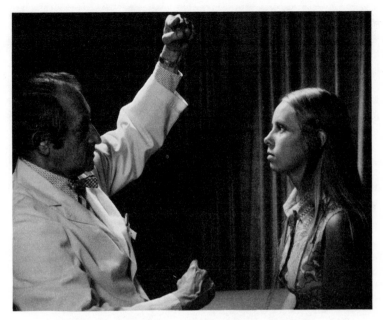

FIG. 9.13: Testing of vertical fields of vision.

If the history has elicited a complaint of diplopia, one additional test for minor degrees of strabismus should be performed. This is the cover test. The patient is instructed to look at a fixed point (mark on the wall, small light source, etc.) and the examiner then covers one eye with a card or his hand. Watch the uncovered eye for movement, for if it does move, it was not looking straight at the fixed point. Repeat the test, covering the other eye. Any move of either eye suggests a small degree of strabismus.

The eyeballs should then be examined in motion. With the examiner directly in front of the patient, ask the patient to follow the movement of a fingertip or point of a pencil without turning his head (Fig. 9.14). A simple rapid test can be done by tracing an imaginary circle in front of the patient, large enough to move the eyes to their full range of motion, horizontally and vertically.

A more precise technique is to trace a large letter "H." Move the target finger horizontally to the left, until the patient's eyes are at extreme gaze in that direction. From that position, trace upward and downward. Next, move the finger horizontally to the extreme right, and then move it up and down on that side. This maneuver will test all of the 6 extraocular muscles of each eye, separately.

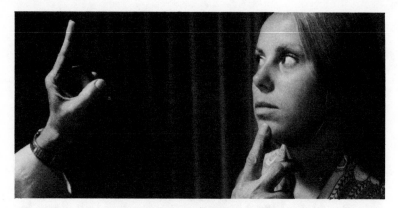

FIG. 9.14: Test for extraocular motion. A fingertip on the patient's chin will prevent motion of the head to follow the target.

Failure of either eye to follow any of these movements smoothly and symmetrically should be carefully recorded. Watch for nystagmus - a rhythmic jerking motion of the eyes - when the eyes are in extreme lateral or upward gaze. Weakness of any of the extraocular muscles or lesions of any of the pertinent cranial nerves will result in divergence and diplopia.

Test for convergence by bringing the fingertip toward the patient's nose. The normal individual should be able to keep both eyes fixed on the target as it is brought to within 15 cm. of the eyes.

OPHTHALMOSCOPY (FUNDOSCOPY)

There is no doubt that ophthalmoscopic examination presents one of the greatest challenges to the student whose aim is skill in physical assessment. Certainly no textbook can provide the beginner with adequate preparation for this objective. Only through the assistance of an instructor and continuous practice can some degree of competence be attained. Practice with specially designed models is useful.

Inspection of the interior of the eye through the ophthalmoscope is of importance in evaluation of local disorders (e.g., cataract, retinal detachment) or of systemic diseases (e.g., diabetes mellitus, hypertension). In the ocular fundus, the examiner can see directly a nerve (the optic disc), arterioles, venules, and a sense organ (the retina) made up of receptors - the rods and cones.

THE OPHTHALMOSCOPE: This is basically a simple instrument which projects a narrow beam of light and has a small aperture through which the examiner can look along the beam (Fig. 9.15).

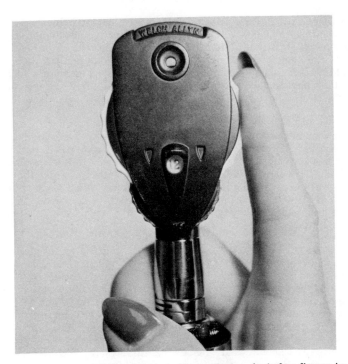

FIG. 9.15: The ophthalmoscope. The examiner's index finger is on
the lens disc and a black +12 diopter lens has been set
in the small viewing aperture above.

There is a set of about 22 lenses (depending on the model) which can
be rotated into the aperture. Usually, there are about 11 convex
lenses, identified by black numerals which range from +20 diopters
(D) to +1D, one zero (plano) lens with no correction, and about 10
concave lenses (red numbers) from -1D to -20D. The lenses are
used to focus on different parts of the patient's eye, and to adjust
for myopia or presbyopia in either the examiner's or the patient's
eye.

Many models have a small wheel below the lens wheel which modifies the projected beam. There are settings for a narrow light beam,
a wider light beam, a grid, a very narrow slit, and a red-free fil-
ter. The beginning practitioner is advised by most experts to ignore
all but the wide light beam.

TECHNIQUE OF EXAMINATION

INTRODUCTION: The student should understand the principles of the examination at this point, although examination should not actually be tried until he is familiar with the structures of the ocular fundus and some of the major abnormalities. This familiarity should be obtained by examining color photographs or color slides. Excellent photographs and descriptions are available in atlases or texts such as Chester's The Ocular Fundus in System Disease.

The light beam from the ophthalmoscope passes through the cornea, aqueous humor of the anterior chamber, lens, vitreous humor and strikes the retina (see Fig. 9.1). Light is then reflected through the transparent structures to the examiner's eye. In this way the clinician can evaluate the clarity of the media through which the light must pass, and also can see the structures which make up the fundus of the eye. The image of the optic disc, blood vessels, and retina (the fundus or "eyegrounds") is greatly magnified by the lens of the patient's own eye.

THE QUESTION OF EYE GLASSES: If the examiner wears glasses or contact lenses for moderate correction of distant vision, he may either learn to do the examination wearing either of these, or he must find the appropriate correction with the ophthalmoscope lenses. Once having determined the proper setting which allows him to be in sharp focus on the retina of patients with no refractive error, he uses this setting each time an examination is begun. However, if the examiner's glasses correct for astigmatism, or for a large error of refraction, he should wear glasses. Similarly, if the patient requires correction for astigmatism, he should wear his glasses while being examined.

DILATION OF THE PUPILS: A more thorough and careful examination can be done through dilated pupils, and dilation should be done if there is no contraindication. If there is no scarring of the iris, or evidence of glaucoma (i.e., previous diagnosis, history of seeing colored rings when looking at lights, acute attacks of eye pain, or hard eyeballs on palpation), it is safe to dilate the pupils. A drop or two of Tropicamide (Mydriacyl) in 1% strength or phenylephrine (Neo-synephrine) 2.5% solution will produce adequate dilation in most cases.

GENERAL CONDITIONS: The examiner should position himself and his patient so that their eyes are approximately at the same level. One convenient technique is for both to be seated on adjustable stools. The room should be dimly lit - not totally dark.

The patient should be instructed to stare straight ahead at some distant spot at about eye level - a light switch, thermostat, etc., or at a mark or tape specifically placed on the wall at the proper location.

Holding the ophthalmoscope in his right hand, the clinician examines the patient's right eye with his own right eye; he reverses this procedure for examination of the left eye. The index finger should be on the lens wheel, so that different lens settings can be made during the examination. With the head of the scope steadied against his brow or nose, and his free hand stabilizing the patient's head, the examiner begins by directing the beam of light into the patient's eye from a distance of about 30 to 60 centimeters (Fig. 9.16).

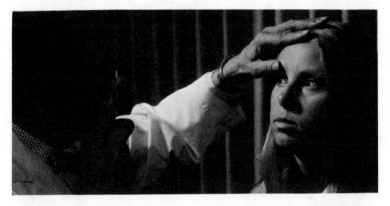

FIG. 9.16: Ophthalmoscopy. Examination of the red reflex.

Here he should pick up the red reflex (see p.111). Following this reflection, the examiner then moves in until the hand holding the scope nearly touches the patient's cheek. If the patient blinks too frequently, the thumb can be used to elevate the upper lid (Fig. 9.17).

If one keeps the red reflex in sight and moves in at about 15° to the patient's line of sight, the optic disc should come into view. If only retina and vessels are seen, the examiner should track vessels back to the disc to start the examination.

If the disc and vessels are not in sharp focus, the lens wheel should be turned in one direction or another until the proper setting is found. Under normal circumstances, all of the fundus should be in sharp focus at one lens setting (Fig. 9.18).

The clinician should learn a pattern of examination in which he examines and notes one portion at a time. The sequence of the following descriptions is a recommended pattern, i.e., red reflex, disc, vessels, and retina (including the macula) in all quadrants. At the completion of the examination, a drop of 1% pilocarpine should be placed in each eye to overcome the dilation.

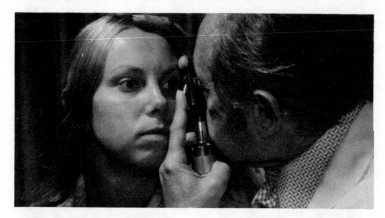

FIG. 9.17: Ophthalmoscopy. Examination of the ocular fundus.

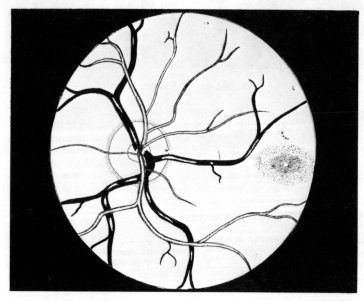

FIG. 9.18: Diagram of normal ocular fundus (O.S.). Arteries are
lighter in color and are about 2/3 the width of veins. At
crossings there are no indentations of veins. The foveal
reflex can be seen about 2 DD from the edge of the disc
at about 3 o'clock (i.e., temporally from the disc) near
the center of the macula.

EXAMINATION OF THE FUNDUS

RED REFLEX: If the cornea, anterior chamber, lens, and posterior chamber are all clear, the examiner should see a red reflection filling the pupil. The color will vary somewhat, depending on the amount of pigment in the fundus, but should be a reddish-orange and bright in intensity (Fig. 9.19).

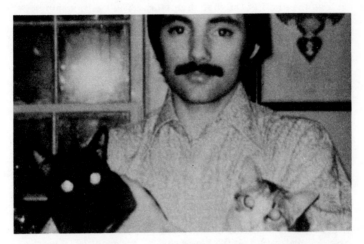

FIG. 9.19: Red reflex. An unplanned red reflex resulting from a photo-flash bulb. Note also the large "green" reflex from the eyes of the black cat, sometimes seen when car headlights are reflected from the retina of an animal on the road at night.

Anything that interferes with light transmission or reflection will change the red reflex. For example, a cataract will produce dark lines or black spots, and other opacities, such as inflammation or hemorrhage, will produce local cloudiness of the reflection or spots in the reflection.

Should such objects be seen interfering with the red reflex, a more detailed view of the opacity may be obtained by using the lens system of the ophthalmoscope. A +20 or +15 lens (black numbers) will enlarge and focus well on lesions of the cornea, anterior chamber and lens. Lens settings from +10 to +4 will focus at different portions of the vitreous, while as noted earlier, a 0 lens should focus on the retina, if both examiner and patient have normal vision or are wearing corrective lenses. The presence of opacities anywhere in the red reflex warrants referral of the patient for special examination.

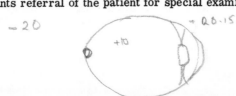

112/ The Eyes

DISC: The flat optic disc (see Fig. 9.18) is the head of the optic nerve and is a prominent landmark. It is round or oval, with a disc diameter (DD) of about 1.5 mm. The temporal margin is quite sharp, while the nasal margin is often less clearly defined. The disc is a pale reddish-yellow in color, a bit darker on the nasal half, and has a small depression near its center - the physiologic cup.

The cup may not be seen in all patients, but is usually present, is lighter in color than the rest of the disc, and should occupy much less than half of the disc diameter. The relationship between the cup and disc diameters is conveniently expressed as a ratio (Fig. 9.20). When the cup enlarges so that the cup/disc ratio is 0.5 or greater, the possibility of glaucoma must be considered, and the patient should be referred to a specialist promptly.

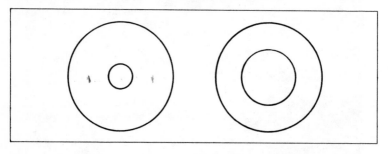

FIG. 9.20: Cup/disc ratios. The diagram on the left has a normal ratio (0.2/1.0), while that on the right is suggestive of a glaucomatous cup with a ratio of 0.5/1.0.

Another significant abnormality of the disc is papilledema (see Fig. 9.22), caused by increased intracranial pressure (often due to brain tumor). As the name suggests, there is edema of the optic disc, causing it to be raised above the level of the retina, and therefore the disc will not be in sharp focus compared to the retina. The margins of the disc are blurred, the disc itself is hyperemic, and the cup may not be clearly visible. Papilledema represents a sign of current danger, requiring immediate referral.

VESSELS: The central retinal artery arises from the cup and spreads out in smaller and smaller branches to all quadrants of the fundus. These branches are arterioles. Venules run roughly parallel to arterioles and reach the retinal vein at the cup. Close observation will often reveal a pulsation of the retinal vein, a normal phenomenon.

Arterioles are smaller in diameter and brighter red in color than venules, which are wider and of a purplish-red color. In the normal state, an arteriole and venule, at the same distance from the cup, will have an arteriole/venule ratio of about 2/3 (see Fig. 9.18).

The reflection of light from arterioles generally produces a narrow light streak, while similar reflections from venules are often patchy. Both arterioles and venules spread across the fundus in wide curves and taper down, more or less evenly, until their caliber is so small that they can no longer be seen. There are frequent crossings, most often with the arteriole crossing above the venule. In a normal crossing, the venule is not kinked, and its outline is not changed; there is no indentation of the venule.

Pathology of the vessels is suggested by changes in size and shape of the vessels and by deformity of the venule at a crossing. In hypertension, the arterioles become spastic - they narrow and become tortuous. With narrowing, the A/V ratio, instead of being about 2/3, changes to about 1/2 or 1/3 (Fig. 9.21). Also, the light streak becomes more prominent so that only a small portion of the arteriole can be seen on either side of the light streak.

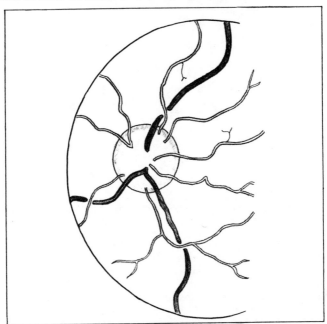

FIG. 9.21: Ocular fundus in moderate arterial hypertension. Note the narrowed, somewhat tortuous arteries compared to the veins and the severe compression of the veins at crossing points.

If narrowing becomes extreme, only the light streak may be seen. As pressure in the arteriole increases, the vessels become more tortuous and, occasionally, they seem to be segmented rather than smoothly tapered.

Kinking or indentation of the venule at a crossing is also abnormal and is referred to as AV nicking. It may become so extreme that the vein seems obliterated (Fig. 9.22). AV nicking is considered to be abnormal only if it occurs at least one DD outside the optic disc. This crossing phenomenon is characteristically seen in hypertensive vascular disease and in generalized arteriosclerosis.

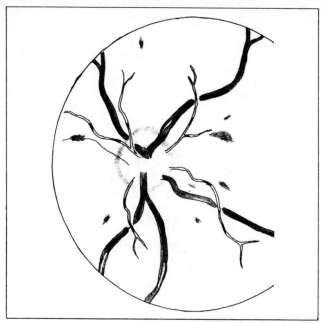

FIG. 9.22: Ocular fundus in severe arterial hypertension. Here, the arteries are extremely narrow, are tortuous, and compress the veins. The edges of the optic disc are blurred, indicating bulging of the disc due to increased intracranial pressure. There are numerous "flame-shaped" hemorrhages visible on the retina.

RETINA: The color of the retina arises from the blood in the underlying choroid vessels and is modified considerably by melanin pigment of the choroid and retina. Thus, the retinal color may vary from a pink-yellow in a light-skinned blonde, to nearly brown in a dark-skinned black individual. The pigment is usually evenly distributed, but occasionally it may be patchy, giving an uneven appearance of the color of the retina. Cyanosis may produce a purplish color, and anemia a paler red tint.

Hemorrhage into the fundus may appear as "flame-shaped" deep red spots (see Fig. 9.22), as round red spots, or, if there is hemorrhage into the vitreous humor, it may produce a hazy medium which

partly obscures the normal sharp appearance of the retina. There
are many other variations in the appearance of hemorrhage, depending on the amount and specific location of the bleeding site.

Exudates are grayish-white patches on the retina and are classified
simply by appearance. "Soft" exudates are often called "cotton-
wool" exudates, since they appear to be fluffy or fuzzy in outline.
"Hard" exudates are somewhat smaller, lighter in color, and have
more discrete borders. Both indicate damage to the retina and
must be reported if present. They occur in various types of diseases such as hypertension, diabetes, and renal disease and, although not diagnostic for any disease, are evidence of general or
local abnormalities.

Macula: The macula is a portion of the retina in which the cones are
collected in greater number, so that this is the area of maximal
visual acuity and of central vision. Due to increased pigmentation,
the macula appears darker than the rest of the retina, with even distribution of the pigment throughout. It lies about 1.5 DD from the
temporal margin of the disc and is about 1 DD in diameter.

During the examination, when the patient is asked to look directly at
the ophthalmoscope light, the macula comes directly into the field,
and a tiny pin-point of bright light can be seen near the center of the
macula. This is a reflection from a small depression in the macula -
the fovea (see Fig. 9.18).

Damage to the macula may appear as a patchy increase in pigment
with loss of the foveal reflex, or as hemorrhage, or as a scar,
obliterating some or all of the area. These are always serious for
they interfere with central vision.

EYEGROUNDS IN HYPERTENSION: Hypertension is a common problem and much useful information about this disorder can be obtained
through fundoscopy. While the level of blood pressure is quite variable from hour to hour or day to day, the retinal changes are relatively permanent. A direct relationship exists between the retinal
changes and the severity of the disease. These changes are graded
by the criteria of Keith, Wagener, and Barker (often abbreviated as
"K-W") as follows:

    K-W Grade 1: Arteriolar constriction, increased tortuosity of
                 arterioles.
    K-W Grade 2: Grade 1 changes plus AV kinking or nicking
                 (see Fig. 9.21).
    K-W Grade 3: Grade 2 changes plus retinal hemorrhages or
                 exudates.
    K-W Grade 4: Grade 3 changes plus papilledema (see Fig.
                 9.22).

Both morbidity and mortality from hypertension are increased as the K-W grade increases. Treatment of severe (i.e., K-W 3 or 4) hypertension may result in slow disappearance of the papilledema and of the exudates and hemorrhages. The arteriolar changes, however, are more or less permanent even with adequate control of the blood pressure.

As indicated at the beginning of the section, fundoscopy is a difficult, complex portion of the physical examination. This section must be considered to be only a brief introduction to the subject and must be pursued by much reading, practice, and instruction.

The references at the end of this chapter are recommended for the student who wishes to develop competence in this examination.

RECORDING

Eyes: Lashes and brows present. No stare or ptosis. Normal ocular tension. Conjunctivae clear. Sclerae white. No defects of cornea or iris. Pupils equal, round, react to light and accommodation (often abbreviated as PERRLA). Snellen: Right eye (OD) 20/20, left eye (OS) 20/20. Color vision intact for red and green. Fields normal by confrontation. Extraocular movements (EOM) normal; no nystagmus or strabismus.

Fundi:

        Red reflex: clear
        Discs: flat with sharp margins. Cup normal
        Vessels: arterioles and venules normal; no AV nicking
        Retina: no hemorrhages or exudates; macula normal,
                foveal reflex present

PATIENT PROBLEM

An 18-year-old woman presents in college infirmary, brought in by roommate because of severe bilateral eye pain and visual disturbances.

Problem: Eye Pain

S: Has been wearing glasses for distant vision since age 12 and hard contact lenses for past 2 years, with no previous difficulty. Because of social commitments, kept lenses in over 18 hours. Awakened from sleep tonight with severe "scratching" pain in both eyes, unable to keep eyes open.

O: Injected conjunctivae; with exam under fluorescein, multiple abrasions noted over both corneas. Excessive lacrimation. PERRLA.

A: Corneal abrasion due to excessive use of contact lenses.

P: Dx - None further.
    Rx - Per protocol: Tetracaine 1% ophthalmic ung. OU. Flush
        with Dacrasol and normal saline.
        Neosporin ophth. ung. OU.
        Patch both eyes - Refer to ophthalmologist promptly
    Pt. Ed. - Review procedures for wearing contact lenses. Re-
    assured re: prognosis. Discussed resumption of use only fol-
    lowing consultation with ophthalmologist.

_____

Signature

SUPPLEMENTAL EXERCISES

1. What are the eye signs that may be found in hyperthyroidism?

2. What is astigmatism? How might it be suspected on the
    examination?

REFERENCES

1. Ballantyne, A.J. and Michaelson, J.C.: Textbook of the Fundus
    of the Eye, 2nd edition. Williams & Wilkins, Baltimore, 1970.

2. Chester, E.M.: The Ocular Fundus in Systemic Disease: A
    Clinical Pathological Correlation. Press of Case Western Re-
    serve University, Ohio, 1973.

3. Mechner, F.: Examination of the Eye - Part I. Am. J. Nurs.
    74:11, November 1974.

4. Mechner, F.: Examination of the Eye - Part II. Am. N. Nurs.
    75:105, January 1975.

5. Rosen, Emanuel and Hannah, Sarir: Basic Ophthalmoscopy,
    Appleton-Century-Crofts, New York, 1971.

CHAPTER 10

THE EAR, NOSE, MOUTH AND PHARYNX

INTRODUCTION

The examination of the ear is principally an inspection of the eardrum, while examination of the nose, mouth, and pharynx is primarily of the mucosa and architecture. Brilliant illumination is essential for viewing these areas which may reflect signs of numerous local afflictions. In addition, the functions of all of these parts must be evaluated carefully.

THE EAR

TOPOGRAPHICAL ANATOMY: The ear is divided into three parts: the external, middle, and inner ear. The external ear consists of the auricle (or pinna) and the external auditory canal. Auricles vary widely in shape and size, but unless very tiny or absent, these variations are usually of no clinical significance. The external auditory canal is about 2.5 to 3 centimeters in length; it narrows toward the mid-portion and widens near the eardrum. Of particular importance is the fact that the first portion of the canal is directed nearly straight into the head, while the remainder of the canal angles medially, anteriorly, and inferiorly. This curve requires the examiner to position the speculum carefully in examination of the eardrum. (It is also the reason for the fact that stethoscope ear pieces must be tailored to each examiner's external auditory canal.)

The middle ear consists of the tympanic membrane (eardrum), the tiny ear bones (ossicles), and an air-filled bony chamber which is connected to the pharynx by the Eustachian tube. The inner ear, which is not accessible to direct examination, is comprised of organs which translate sound waves from the outer world into the language of the "upper world" - nerve impulses - carried by the acoustic branch of cranial nerve VIII. Also here are the semicircular canals which provide the sense of balance, conducted by the vestibular branch of the 8th cranial nerve.

EXAMINATION: The auricles are inspected for abnormally small size or absence, malpositioning, skin lesions, and the presence of nodules. The auricle should also be palpated for nodules - in particular for tophi which are hard, pale, non-tender nodules usually found in or near the outer fold (helix) or near the lobe of the auricle. These tophi are collections of urate crystals associated with gout. Occasionally these tophi rupture, in which case the examiner will see the

118

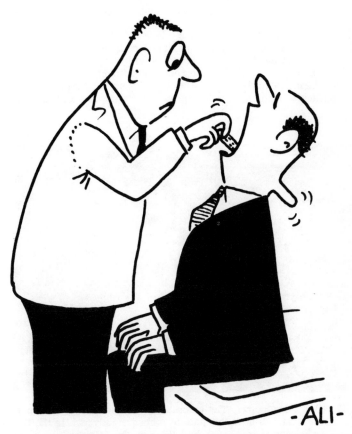

chalk-like crystals which make up these nodules. Crystals should be taken for laboratory examination since gout may be diagnosed definitely if uric acid is identified.

The external auditory canal should be carefully inspected for the presence of blood or discharge of pus or serous fluid before using the otoscope. If present, such discharge should be carefully collected on a cotton-tipped applicator and its character recorded.

For examination with the otoscope (Fig. 10.1), the patient's head should be tilted and the otoscope held firmly between the thumb and fingers of one hand. The auricle is held by the thumb and index finger of the other hand, with the remaining fingers placed on the patient's head. This latter positioning allows the examiner to steady the patient's head and to pull on the auricle upward and backward.

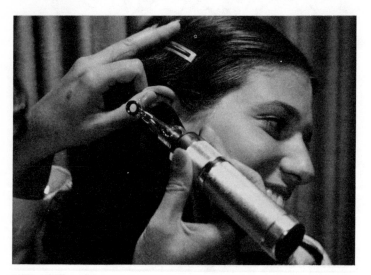

FIG. 10.1: Otoscopy. The examiner's left hand is used to position and to hold the patient's head steady, while the thumb and index finger pull the auricle. Holding the otoscope in the fingers prevents too much force from being applied as the speculum is inserted.

Pulling the auricle serves two purposes: it tends to straighten the curve of the external auditory canal, making insertion of the otoscope speculum easier, and it may produce tenderness in the ear. The presence of tenderness will alert the examiner to the possibility of infection in the canal or the middle ear. The speculum is then inserted slowly and carefully in the direction of the axis of the canal while the examiner "watches his way in." Blind insertion of the speculum is <u>always</u> to be avoided. Cerumen in the external canal which often appears to be red under the bright light is a common and normal finding. Unless the wax obstructs too much of the canal for adequate visualization, it may be ignored. Unless you have had special instruction, do not attempt removal of hard, impacted cerumen - simply report that the examination was incomplete.

Watch for the presence of blood, tumors, or foreign bodies as the speculum is pushed gently toward the eardrum. If difficulty is found in inserting the speculum through the canal, pulling slightly more or less on the auricle and varying the angle of tilt of the patient's head may assist in passage.

Only a portion of the tympanic membrane (TM) may be seen from one position, so the angle of the otoscope will need to be changed, being rotated so that the entire drum and annulus can be visualized completely. The drum normally appears as an oval, thin, partly transparent, gray membrane (Fig. 10.2). There are three important landmarks of the TM - the annulus, the malleus, and the light reflex. The <u>annulus</u> forms the outer border of the drum and is normally much <u>paler in</u> color than the membrane itself.

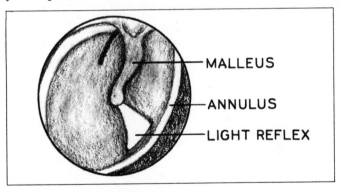

FIG. 10.2: Major landmarks of the oval tympanic membrane as seen through the speculum. The dark crescent seen at the right is the wall of the auditory canal.

At the superior portion of the <u>malleus</u>, a bright, small knob is readily seen. This is the <u>short process</u> of malleus. The handle of malleus - largest of the ear bones - angles downward and posteriorly from the annulus to a point (the umbo) at the center of the tympanic membrane. From the umbo a bright cone-shaped reflection of light can be seen - the <u>light reflex</u>. In cases where the membrane is quite transparent, a portion of another bone - the incus - may be seen extending downward from the annulus, slightly posterior to the malleus.

INSPECTION OF THE EARDRUM: Some common abnormal findings are listed in Table 10.1.

TABLE 10.1		
SOME ABNORMALITIES ON OTOSCOPY		
FINDING	INTERPRETATION	EXAMPLES
Bright red drum	Inflammation	Acute middle ear infection (otitis media)
Yellowish drum	Pus or serum behind drum	Acute or chronic otitis media
Bluish drum	Blood behind drum	Skull fracture
Bubbles behind drum	Serous fluid in middle ear	Chronic otitis media
Absent light reflex	Bulging of drum	Acute otitis media
Absent or diminished landmarks	Thickening of drum	Chronic otitis media or otitis externa
Oval dark areas	Perforation	Recent or old rupture of drum
Malleus very prominent	Retraction of drum	Obstruction of Eustachian tube

HEARING TESTS: Despite the fact that the examiner has had much conversation with the patient up to this point, he should perform one specific clinical hearing test. Some patients with hearing loss will, consciously or unconsciously, deny such a loss, or may have been able to compensate for a unilateral loss by a combination of use of the good ear and some basic lip-reading.

Clinical tests to evaluate the patient's ability to hear are rather crude in that they can give evidence of a hearing loss but are not adequate to measure the degree of loss.

It is our opinion that, if the patient has difficulty with any of these simple, nonquantitative, clinical tests, he should be referred for further examination. All of these will test hearing somewhere in the conversational range of hearing (roughly 100-2000 cps), and a defect here may definitely impair a patient's daily life style.

Any one of the following is an adequate screening test but the examiner should become familiar with all of them so that he can select one, depending upon the circumstances. All should be done in a quiet environment, however.

Simplest is the watch test if the examiner carries a watch which ticks loudly enough. Here, the examiner tests one ear at a time by moving the watch toward the patient's ear and estimating the distance at which the ticking begins to be heard. Knowing the distance at which the normal can just hear the ticking, the examiner can judge the presence or absence of hearing loss. Simply record normal or diminished hearing for each ear.

Another method is to use your tuning fork as the sound source. Stand at the patient's side, set the fork vibrating gently and hold it at an equal distance between your ear and the patient's. Testing each ear separately, ask the patient to let you know when he no longer hears the sound.

Should you still be able to hear the hum distinctly when the patient no longer hears it, you have identified some degree of loss for the tested ear. On the other hand, if you no longer can hear the sound and the patient still has not signalled that the sound is gone, it may suggest that the patient is not being truthful. Of course, this test assumes that you have normal hearing.

The whispered voice test is somewhat better than the others and is useful if no suitable watch is available, or if the examiner's own hearing is not normal. Position the patient about 6 meters (20 ft.) away, turned so that one ear is facing the examiner and have the patient plug the other ear with a fingertip; whisper a few words slowly and clearly, asking the patient to repeat each word as he hears it. Use two syllables such as "baseball," "forty-six," "hot dog," "textbook," etc. Two or three such words are adequate. Have the patient face in the opposite direction and test the other ear in similar fashion, using different words.

If the patient hears these words well, his hearing can be reported as normal. If he cannot hear at that distance, simply report a loss for the affected ear, or ears. Do not waste time by continuing to repeat this test by moving closer and closer to the patient, as this is still a rough, clinical test for the presence of enough hearing loss to warrant referral.

It is obviously necessary for the examiner to practice on a normal subject so that he learns just how loudly to project his voice to be heard clearly at about 6 meters, but not much further. It is also

obvious that hearing should be tested after otoscopy, for if a patient
has one or both canals completely obstructed by cerumen, no proper
evaluation of hearing function in a blocked ear can be performed.

The Weber test is routinely performed. Strike the tuning fork, hold
it by its stem, and press the stem firmly against the skull or forehead in the mid-line (Fig. 10.3). The sound should be heard equally
well in both ears, or nearly so; a distinct difference is abnormal.
The Weber test should be reported as "normal" if the sound is equal
in both ears, and as "heard best in the _____ ear" or "lateralized to
the _____ ear," if abnormal.

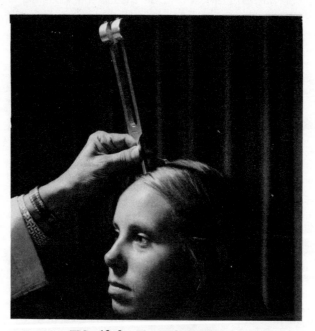

FIG. 10.3: The Weber test

While the Rinné test is described in almost all other textbooks, we
suggest that it be eliminated from the routine examination. A defect
in hearing by the watch or whispered voice test, and/or a lateralization in the Weber test is sufficient to determine that the patient should
be referred to a specialist.

Vestibular function is not tested in this examination, as specialized
equipment is required.

THE NOSE

The functions of the nose are to serve as an organ of smell, as a passageway for air into the sinuses and the respiratory tract, as an accessory organ in speech production, and as part of the disposal system for tears which reach it via the lacrimonasal duct. In addition, the nose, as the most prominent feature of the face, is extremely important to the individual's appearance. Deformities, supposed deformities, or disfigurements, are therefore frequently disturbing to the person's self-image.

TOPOGRAPHICAL ANATOMY: Internally, the nasal septum divides the nose into right and left nasal cavities. The septum, which is composed of a lower cartilaginous portion and a superior bony portion, is frequently not perfectly straight. Septal deviations are of little importance unless they obstruct the flow of air through the cavity. The lateral wall includes three bony structures - the inferior, middle, and superior turbinates. The septum and outer walls are covered by a specialized mucous membrane often of a slightly redder color than the oral mucosa. The frontal, maxillary, ethmoidal, and sphenoidal sinuses all open into the nasal cavity.

EXAMINATION: Simple inspection of the external nose is generally adequate unless there has been recent facial trauma or a complaint of pain, in which case palpation for tenderness should be performed.

Before use of the nasal speculum, a brief check for patency of each nasal passage should be performed. Obstruct one nostril, have the patient exhale with the mouth closed, and feel the puff of air with the fingertips several inches away from the other nostril. Significant degrees of obstruction can be detected and will alert the observer to identify the cause of the obstruction as he inspects the nasal cavities.

The examination of the nasal cavities is carried out with a nasal speculum (Fig. 10.4). This instrument, like the ear speculum, is inserted gently while the examiner "watches his way in." The presence and character of any discharge should be noted. The septum is inspected for perforation, tumor, and significant deviation. On the lateral wall, the large inferior turbinate is readily seen and the middle turbinate should ordinarily be seen. Difficulty in visualizing the cavity up to the level of the middle turbinate is often due to swelling of the mucosa of the inferior turbinate - a common finding in our modern environment. No attempt should be made to push the speculum past a swollen turbinate. The upper or superior turbinate is almost never seen since it is small and lies in the deep posterior portion of the wall.

The color of the mucosa varies from the bright, fiery red of inflammation to normal pink to a pale grayish color often associated with allergic rhinitis.

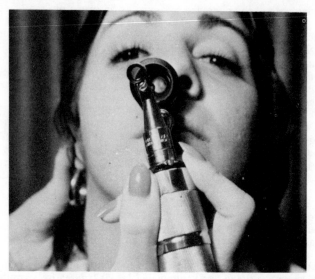

FIG. 10.4: Use of nasal speculum. The patient's head is tilted
backward to allow for easy viewing of the nasal passage.

If the patient's history or the finding of pus in the nasal cavity suggests sinusitis, palpation over the sinuses may produce useful information. Here, palpation is in the form of firm pressure on the
right and left sides simultaneously to detect tenderness - just above
the supraorbital ridge (frontal sinuses) and just below the orbits and
across the cheek bones (maxillary sinuses). Percussion over the
frontal or maxillary sinuses may elicit pain in the presence of acute
sinusitis.

With his eyes closed, the patient should be able to identify the odor
of a common substance such as alcohol, chocolate, or tobacco.

MOUTH AND PHARYNX

The oral cavity and pharynx with their associated structures are
highly complex organ systems which function in numerous important
somatic and psychic activities. The mouth is only rarely used as a
weapon of offense but serves to bite, chew, taste, mix, and propel
food; it is used constantly to express emotions; and together with the
pharynx, it is a major passageway for respiratory air and for speech.
In such a complex system there is much for the practitioner to
examine.

Early detection of malignant lesions is of critical importance because of the tendency for rapid spread of squamous cell carcinomas of the tongue, floor of the mouth and tonsils.

ANATOMY: The roof of the mouth consists of an anterior, pale, hard palate and a smaller, pink, mobile, soft palate posteriorly. The uvula hangs downward in the midline from the posterior border of the soft palate (Fig. 10.5).

The floor is made up of the tongue and underlying muscles. Posterolaterally, on either side, the anterior and posterior tonsillar pillars frame the passageway to the oropharynx (Fig. 10.6). Between these pillars lie the palatine tonsils. At the back of the oropharynx is the posterior pharyngeal wall.

The tongue is a muscular organ with small taste buds in the anterior two-thirds of its surface, and larger taste buds - the circumvallate papillae-posteriorly (Fig. 10.7). When the tongue is raised, a fold of oral mucosa called the frenum can be seen, attaching the lower surface of the tongue to the floor of the mouth (Fig. 10.8). It is congenital shortening of this frenum which causes "tongue-tie." The ducts of both the sublingual and the submandibular salivary glands open into the mouth along the frenum. Lateral to the frenum near its attachment to the tongue, the sublingual veins can be seen.

The openings of the ducts of the main salivary glands - the parotids - can be seen on the lateral (buccal) surfaces of the cheeks opposite the upper second molar teeth. These ducts usually open on a small raised pad on the buccal surface.

The mouth contains 32 teeth in the adult with complete dentition. These are set in spongy tissue - the gingivae (gums).

EXAMINATION: The external portions of the mouth and lips are inspected for color changes (i.e., cyanosis, pallor), for clusters of darkly pigmented freckles, for ulcerative lesions, for incomplete fusion (i.e., cleft lip), and for symmetry. The corners of the mouth are observed carefully for cracks or fissures. If present, the condition is called cheilosis, commonly due to poor dental hygiene, ill-fitting dentures, or vitamin deficiency.

An acute vesicular eruption referred to as "fever blister" or "cold sore" may be found on or around the lips. Known as herpes simplex, this condition is due to a viral infection, and is frequently associated with prolonged exposure to the sun, the common cold, menstruation, or high fevers in bacterial infections.

If any drooping of one side of the mouth is noted on preliminary inspection, it may be evidence of paralysis of the seventh cranial nerve. Since minor degrees of paralysis may not be evident, all patients should be asked to clench the teeth tightly together while

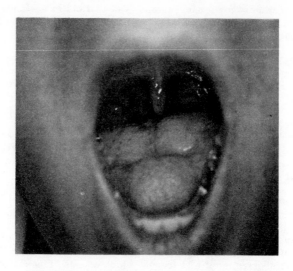

FIG. 10.5: View of the mouth showing the uvula hanging in the mid-
line from the soft palate, the tongue, and enlarged
tonsils.

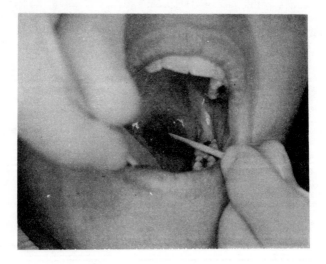

FIG. 10.6: Tonsillar area. The pointer is on the anterior pillar,
and the posterior pillar is seen directly behind it. The
space between the pillars is the tonsillar fossa. This
patient has had a tonsillectomy.

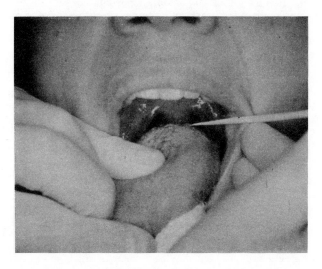

FIG. 10.7: The large, circumvallate papillae of the tongue are indicated by the pointer.

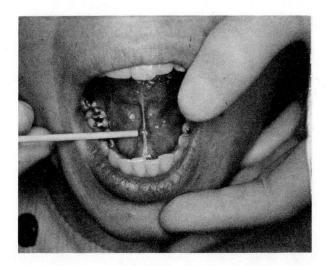

FIG. 10.8: The frenum of the tongue (lingual frenum). The pointer indicates the location of the outlets of the ducts of the sublingual and submaxillary salivary glands.

opening the lips as widely as possible. Seventh nerve weakness
may become evident with distinct asymmetry of the corners of the
mouth. Failure to be able to clench the teeth tightly is evidence of
weakness of the jaw muscles or of the motor nerve to those muscles (see p. 258). The upper and lower teeth should be aligned
when the jaw is clenched.

Next, the oral cavity and pharynx should be examined. If the patient has dentures or removable bridges, ask him to place these on
a paper towel or some other clean surface. The human mouth is
teeming with bacteria, so the examiner is well-advised not to touch
dentures or portions of the oral cavity with ungloved fingers. Use
the tongue blade to retract the lips and to push the sides of the
mouth open wide to visualize all of the oral mucosa, the teeth, and
the gums, leaving the tongue and pharynx for last.

With the tongue blade and a penlight, or other good source of light,
inspect the teeth and gums, including the biting and chewing surfaces of the teeth, and both the buccal (cheek) and lingual (tongue)
aspects of all of the teeth and gums. The teeth are inspected for
obvious defects such as large cavities, cracks or chips, looseness
in their sockets, discoloration, or loose appliances such as bridges
or crowns on the teeth. The gums are examined for bleeding, swelling, pus, or discoloration.

Then the oral mucosa of the floor, cheeks, and palate is inspected
for color, pigmented spots, vascular lesions such as telangiectases
(see p. 73), ulceration, firm white plaques, or tumors.

Any lesions of the lip or buccal mucosa seen on inspection should be
palpated (Fig. 10.9). The floor of the mouth is routinely palpated.
This is best done bimanually with one finger in the mouth and the
other hand outside; masses or tenderness are reported in detail.

The tongue is inspected by having the patient stick it out as far as
he can. It should protrude in the midline, and there should be no
tremor. The upper surface, the sides, and the under-surface of the
tongue should then be inspected for color, texture, size, symmetry,
and the presence of lesions. The color of the tongue is ordinarily
not much different from that of the oral mucosa, and its surface is
slightly irregular due to taste-buds and small furrows. Its size
must be evaluated in proportion to the mouth. Only experience will
teach the student what represents an enlarged tongue, but the presence of deep furrows running from the back toward the front of the
tongue is a sign of reduced size of that organ. This is frequently due
to dehydration of the patient. Palpation of the tongue should then be
performed to detect masses or tenderness.

Since the lateral posterior third of the tongue at the junction with the
floor of the mouth cannot be seen readily, and since it is a location
in which squamous cell carcinoma can remain hidden, it is necessary

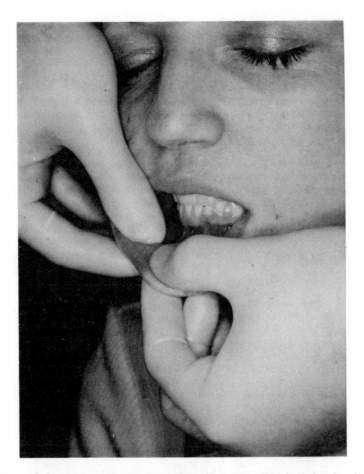

FIG. 10.9: Bimanual palpation of the lip. Note that both hands of
the examiner are gloved.

to pull the tongue aside for a proper view. A recommended technique is to fold a 4 x 4 gauze pad into a 1 x 4 strip and have the patient place his tongue on the middle of the strip (Fig. 10.10). The
gauze is then wrapped around the tongue, firmly but not tightly, making a thick, nonslippery, protective pad. This pad is then grasped
by one hand, and the tongue can be pulled gently outward and laterally,
exposing the lateral posterior portion of the tongue (Figs. 10.11,
10.12). A tongue blade or gloved finger can then pull the cheek outward to provide a good view.

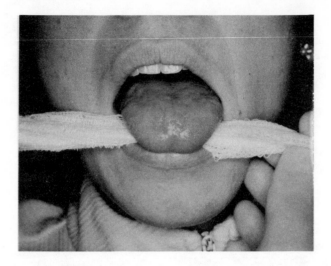

FIG. 10.10: Placement of gauze pad.

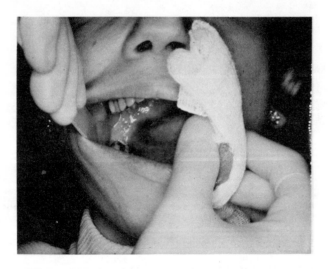

FIG. 10.11: View of the postero-lateral portion of the tongue.

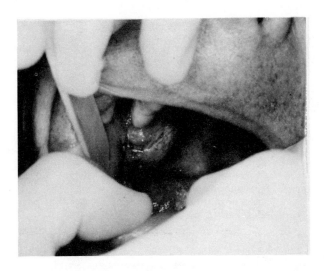

FIG. 10.12: Carcinoma of the postero-lateral portion of the tongue.
This is a large lesion, seen late in its growth.

Prompt referral to a dentist is indicated for any significant abnormalities noted on the inspection or palpation of the oral cavity.

After this, the pharynx is examined. Since many patients gag readily, it is often easier to examine one side at a time. Have the patient protrude his tongue and breathe rapidly. Place the tongue blade on the right or left half of the tongue, with its tip no further back than the level of the uvula, and press downward and medially. This will give good exposure of the tonsillar pillars, the tonsil, and a portion of the posterior pharyngeal wall of one side. The presence of pus or large amounts of mucus on the posterior pharyngeal wall is evidence of inflammation or infection of the nasopharynx or sinuses.

After repeating this procedure on the other side, ask the patient to say a prolonged "ah." This act of phonation should cause the soft palate to elevate, providing a better view of the posterior pharyngeal wall. Both sides of the soft palate should rise equally, carrying the uvula upward in the mid-line. Deviation of the uvula to one side or the other is evidence of probable involvement of the 9th or 10th cranial nerve on one side. Absence of upward motion of the soft palate is indicative of probable damage to these nerves bilaterally.

As a final test, touch the tonsillar pillar on each side to produce a gag reflex. Watch carefully to see if both sides of the soft palate rise equally.

RECORDING

Ears: No masses or lesions of auricles or canals. No dis-
       charge. Both TM pearly-gray, no perforations; light
       reflex present. Watch ticking heard bilaterally.
       Weber test normal.

Nose: Patient bilaterally. No septal deviation or perfora-
       tion. Mucosa pink. Can identify alcohol.

Mouth: Can clench teeth. Mucosa and gingivae pink, no le-
       sions or masses. Teeth in good repair. Tongue pro-
       trudes in midline, no tremor.

Pharynx: Mucosa pink, no lesions. Tonsils absent. Uvula
         rises in midline on phonation. Gag reflex present
         bilaterally.

PATIENT PROBLEM

Liz A. is a four-month-old, alert, well-developed girl infant brought
to the Health Center by her anxious mother because she has been irritable, crying, sleeping and eating poorly for the past week.

Problem: Fever and Irritability

S: Health record indicates infant low forceps delivery of primipar-
    ous mother, age 21. Pregnancy normal except for urinary
    tract infection in the fifth month. Labor 16 hours, mother re-
    ceived general anesthesia. Apgar score of infant 8. Birth
    weight 3350 Gm. Uneventful neonatal period. Growth and de-
    velopment patterns normal. Mother states infant has been
    sleeping through night, taking soybean formula well (eczema
    since 2 weeks) and eating prepared fruits and cereals well until
    one week ago when she developed cold symptoms, temp. 38.3°C
    (101°F.), Rx with liquid aspirin, steam vaporizer. Condition
    improved and no respiratory problem persists. Two days ago,
    began to cry during feeding and refused formula. Has been dif-
    ficult to feed and sleeps poorly, awakening for formula appar-
    ently hungry, yet refusing to suck more than an ounce or so.
    Has never had penicillin.

O: Well-developed, weight and length appropriate to age and birth
    weight. Skin flushed, temp. 38.3°C., crying throughout exam.
    Mouth: lower right central incisor erupting, gums red. No le-
    sions. Pharynx: Mucosa reddened with thin film of white exu-
    date. Tonsils enlarged bilaterally. Ears: Normal placement.
    Right canal with discharge (yellowed). Right TM - deep red and
    bulging. Light reflex not visible. Left TM pink - increased
    vascular markings. Light reflex not visible.

A: Acute otitis media both ears. Possible streptococcal infection pharynx.

P: Dx - Nose and throat culture stat.
Rx - Per protocol. Liquiprin 2 ml. qid. Erythrocin 125 mg. p.o. Qid x 3 da. Encourage feeding q2h if possible.
Pt. Ed. - Mother advised to call Center in AM for throat culture report. Reviewed need to increase fluid intake and procedure for direct administration of medications - not in formula.

_____
Signature

SUPPLEMENTAL EXERCISES

1. What is the significance of the Rinné test? Why should it be performed with a C-512 or higher-pitched tuning fork?

2. List several common causes of epistaxis.

REFERENCES

1. De Weese, D.D. and Saunders, W.H.: Textbook of Otolaryngology, 5th edition. C.V. Mosby Co., St. Louis, 1977.

2. Brown, M.S. and Alexander, M.M.: Physical Examination, Part 7: Examining the Ear. Nursing '74 4:48, Feb. 1974.

3. Brown, M.S. and Alexander, M.M.: Physical Examination, Part 9: Examining the Nose. Nursing '74 4:35, July 1974.

4. Mechner, F.: Examination of the Ear. Am. J. Nurs. 75:457, March 1975.

CHAPTER 11

THE THORAX AND LUNGS

INTRODUCTION

Although x-ray study of the chest is considered a major tool in
health screening and evaluation of respiratory problems, it is not
intended to replace careful physical examination. Both these types
of examination contribute to the total examination of the chest wall
and its contents, since each can detect abnormalities not able to be
picked up by the other. Certain abnormalities of respiratory disease may be detected only by physical examination (i.e., asthma),
while deep-lying tumors can be found only by x-ray examination.

Within the bony framework of the thorax lie the bronchi, lungs and
heart. The domes of the right and left portions of the diaphragm
rise high into the thoracic cage, so that the upper abdominal contents are also enclosed within the chest (see Fig. 11.18). Although
all of these structures, as well as the breasts, will be eventually
examined as a unit, this chapter will consider only the examination
of the thorax and the lungs.

TOPOGRAPHICAL ANATOMY

The bony thorax (Fig. 11.1) includes twelve pairs of ribs and twelve
thoracic vertebrae.

Anteriorly the sternum is seen in the center of the chest as a vertical flat bone consisting of a manubrium, body, and xiphoid cartilage.
At the superior edge of the manubrium is a depression which is referred to as the suprasternal notch. The junction of the manubrium
and the body forms a slight angle protruding forward which is known
as the angle of Louis. Since the second ribs articulate at the level
of this angle, it serves as a reference point for counting the ribs.

The shape of the thorax is essentially elliptical in adults with a wider
diameter at the base than at the top, but in infants it is cylindrical
with a more nearly equal diameter from top to base.

The antero-posterior (A-P) diameter of the thorax is clearly smaller
than the transverse diameter in normal individuals. Each rib is a
flattened arched bone, arising at approximately a 45 degree angle
from its junction with the vertebra, and continuing as a costal cartilage in its attachment anteriorly to the sternum. It is separated
from the next rib by an intercostal space which takes its number

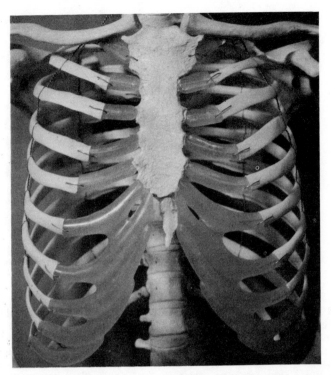

FIG. 11.1: Bony thorax. The first ribs are barely visible. The second ribs articulate at the junction of the wide manubrium with the narrower body of the sternum where the angle of Louis is formed.

from the rib above. There is a downward and forward slope of each rib which increases progressively, so that the width of the intercostal spaces increases toward the inferior edge of the rib cage.

The first seven ribs (true ribs) articulate directly with the sternum. The eighth, ninth, and tenth (false) join with the cartilage of the rib above. The eleventh and twelfth are free (floating ribs), and do not articulate at their anterior ends. The tenth is the lowest seen anteriorly, while the eleventh may be seen laterally and the twelfth rib is seen posteriorly only. The subcostal angle, formed by the lower anterior rib margin with the xiphoid process, is normally less than 90 degrees.

The thorax includes this bony cage, the scapulae, and the soft tissues. For purposes of reference, several vertical lines are used (Figs. 11.2,

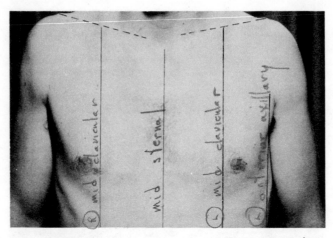

FIG. 11.2: Reference lines. From the left of the picture these are the right mid-clavicular line, the mid-sternal line, the left mid-clavicular line, and (barely visible) the left anterior axillary line.

and 11.3). The mid-sternal line passes from the suprasternal notch to the xiphoid and the mid-clavicular lines are drawn from the centers of each clavicle. The anterior and posterior axillary lines are dropped vertically from the anterior and posterior axillary folds respectively and a mid-axillary line lies between these. Posteriorly, the mid-spinal line runs vertically down through the spinous processes of the vertebrae. The space between the medial borders of the scapulae is referred to as the interscapular area (see Fig. 11. 16). Imaginary horizontal lines are not necessary, since the ribs and interspaces are used as reference lines.

The trachea, as pointed out in the section on neck examination, should be in the mid-line directly posterior to the suprasternal notch. It bifurcates into the right and left mainstem bronchi at about the level of the angle of Louis. Thus, physical findings related to the major bronchi occur in the upper mid-portion of the chest.

Fig. 11.4 illustrates the projection of the right and left lungs as they appear in different phases of respiration.

PHYSIOLOGY

In the normal adult, the resting rate of respiration is approximately sixteen to twenty cycles per minute, regular in rate and rhythm. The normal respiratory cycle consists of an inspiratory phase requiring muscular activity, and a shorter, passive expiratory phase.

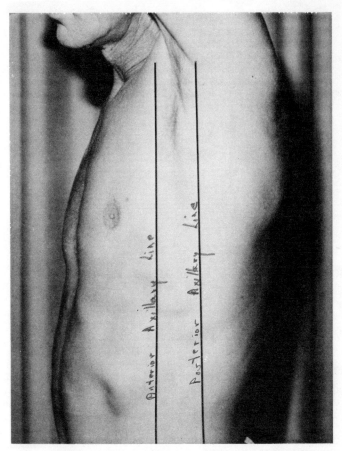

FIG. 11.3: Reference lines. Anterior axillary line and posterior axillary line are shown. The mid-axillary line falls midway between these.

During inspiration the ribs are elevated primarily by action of the intercostal muscles. This serves to increase the antero-posterior diameter of the chest. Also during inspiration the diaphragm descends. This coordinated action increases the volume of the thorax, allowing for the free entry of respiratory air into the lungs. Expiration, on the other hand, is a passive and more rapid action in which the air is expelled by a recoil of the expanded thoracic cavity in a return to its resting state.

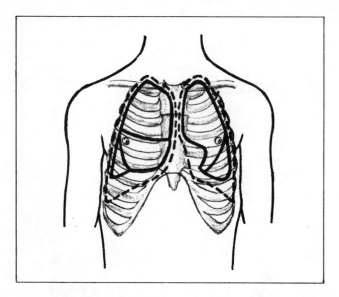

FIG. 11.4: Projection of the lungs on the thoracic wall. The solid
lines represent the lungs in expiration; the dashed line
shows the expansion of lungs during inspiration. The
right lung is shown divided into a right upper, a right
middle, and right lower lobe, while the left has only an
upper and lower lobe.

Normally the entire chest wall moves together and expands equally
with a 5-8 centimeter expansion from maximum expiration to maximum inspiration. Males characteristically use the chest wall less
than females in normal respiration, depending more on diaphragmatic breathing.

BREATH SOUNDS: As a result of the movement of air through various portions of the respiratory system during respiration, soft audi-
ble vibrations are produced - the breath sounds. The quality and
intensity of the sounds depend upon the location of their production
and the tissues through which they are transmitted to the examiner's
stethoscope. There are three types of normal breath sounds (Fig.
11.5):

1. Vesicular sounds: soft, low-pitched (100-300 cps) fine rustling
   or swishing sounds, like a sigh, heard from early inspiration to
   early expiration. In quiet respiration the expiratory sound may
   not be heard at all. These sounds are produced by air movement in the terminal bronchioles and alveoli and are heard over
   most of the chest.

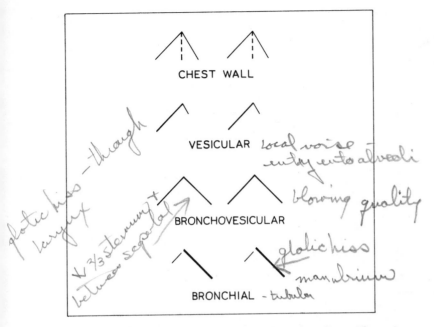

FIG. 11.5: Diagrammatic representation of two breaths. The upper
diagram represents chest wall motion during inspiration
(upstroke) and the shorter expiratory period (down-
stroke). For purposes of clarity, bronchovesicular
sounds are illustrated between vesicular and bronchial
sounds to show the mixed character of these sounds.

2. Bronchial sounds: loud, high-pitched (over 500 cps) "tubular"
   sounds, louder and longer in expiration with a brief pause between the inspiratory and expiratory components. These are
   normally heard only anteriorly over the trachea and major bronchi (see Fig. 11.14).

3. Broncho-vesicular sounds: a combination of the above two
   sounds, since they represent a mixture of sounds being produced by both bronchial and alveolar air vibrations. Note that
   there is no pause between the inspiratory and expiratory sound.
   These are characteristically heard over portions of the chest
   where a bronchus is near lung parenchyma, i.e., over the upper
   anterior chest, the apex of the right lung and in the interscapular
   space (see Fig. 11.15).

Vocal fremitus: Speaking produces vibrations in the larynx which are
transmitted through the respiratory system to the chest wall. These
vibrations, known as fremitus, can be felt with the hands ("tactile

fremitus") or heard with the stethoscope ("vocal resonance"). Fremitus varies from individual to individual, being better transmitted in males and in thin-chested persons. Fremitus is also better felt or heard in the upper portion of the chest wall than near the base.

EXAMINATION

Adequate examination of the thorax requires that the patient have all clothing removed to the waist and that, if possible, he be sitting on an examining table or standing.

AXILLA

The axilla is a pyramid-shaped space in which the examination is directed toward the sebaceous glands of the apex and the lymph nodes of the apex and thoracic wall of the pyramid. The patient's arm should be raised to allow for inspection. Lymph nodes may be enlarged enough to be visualized, and occasionally the development of infection of the sebaceous glands will be evidenced by reddening and edema of the skin near the apex.

Following inspection with the patient's arm still raised, the fingertips are placed at the apex. When the patient's arm is lowered, the muscles of the area are relaxed and deep palpation of the apex can be accomplished (Fig. 11.6). Lymph nodes should be felt for here and down the thoracic side of the pyramid. If nodes are palpable, they should be described as masses using the criteria described in Chapter 7.

THE THORAX AND LUNGS

General: The thorax and lungs are examined as a unit because of the intimate relationship between the bony cage of the thorax and the chest motions in ventilation of the lungs. For purposes of clarity, the breast and the heart are described separately.

The sequence of examination of the chest should be Inspection - Palpation - Percussion - Auscultation.

Inspection: Consideration should be given first to posture, contour, general development, and motion of the thorax. It is important to note the patient's posture, since individuals with chronic obstructive lung disease often sit up and prop themselves on their arms (Fig. 11.7) or lean forward with their elbows on a desk, in an attempt to fix their clavicles and gain greater ability to expand the chest.

The contour of the chest is often abnormal due to an increase in the A-P diameter so that it approaches the transverse diameter. The sternum appears pushed forward and the ribs are more horizontal. The patient seems to be in a constant state of full inspiration with

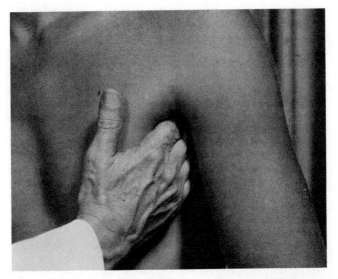

FIG. 11.6: Palpation of the left axilla. Note the examiner's hand flat against the chest wall and the relaxed arm of the patient.

little motion during the respiratory cycle. This is called "barrel chest" and is characteristic of advanced chronic obstructive pulmonary disease (see Fig. 11.7).

Other deformities of the chest contour may be caused by unilateral lung disease or structural deformities of the bony framework. Pigeon Breast or Chicken Breast is a permanent deformity, usually caused by rickets, in which the A-P diameter is increased, the transverse diameter is narrowed, and vertical grooves are formed in the line of the costochondral junctions.

Funnel Breast (Pectus Excavatum) is the reverse of Pigeon Breast. The softened ribs of the lower part of the sternum sink posteriorly, creating a pit or depression which decreases the A-P diameter (Fig. 11.8). Other thoracic deformities include bulges on the chest wall caused by cardiac enlargement, aortic aneurysm, xneoplasm, or depressions caused by retractions due to underlying fibrosis, or surgical removal of ribs.

Inspection of the profile of the thoracic wall from the side and from the back may identify several spinal deformities which modify the contour. In the long thoracic spine, several abnormalities are of

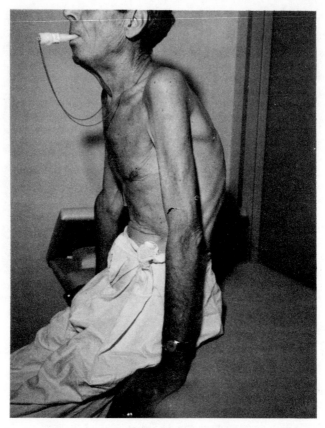

FIG. 11.7: Patient with chronic emphysema. Note the use of his
arms to fix the clavicles and the increased anteroposterior thoracic diameter ("barrel chest"). He is using an
"emphysema whistle" which assists in controlling his
forced expiration.

importance. Both an increase in the normal curve, or kyphosis,
(Fig. 11.9) as well as straightening of the normal curve with rigidity
(poker spine) interfere with free movement of the ribs and thus with
good ventilation. If either deformity is observed, the patient's chest
expansion should be measured to determine the degree of limitation
of motion of the chest wall. Scoliosis (Fig. 11.10) or lateral curvature, of significant degree, will cause one side of the chest to be
compressed and the other to be abnormally expanded, thus also interfering with normal respiratory motion.

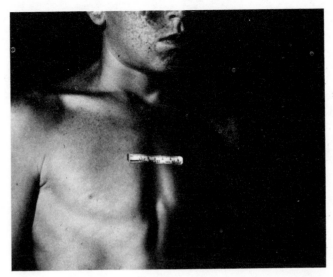

FIG. 11.8: Young man with moderate degree of pectus excavatum.

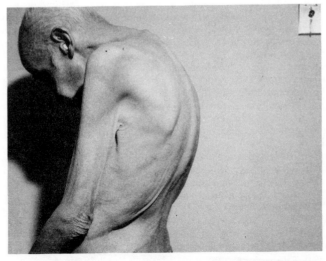

FIG. 11.9: Elderly man with severe degree of thoracic kyphosis.

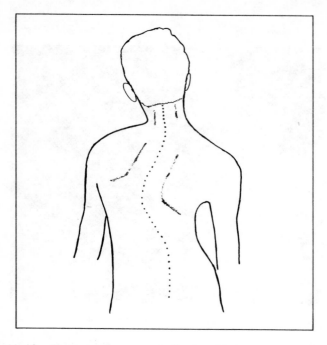

FIG. 11.10: Diagram of severe scoliosis with the concavity directed toward the left.

Respiratory Motion: The motion of the thoracic wall should be observed during quiet normal breathing and then during deep inspiration. It is important to note the type, rate, rhythm, and depth of the respiratory effort as well as the use of accessory respiratory muscles of the neck. The rhythm of a single respiratory cycle should have a longer inspiratory phase and a shorter expiratory phase (see Fig. 11.5, upper diagram). Irregularities in rhythm should be noted, such as Cheyne-Stokes breathing in which there are alternating periods of apnea and respiration with variable rate. The depth of respiration is as meaningful as the rate, for it may help to distinguish between pulmonary, metabolic, or neurological causes of rapid or slow breathing. Rapid, deep respirations may indicate Kussmaul Respiration of diabetic acidosis, while rapid, shallow breathing may signify obstructive or restrictive lung disease. The duration of inspiration versus expiration is important in determining whether or not there is airway obstruction. In patients with obstructive lung disease, expiration is prolonged and requires the use of muscular effort, an important diagnostic sign.

The chest should also be observed for symmetrical expansion. Unilateral diminished expansion may be due to acute pleurisy, pleural

fibrosis, or massive atelectasis. A pulmonary embolus, pneumonia, pleural effusion, pneumothorax, or any cause of chest pain
such as fractured ribs may lead to diminished chest expansion. In
addition, general chest expansion may be limited in ankylosing
spondylitis, since the ribs cannot rotate at their joints with the
spine.

A comparison should be made of expansion of the upper chest to that
of the lower chest. If the examiner suspects that there is a significant difference, he should use the tape measure to verify his
suspicions.

The examiner should also look for bulging or retraction of the interspaces. Bulging of interspaces may occur in a massive pleural
effusion, with tension pneumothorax, or during the forced expiration of the patient with emphysema or asthma.

Palpation: Although palpation may be conducted together with inspection in the process of examination of the chest, the beginning
student should approach the technique as a separate entity. Initially,
he will be concerned with validating the data found upon inspection,
particularly in relation to symmetry of expansion of the chest wall
during respiration.

Symmetrical areas of the thorax should be palpated with the fingertips and the palms. With the patient upright, the anterior lower
lateral and posterior thorax can all be examined for symmetry of
onset and depth of inspiration. The movement of the chest can be
seen particularly well by placing the hands on the lower portion of
the postero-lateral wall with the thumbs adjacent near the spine
(Fig. 11.11). During deep inspiration the thumbs should move apart
at the same time and equally in distance from the mid-spinal line.

General palpation of the chest wall should also give attention to the
temperature, moisture, and general turgor of the skin, as well as to
the presence of edema. Any evidence of masses or tenderness
should receive special consideration.

In the event that patient is complaining of chest pain, bones and
joints of the thorax should be palpated for presence of tenderness.

Feel for fremitus with the palms, or the ulnar aspect of the hands
(Fig. 11.12) and ask the patient to say, "1, 2, 3" or "99." A mild
purr-like sensation should be felt, similar to the sensation one would
feel if hands were placed on the sides of a cat while it was purring.
Fremitus should not be palpable unless the patient is vocalizing.

A satisfactory technique is to use both hands simultaneously on corresponding areas of the chest so that comparison of one side to the
other can be made. Since, in general, only large lesions of the

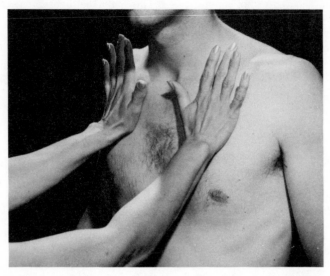

FIG. 11.11: Palpation for equality of lower posterior chest expansion. Note the positions of the thumbs and fingers.

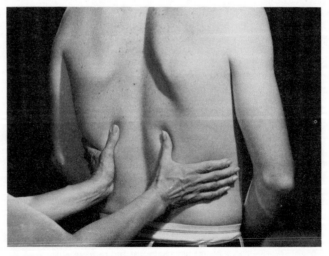

FIG. 11.12: Palpation for fremitus using the palms of the hands on symmetrical portions of the chest wall.

chest produce changes of fremitus, one can examine about three areas anteriorly, two laterally, and three areas of the back for fremitus - each square centimeter need not be tested.

A solid medium of uniform consistency will conduct vibrations from the larynx to the chest wall better than one containing air, such as normal lung tissue. Therefore, one can expect increased fremitus in conditions such as pneumonia, where there is consolidation of the lung, especially when that consolidation is close to the lung surface. When a major bronchus is obstructed, vibrations will not be able to be transported, and fremitus will be absent over the lung area served by that bronchus.

Decreased fremitus will occur when abnormalities involving the pleura interfere with the normal transmission of laryngeal sounds. Thus, fibrous thickening of the pleura, pleural effusion, or pneumothorax will all lead to either decreased or absent fremitus.

An unusual finding on palpation of the neck or chest is crepitation ("crackling"), produced when the fingertips press on and move tiny air bubbles in the subcutaneous tissues. This is most often secondary to trauma which allows escape of air from the lung and pleural space. Such trauma may arise from a fractured rib, a chest wound, or following surgery.

Crepitation may infrequently be felt in the abdomen or in an extremity - and in rare instances it may be due to gas gangrene. The term is also used to describe the grating sensation when a damaged joint is moved, or when the rough ends of a fractured bone are moved against each other. Some authors describe fine rales (see p. 154) as crepitant rales. Thus, the student must be prepared to understand that when the term appears it means "crackling" or "grating" either on palpation or auscultation from any source.

Percussion: The general procedure for percussion which was described in Chapter 5 assumes special significance during examination of the chest.

The normal percussion note, heard as a result of the vibration of underlying chest wall and organs, varies with the thickness of the chest wall, the muscular development, and the location of underlying organs, as well as the force applied by the examiner. The clear, long, medium-pitched sound usually heard over the normal lung is called resonance. The sound can be appreciated fully only through the experience of percussion of many normal chests.

Where the air content of the underlying tissue is decreased and its solidity increased, such as over the heart, dullness is heard. This is a short, higher-pitched, soft thud which fails to demonstrate the vibratory quality of a resonant sound. The high-pitched, clear, longer drum-like sound over the air-filled stomach or over any hollow intestine is a musical note referred to as tympany. Naturally, the changes in sounds from one area to another are gradual so that there are zones of transition.

Proceed to percuss the anterior and lateral chest in a systematic manner from top to bottom. At each level, parallel areas of both sides are percussed, each interspace being compared with the corresponding space, keeping in mind the normal changes in sound expected over the heart, the liver, and the stomach and colon (Fig. 11.13).

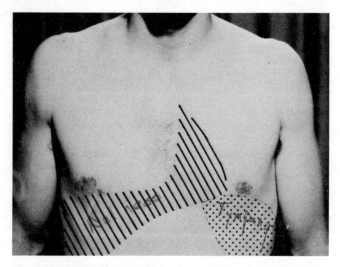

FIG. 11.13: Normal percussion areas. Dullness will normally be found in the hatched areas. On the patient's left, dullness is due to the underlying heart while the area on the right represents liver dullness. The dotted area, somewhat variable in actual size, is tympanitic. This is Traube's space, lying over air in the stomach and splenic flexure of the colon. See also Figs. 13.2 and 11.18.

On the right chest, percussion down the mid-clavicular line will identify the location of the upper edge of the liver. The transition is quite distinct here between lung resonance and liver dullness. The upper border of the liver is ordinarily found at about the 4th or 5th intercostal space. With the patient's head flexed forward and the forearms crossed at the waist to separate the scapulae, the posterior chest should be percussed starting at the apices and continuing downward to the bases where the location and range of motion of the diaphragm are determined (Fig. 11.14). The method used to locate and measure the respiratory excursion of the diaphragm requires instructing the patient to take and hold a deep breath. The lowest level of resonance is identified by percussing downward until the tone changes to dullness. The patient is then instructed to exhale and hold, while the procedure is once again accomplished. The range of motion of the diaphragm is determined by the distance between the two levels, which is normally about three to five centimeters in females and five to six centimeters in males. Reduced movement of the diaphragm is often seen in pleurisy or emphysema.

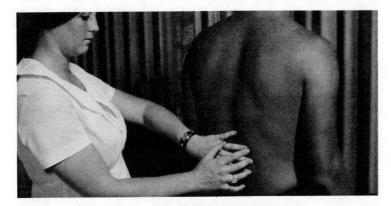

FIG. 11.14: Percussion of the diaphragm.

Abnormal findings identified through percussion are created when there is an increased amount of air or when fluid or pleural thickening is present in the underlying structure. For example, in emphysema and in extensive pneumothorax, increased air creates a "booming" well-sustained, and easily heard sound referred to as hyperresonance. When there is a considerable amount of fluid in the lung, dullness will be located where there should normally be resonance. Consolidation or filling of alveolar spaces by fluid, pus, or blood due to pneumonia, tuberculosis, tumor process, lung abscess, infarction, and pulmonary edema are examples of situations which produce dullness. The presence of some fluid in the pleural space over underlying air-containing lung will also create abnormal dullness. Absolute dullness or flatness will occur when there is a large amount of fluid over an area, with little underlying air-containing lung remaining, as with pleural effusion.

Auscultation: Much of what has been learned through inspection, palpation, and percussion of the chest, as well as from the history, can be appreciated further when the examiner goes one step beyond and uses the stethoscope.

Auscultation determines the character of the breath sounds, the character of the whispered voice, and the presence of abnormal (adventitious) sounds heard over the chest wall during respiration.

Breath Sounds: If ever the beginning practitioner needs a quiet room, it is when he is learning to listen for breath sounds. The patient should be as comfortable as possible to avoid any unnecessary movement. With the diaphragm of the stethoscope, (warmed, if necessary), placed firmly against the chest wall, the patient is directed to breathe quietly with his mouth open. Concentrate first on the quality of the breath sounds. Once again, as in palpation and percussion, corresponding regions of each side of the anterior chest from the apex to the base of the lung are auscinted. Symmetrical regions should be compared in relation to pitch, intensity, quality, and duration of breath sounds, and the presence of abnormal sounds noted. Figs. 11.15 and 11.16 illustrate the areas in which the three types of breath sounds are heard in the normal person. Note again that vesicular breathing is heard over most of the chest.

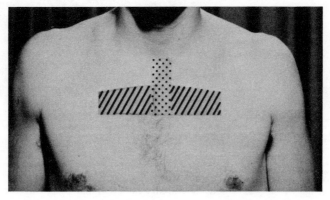

FIG. 11.15: Location of normal breath sounds. Bronchial breathing may be heard in the area over the trachea and major bronchi (dotted area). Broncho-vesicular sounds may be heard normally within the hatched area.

It should be noted well that deep breathing will convert the fine vesicular sounds into bronchovesicular sounds, so a portion of the auscultation should be done with quiet respiration on the part of the patient. Breathing through the mouth will avoid the production of sounds in the nasopharynx and nares and is, therefore, preferred.

In pathological conditions, such as early pneumonia or minimal pulmonary edema, fluid begins to fill some of the alveoli, converting vesicular sounds into broncho-vesicular sounds. Thus, the presence

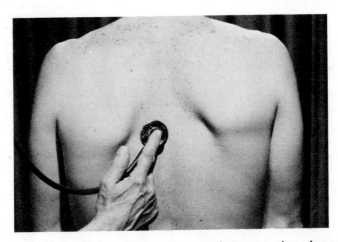

FIG. 11.16: Auscultation in the interscapular space where broncho-vesicular sounds are normally present.

of broncho-vesicular sounds is <u>abnormal</u> in an area where only vesicular sounds should be heard. This finding will be detected in the early stage of disease when the chest x-ray is still unchanged. As larger amounts of fluid collect, such as in lobar pneumonia, the involved area becomes much more solid, no vesicular component is present, and the sounds produced by underlying bronchi are well transmitted, producing bronchial sounds in an abnormal location (see Patient Problem, p. 156). This is a classical sign of consolidation of the lung.

If a large bronchus becomes obstructed, no air will pass in or out of a portion of the lung. Listening over such an area, the clinician will hear no breath sounds of any type.

The absence of breath sounds, in addition to indicating obstruction of a bronchus, may also be found over an area of lung collapse such as in pneumothorax. In both situations, no air is passing to the area under the stethoscope and, therefore, no breath sounds are produced. Conditions in which there is very little air moving, (severe emphysema, fractured ribs with a splinted chest, etc.), will cause the breath sounds to be diminished or absent. Another reason for diminished sounds is the presence of air or fluid in the pleural space which separates the underlying lung from the stethoscope. Thickened pleura will also prevent good transmission of breath sounds.

<u>Whispered Voice Sounds</u>: As noted earlier, speaking produces vibrations in the respiratory system which are transmitted to the chest

wall. Place the stethoscope on the chest in various locations and ask the patient to whisper a few words or numbers. In the normal situation, the examiner should hear the sounds as a muffled hum with the words not clearly distinguishable. Increased transmission, which makes the whispered voice sound louder and the syllables clear, is evidence of consolidation of the underlying lung. This abnormality may be detected quite early in the course of pneumonia or other diseases causing the lung to become more solid. Increased transmission of the whispered voice is referred to as whispered pectoriloquy. This is a more sensitive index of consolidation than bronchophony in which the spoken voice is transmitted more loudly than normally.

Adventitious Sounds: These are abnormal sounds superimposed on the basic breath sounds. They consist of rales, rhonchi, and rubs. Unfortunately, there are several definitions and classifications, leading to some confusion in terminology.

Rales are clusters or showers of sounds produced by the bubbling of air through fluid in the alveoli, bronchioles, or bronchi. In general, they vary in quality, depending upon the location of the abnormal fluid. Thus, fine rales are produced by bubbling in the alveoli and terminal bronchioles. They are not loud, are high-pitched, and seem to the listener to be heard quite close to the ear. A classical analogy is that fine rales sound somewhat like the sound of several strands of hair being rubbed between the fingers close to the ear.

Subcrepitant —

Medium rales result from air passing through larger amounts of fluid in larger air passages, usually the bronchioles. They are lower pitched and crackling, not unlike the bubbling sound of a freshly-opened bottle of a carbonated beverage.

When showers of rales are heard, the patient should be instructed to cough. If the rales do not disappear, or if they are accentuated by the cough, they are significant and are evidence of fluid in the lung due to left heart failure (pulmonary edema), pneumonia, or other inflammatory diseases such as tuberculosis. Deep breathing may help to accentuate rales.

Rhonchi are coarser sounds, probably produced in the larger bronchi by passage of air through mucus or through a narrowing of the air passage.

Coarse (or sonorous) rhonchi are low-pitched, "snoring" sounds resulting from vibrations of mucus strands in the bronchi. They are generally continuous through one or both phases of the respiratory cycle, are often variable in pitch and loudness from one breath to another, and tend to change in character after a cough. These are typical of bronchitis with accumulations of mucus.

Sibilant rhonchi (wheezes) are musical, whistling, or hissing sounds, of distinctly higher pitch than coarse rhonchi. Wheezes are produced by narrowing of bronchioles (as in asthma) or by partial obstruction of larger bronchi due to edema of the mucosa, a tumor, or other lesions which reduce the normal diameter of the bronchi. A <u>unilateral</u> wheeze is highly significant, suggesting localized compression or obstruction of a bronchus. This is often the first sign of carcinoma of the lung or of obstruction due to aspiration.

If rales or rhonchi are detected, the observer should report where they are heard in the respiratory cycle. This is an important distinction since they have quite a different significance in the inspiratory phase from those heard during expiration. A sketch may be drawn to illustrate the examiner's findings. Fig. 11.17 shows several examples.

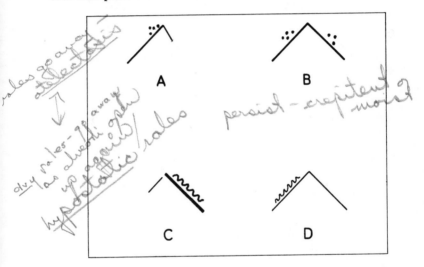

FIG. 11.17: Sketches of breath sounds and adventitious sounds.
   a) Vesicular sound with rales at the <u>end of inspiration</u>
   b) Bronchovesicular sound with rales in mid-inspiration and mid-expiration
   c) Bronchial sound with rhonchi in expiration
   d) Bronchovesicular sound with inspiratory rhonchi

<u>Friction rub</u> is a coarse, grating sound which results when two inflamed surfaces of pleura are rubbing against each other as in pleurisy. It is similar to the sound elicited when the palm of one hand is placed over the ear and the finger of the other hand is used to rub the back of that hand. Most of the time it is heard over the anterolateral chest throughout the respiratory cycle. The practitioner should hold the stethoscope firmly over the chest so that sliding on the skin does not artificially produce sounds similar to a rub.

RECORDING

Thorax:

Insp: Symmetrical, full expansion equal bilaterally,
A-P diameter not increased
Palp: No axillary adenopathy

Lungs:

Palp: Fremitus equal bilaterally
Perc: Lung fields resonant throughout
Ausc: Breath sounds normal. Voice sounds normal. No
rales, rhonchi, or rubs

PATIENT PROBLEM

Mr. L.A., 36-year-old black man with CC of chest pain, cough,
chill and fever of 6 hrs. duration (Fig. 11.18)

Problem: Chill, Fever, Cough, Chest Pain

S: Four days ago pt. noted mild sore throat and "sniffles" for
which he took aspirin with some relief. At about 6 a.m. today,
awakened by a severe shaking chill which lasted for about 20
minutes. Felt sick but was able to fall back to sleep. Awakened about 2 hours later with right chest pain, began coughing,
produced small amounts of "rusty" sputum and came to clinic
as an emergency. Major complaint now is chest pain and
malaise.

O: T 39.4°C (103°F), P 120 R 26 BP 140/60
Insp. Face flushed, skin hot and sweaty, labored respiration,
right chest spinted.
Palp. Confirms splinting of R chest, increased fremitus R
chest above 4th ICS.
Perc. Diminished resonance R chest from clavicle to 5th ICS,
from mid-axillary line to sternum.
Ausc. Bronchial breath sounds, crackling rales, whispered
pectoriloquy over involved area. Remainder of chest
clear.

A: These findings on history and P.E. are characteristic of lobar
pneumonia. Patient is acutely ill.

P: Dx - Stat PA chest x-ray
Present to Dr. _____ at once
Rx - None
Pt. Ed: Advised that he probably has pneumonia, that he will be
seen promptly by MD, and that hospitalization is probable.

_____
Signature

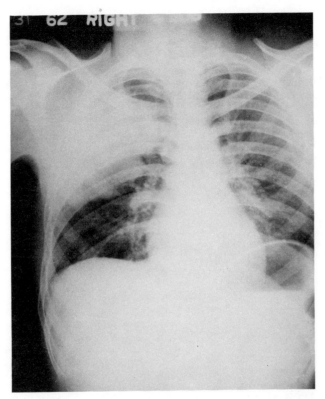

FIG. 11.18: Chest x-ray showing characteristic consolidation due to pneumonia of the right upper lobe. The relationships of the heart to the chest and the diaphragm are well illustrated. Note that the left leaf of the diaphragm is above the gas bubble of the stomach. Percussion over this area would produce tympany while resonance would be found above the diaphragm.

SUPPLEMENTAL EXERCISES

1. Sketch representations of respiratory motions in Kussmaul breathing, Cheyne-Stokes respiration, Biot's breathing.

2. Chronic Obstructive Pulmonary Disease is a combination of obstructive emphysema and chronic bronchitis. What abnormalities should be anticipated in the history and physical examination of a patient with COPD?

3. What symptoms and what signs are expected with a large unilateral pneumothorax?

REFERENCES

1. Traver, G.: Assessment of Thorax and Lungs. Am. J. Nurs.
73:466, March 1973.

2. Delaney, M.T.: Examining the Chest, Part 1: The Lungs.
Nursing '75 5:12, August 1975.

3. Sherman, J.L. and Fields, S.K.: Health Assessment Techniques: Examination of the Thorax and Lungs. A multimedia
program. Westinghouse Learning Corporation, New York,
1974.

CHAPTER 12

THE BREAST

INTRODUCTION

It is indeed an unfortunate commentary on the American health delivery system, when one realizes that the mortality rate due to cancer of the breast has not decreased at all in the past 40 years.
Meanwhile, the basic method of examination of the breast can reveal the presence of the disease in its still curable state and is essentially a simple technique, easy enough for women to learn themselves. For the primary health practitioner, the mastery of this
technique and subsequent teaching to large groups, as well as individual patients, may become one of the most important tasks for
which he can assume responsibility. In any event, the significance
of careful, thorough, systematic inspection and palpation of the breast
in all patients cannot be overemphasized.

TOPOGRAPHICAL ANATOMY

The breasts, or mammary glands, two highly specialized glands,
are located on either side of the anterior wall of the chest between
the third and the seventh ribs, from the edge of the sternum to the
anterior axillary line with an extension to the anterior axillary fold.
Each organ is divided into 15-20 lobes which are separated from
each other by fibroelastic tissue. The external surface is made up
of a soft area of skin extending from the circumference of the gland
to the areola, which is a pigmented circle surrounding the nipple.
The areola, which has a pinkish hue in blondes and a darker rose
color in brunettes, has a more or less roughened surface with small
fine papillae, known as the glands of Montgomery.

The nipple is composed of sensitive, erectile tissue and forms a
large conic projection in the center of the areola, its summit holding multiple openings of the milk ducts.

The breasts are particularly well supplied with lymphatic channels,
especially toward the axilla, which are also included in the examination of the breast.

PHYSIOLOGY

The breasts lie close to the skin between the superficial and deep
layers of the superficial fascia supported by the suspensory
ligaments.

During the developing years, and in young women, especially those who have not borne children, the breasts are soft and almost homogenous in consistency despite their lobular characteristic, but as the years progress and pregnancies occur, they become more nodular and stringy in consistency.

Since the breasts are the organs of lactation, there are changes which occur during pregnancy, in anticipation of lactation. In the early months, the changes are similar to those which occur monthly under cyclic influence of pituitary and ovarian hormones - tenderness and slight enlargement. As pregnancy continues, the breasts themselves enlarge, while the Montgomery glands, particularly, become more marked, the areola becomes darkened, and the nipples become larger and more mobile. A yellowish secretion, colostrum, is formed and is maintained until several days following delivery, when milk is formed.

During lactation, the breasts continue in their enlarged state and, in addition, present multiple prominent vascular markings.

EXAMINATION TECHNIQUE

In order to conduct a thorough examination of the breast, the patient's gown must be removed and a good light and screen provided.

Despite the Madison Avenue attention given to the female breast in the United States, and the fashionable acceptance of the bikini on the beaches around the world, it must be remembered that, perhaps because of its role as a sexual organ, many women, both young and old, respond to the need for this examination and its possible pathological implication with fear and anxiety. Certainly, the examiner's approach must be gentle, supportive, and reflective of such understanding, for without a doubt, the high incidence of neglected medical consultation for early breast lesions is directly related to the poor rate of cure mentioned earlier in this chapter.

The breasts, nipples, and lymph nodes in the axillary and supraclavicular region should be carefully inspected and then palpated with the patient first sitting, hands at the sides and then over the head, and later, in the supine position. The details to be noted are included in the next sections under the specific technique.

INSPECTION: Since the size, shape, and position of the breasts vary markedly depending upon age, heredity, endocrine function, and presence of adipose tissue, it is impossible to provide data here which can classify normal breasts in relation to these factors beyond the illustrations we have included.

Even the beginning practitioner should have little difficulty in recognizing deviations from normal once a variety of breasts have been examined.

The examination should begin by inspecting and comparing both breasts for (1) size; (2) shape; (3) symmetry and (4) position. Asymmetrical development is not uncommon, but may be a source of emotional distress to the patient. It is also important to consider that any unilateral increase in size may indicate cyst formation, inflammation, or tumor, as well as congenital anomaly.

The position of breast and nipple should be observed and then compared by having the patient raise her arms above the head, making note of any unilateral shift in position.

Edema may be noted upon inspection when there is underlying disease process. This causes the hair follicles and their openings to be more pronounced and is usually due to obstruction of lymphatic drainage (lymphedema), or leakage of serum into intercellular spaces (inflammatory carcinoma). This condition is commonly referred to as "orange peel" or "pig skin" (Fig. 12.1).

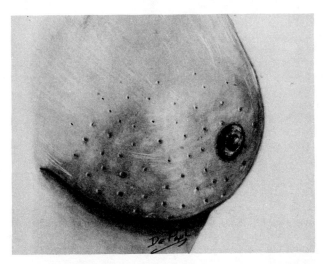

FIG. 12.1: "Orange peel" defect of skin of breast due to edema or carcinoma.

Attention should then be paid specifically to the nipples themselves. The areola and nipple are carefully inspected for pigment change, erosions, crusting, scaling, discharge, and edema. Although many women have inverted nipples without evidence of disease, any retraction should be noted, especially when it is unilateral. Paget's disease, a malignant condition of the breast, may give rise to unilateral ulceration of one nipple, while bilateral ulceration may be a benign process. Any discharge from the nipple should, of course, be described according to color, amount, and consistency.

Skin retraction is one of the most significant findings to note in examination of the breast (Fig. 12.2). Any disease process may infiltrate the tissue enough to apply abnormal traction on the suspensory ligaments, pulling with it a portion of the skin overlying the lesion and even the nipple itself, usually toward the side of the lesion.

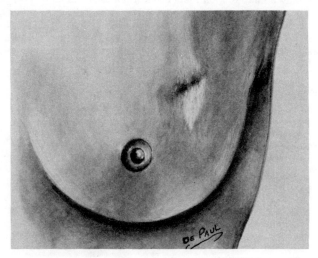

FIG. 12.2: Skin retraction, or "dimpling" of the breast. An early sign of underlying carcinoma which has invaded the skin.

The examiner should first inspect for retraction with the patient's hands at her side and then overhead. Since contraction of the pectoral muscles will exaggerate any retraction, it may be better seen when the patient presses her palms together or applies pressure to both hips (see Fig. 12.3).

It is important to remember that even when evidence of acute inflammation is not present, skin retraction may be one of the earliest physical findings of malignant tumor.

Inspection is not complete, however, unless attention is given to the axillary and supraclavicular regions where retractions, bulging, discoloration, and edema may also provide clues to underlying disease processes. Each arm should be put through a full range of motion, in order to fully visualize problem areas.

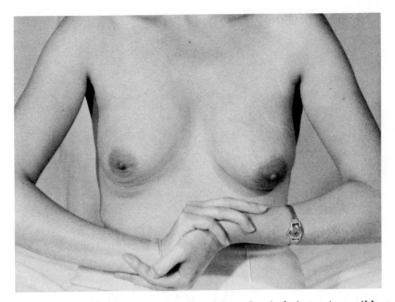

FIG. 12.3: Tightening of the pectoral muscles to bring out possible dimpling of the skin of the breast.

PALPATION: The examiner should now proceed to palpate the dependent breast with the patient still sitting up, first with the arms at the side, and then with the arms raised over the head.

For purposes of examination and identification of location of lesions, the breast may conveniently be divided into quadrants - the upper outer, upper inner, lower inner, and lower outer quadrants. It is extremely important to recognize the fact that breast tissue of the upper outer quadrant extends laterally upward to the anterior axillary fold. This portion must not be neglected in the examination of the breast.

With the fingers and thumb, the areola and nipples are examined and then gently compressed in order to elicit the presence of tenderness, nodules, and nipple discharge. Then, each quadrant is carefully examined for consistency, elasticity, tenderness, and masses. A preferred technique is to place the palmar surface of the fingers gently but firmly against each quadrant of the breast, and to move the hand in a rotary motion, pressing the breast tissue against the chest wall (see Figs. 12.4 to 12.6).

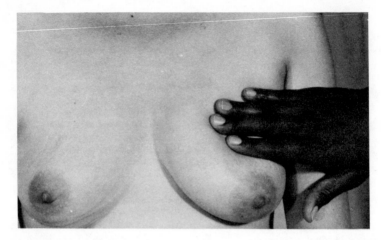

FIG. 12.4: Examination of the breast. Palpation of the breast in the upright position.

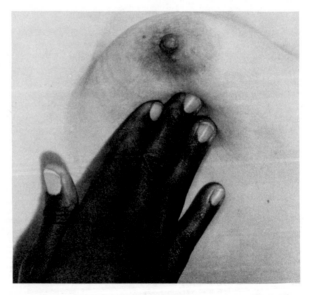

FIG. 12.5: Examination of the breast. Palpation of the lateral breast in the supine position.

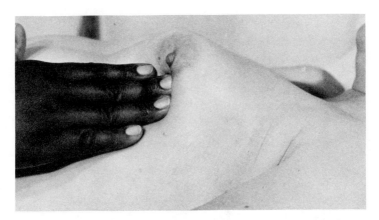

FIG. 12.6: Examination of the breast.   Palpation of the inferior portion.

Another useful technique is bimanual palpation, in which one hand
raises the breast and the other presses breast tissue between the
two sets of fingers (Fig. 12.7).   This may detect small dimples or
mobile masses not picked up by other techniques.

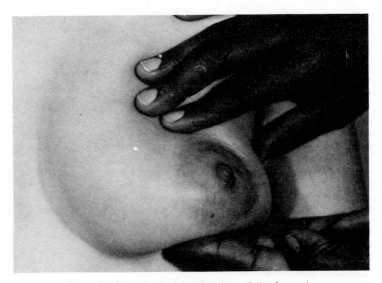

FIG. 12.7: Bimanual palpation of the breast.

The presence of a mass should be described according to criteria outlined in Chapter 7 and the patient immediately referred to a specialist. Since all masses are not malignant, the patient should not be unduly frightened by such a referral, but must be impressed with the importance of prompt consultation.

Once the breast and nipples themselves have been palpated, attention must be given to the axillae (Fig. 12.8), the supraclavicular area (Fig. 12.9), and the neck, in a search for lymph nodes, if these areas have not been examined up to this point.

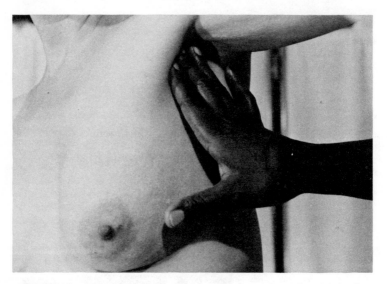

FIG. 12.8: Palpation of the upper outer breast quadrant into the axilla.

SELF-EXAMINATION

As health educators as well as practitioners, we have obligations for teaching self-examination to all women past their menarche. It is reliably estimated that 88,000 new cases of breast cancer will be discovered this year, and many should be first detected by the woman herself. This will enable early detection and can have the important result of initiating diagnosis and treatment soon enough to prevent unnecessary death from this epidemic disease.

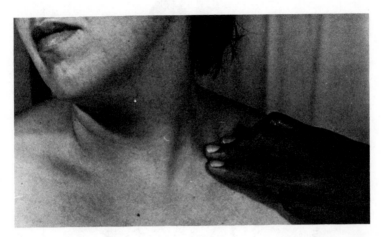

FIG. 12.9: Palpation of the supraclavicular region for lymph nodes.

For the development of a common technique which should be taught to all American women, there is no better source than the brochure published, at no cost to the recipient, by the American Cancer Society (Reference 4). Provision of one technique to all will avoid confusion on the part of the female population, who otherwise might get several sets of instruction from different practitioners.

All practitioners should obtain copies of this brochure, and should advise their female patients to perform the examination as specified in the brochure. The technique should be reviewed with the patient, who should then perform the examination under observation, so that the clinician can evaluate the patient's ability to do it fully and properly, even if she claims to know the technique.

Advise the patient to examine her breasts at a regular time each month, preferably after her menstrual period. Figs. 12.10 through 12.15 are offered to illustrate the appropriate self-examination technique.

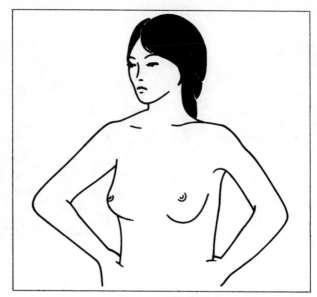

FIG. 12.10: Advise the patient to stand in front of a mirror with her hands at her sides and look for any changes in size, shape and position, as well as for areas of indentation or dimpling, redness or irritation.

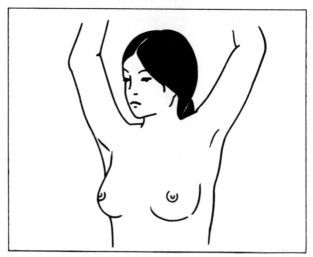

FIG. 12.11: Tell her to then inspect with her hands raised over her head. Have her do a self-examination in front of a mirror under your directions so you can point out what to look for, as well as the technique of examination.

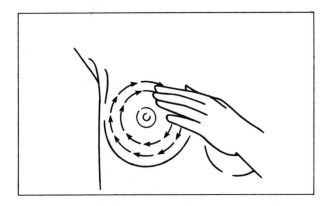

FIG. 12.12: She should systematically palpate all four quadrants of the breast with the palmar surfaces of her fingertips.

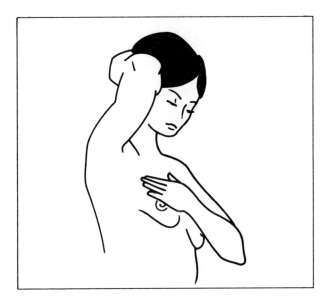

FIG. 12.13: Show her how to examine the axillary area for any sensations of tenderness, nodules or masses. Have her palpate while you observe her technique. Explain what she is feeling.

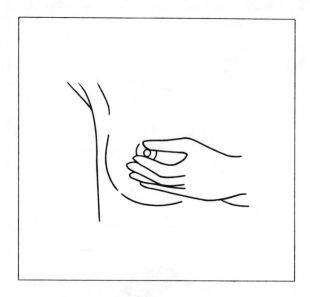

FIG. 12.14: Demonstrate how to compress the nipples for discharge.

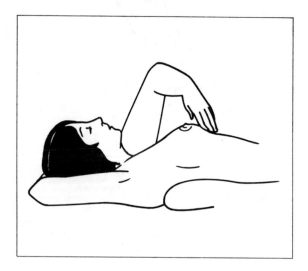

FIG. 12.15: Show her how to examine all areas again while lying
down so the breast is spread against the chest wall.

EXAMINATION OF THE MALE BREAST

Although significant lesions of the male breast are rare compared
to those of the female breast, this organ must not be neglected.
The normal male breast is flat and smaller than the female breast.
If slightly or moderately prominent, it is usually because there is
underlying fat, not breast tissue.

Inspection and palpation may be much briefer in the male, but discharge from the nipples, swelling, tenderness, or masses must be
searched for. If the breast is prominent, palpation should be used
to distinguish between the soft, mushy feeling of fat and the presence
of true breast tissue underneath the nipple with its firmer, slightly
nodular, and stringy characteristics. If true breast tissue is present,
the condition is referred to as gynecomastia and may represent an
endocrine disorder.

RECORDING (Female)

> Breasts: Symmetrical. Contour and consistency appropriate
> for age and parity. No retraction, no nipple discharge. No
> masses or tenderness.

RECORDING (Male)

> Breasts: Symmetrical. No nipple discharge, masses or ten-
> derness. No breast tissue.

PATIENT PROBLEM

Mrs. J., a 75-year-old alert, well-developed, well-nourished black
woman, is brought to the health center by her daughter, who is concerned that her mother may have cancer of the breast.

Problem: Breast Lesion

S: Mrs. J has been generally well, except for mild hypertension,
    and able to care for herself in her own apartment in another
    city. She is now visiting her daughter for the summer. While
    assisting her mother to dress, Mrs. J's daughter noted that the
    nipple of Mrs. J's right breast was deeply retracted. Mrs. J
    said she noticed it several months ago but thought it was due to
    age.

O: Inspection: breasts are pendulous and not symmetrical. Right
    breast is larger than left, with nipple deeply retracted. Areola
    of right nipple is darker than left, with crusting at 9 o'clock.
    Surrounding skin is reddened, with increased vascular markings.

    Palpation: hard, irregular, slightly tender mass 2 cm. x 2 cm.,
    about 3 cm. deep behind the retraction. Mass is mobile within

the breast but skin is adherent to mass. Several matted lymph nodes palpable in right axilla. No other masses palpable in left breast or left axilla.

A: Mass of right breast with retraction, apparently carcinoma.

P: Dx - Refer to M.D. immediately.
Rx - None at this time.
Pt. Ed. - Mother and daughter advised that there is need for medical evaluation. Discussions of strong possibility that mass is carcinoma and that surgical intervention will be necessary. Appointment made for consultation today to avoid prolonged delay in evaluation. Will follow up after medical consultation to provide continued support and counseling to both mother and daughter.

SUPPLEMENTAL EXERCISES

1. Draw a diagram outlining the lymphatic drainage of the breast.

2. What is the purpose of placing a small pillow under the shoulder of the side being examined when the patient is supine?

REFERENCES

1. Leis, H.P.: Diagnosis and Treatment of Breast Lesions. Medical Examination Publishing Co., Inc., New York, 1970.

2. Haagensen, C.D.: Diseases of the Breast. W.B. Saunders Co., Philadelphia, 1971.

3. How to Examine Your Breasts. American Cancer Society, 1975.

4. Omni: Breast Examination. Ortho Pharmaceutical Corp., Raritan, New Jersey, 1974.

CHAPTER 13

THE HEART

INTRODUCTION

This chapter will deal with direct examination of the heart, for the sake of concentrating the student's attention on this facet of physical diagnosis. However, the student must be aware that full appreciation of the state of the heart's function must be obtained by combining what is found here with all that is learned elsewhere. Thus, peripheral cyanosis, edema of the eyelids, dilation of neck veins, splinter hemorrhages of the finger-nail beds, clubbing, cough, shortness of breath, enlarged liver, ankle edema, and many other findings on history and physical examination may all provide evidence of cardiac disease.

TOPOGRAPHICAL ANATOMY

The heart lies in the thorax as if it were hung from the top - as, in fact, it is (Fig. 13.1). The aorta, pulmonary arteries, and great veins are all at the upper (superior) portion of the heart, called the base, while the lower portion, the apex, hangs free. The organ is a wedge-shaped muscle with its base (the right and left atria) facing backward and to the right, and its apex (formed by the left ventricle) pointing forward and to the left. In the average adult, the base extends slightly to the right of the sternum while the apex comes into contact with the anterior chest wall at or near the fifth left intercostal space (ICS), usually just medial to the mid-clavicular line.

The right ventricle is anterior and thus lies directly under the sternum while the left ventricle is posterior and lateral, making up a large portion of the left cardiac border and the apex. The area of the chest overlying the heart bears the name precordium.

Except for the portion of right ventricle which lies against the sternum, the heart is separated from the chest wall by lung. The deeper portions of the heart are, therefore, covered by more lung tissue than the more superficial parts. Thus, in doing percussion and auscultation over the precordium, the examiner will elicit signs from both organs to a greater or lesser degree.

Pericardium: The heart is encased in a tough, double-walled fibrous sac - the pericardium - which protects the heart from trauma. The outer layer of pericardium is firmly attached within the thorax to the esophagus, the aorta, the pleura, the sternum, and the diaphragm. A few cubic entimeters of fluid are present between the inner and outer layers of pericardium.

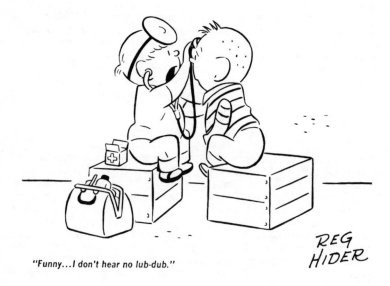

"Funny...I don't hear no lub-dub."

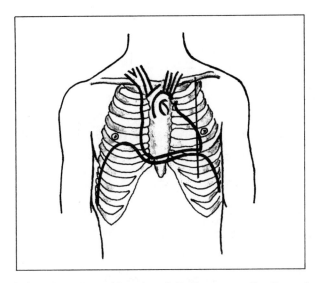

FIG. 13.1: Projection of heart and diaphragm on the thoracic wall.
Note the landmark of the left mid-clavicular line.

PHYSIOLOGY

As William Harvey said in 1628, "When the ventricle is full, the
heart raises itself, forthwith tenses all its fibers, contracts the
ventricles, and gives a beat." This single event - and the relaxation which follows - is the source of the point of maximum intensity,
sternal heave, thrills, and the first and second (and other) heart
sounds. Murmurs, clicks, snaps, pericardial friction rubs, as well
as the pulse, the systolic blood pressure and venous pulse waves are
all related to this event.

Keep firmly in mind that the normal heart sounds are produced principally by valve closure. There is much argument still going on today about exactly what events contribute to heart sounds, but for a
clear understanding of physical findings, remember that valve closure produces the first and second heart sounds.

For convenience, the cycle of events will be described beginning with
blood flowing into the atria. Venous blood from the systemic circulation and oxygenated blood from the lungs flow into the atria and
through the open atrioventricular valves (mitral and tricuspid) into
the relaxed ventricle under very low pressure. When the atria are
stimulated to contract, they squeeze the blood in them into the ventricles which are then filled. Now the ventricles become tense and
the pressure, rising rapidly, snaps the atrioventricular (A-V) valves
shut (Fig. 13.2). Although both A-V valves do not snap shut

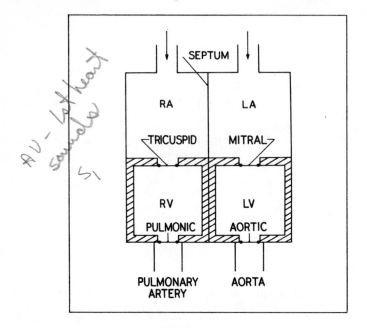

FIG. 13.2: Diagram of position of valves. The A-V valves have
just shut producing the first heart sound. This is the
beginning of systole.

simultaneously, the closures occur so closely together that the result is ordinarily heard as a single sound - the first heart sound (S1).

As pressure continues to rise rapidly in both ventricles, the semi-
lunar (aortic and pulmonic) valves are forced open and blood begins
to flow out into the aorta and pulmonary artery. When the ventricles
have emptied themselves of blood, the pressure in the aorta and
pulmonary arteries forces the semi-lunar valves shut (Fig. 13.3).
This shutting of the valves produces the second heart sound (S2).

Blood then flows through both the systemic and pulmonary systems,
the ventricles relax, blood returns through the veins, and the A-V
valves open, letting blood flow again into the ventricles, completing
a single cardiac cycle. The entire sequence just described takes one
second at a heart rate of sixty beats per minute, or one half a second
at 120 per minute. Pause for a moment in awe as you review this
remarkable phenomenon before going on!

Systole begins with the first heart sound and ends at the second heart
sound. During this period the ventricles have contracted and the
apical portion of the heart has swung forward and upward striking the
anterior chest wall.

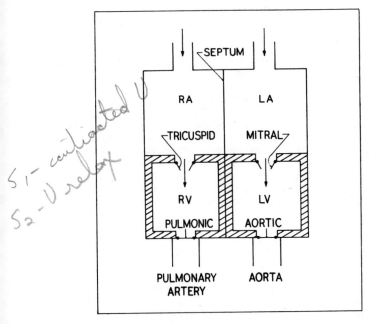

S₁ - contracted V
S₂ - U relax

FIG. 13.3: Diagram of position of valves. The semi-lunar valves, which opened during systole, have just snapped shut producing the second heart sound marking the end of systole.

Diastole is the period which begins with the second sound and ends at the next first sound. This is the period of relaxation of the ventricles and it is usually longer than systole (see Fig. 13.6, p. 183).

EXAMINATION

The cardiac examination is carried out in the same sequence used for the thorax and lung - inspection, palpation, percussion, and auscultation. While the examiner often is in a hurry to get his stethoscope on the chest, he should not do so. Auscultation is deliberately done last so that the clinician will have had time to obtain clues from other modes of examination. He frequently will have a considerable amount of diagnostic information before listening, so that he can listen with more understanding.

INSPECTION:

The principal purpose of inspection is to see the effect of ventricular contraction on the precordium. The normal findings are an apical impulse and slight retraction, medial to this impulse. These occur synchronously with cardiac systole and may be timed by palpating the carotid pulse while watching the chest.

Apical Impulse: The apical impulse may be found somewhere in the fourth, fifth, or sixth left intercostal spaces, normally at or medial to the mid-clavicular line. An apical impulse will not be seen (or palpated) in nearly half of the normal adult population.

When present, the apical impulse identifies an area very near the cardiac apex and is the best index of cardiac size on physical examination. Reports its location carefully by interspace and relationship to the mid-sternal line (MSL) or mid-clavicular line (MCL). (See Fig. 13.1.) Both methods of reporting the horizontal location of the apex are used. Normally, the apical impulse is no more than ten centimeters to the left of the MSL. However, considering the great variation in body build, our preference is to use the MCL for reference, since this line lies approximately half-way across the left chest wall no matter what the patient's size or shape. The apical impulse is normally found at or medial to the MCL, and if the heart is enlarged - or displaced - the impulse may be found lateral to that line. Thus, a normal location might be described as follows: "Apical impulse in fifth LICS at the MCL." If laterally displaced, the location should be reported by measurement, viz., "Apical impulse in sixth LICS four centimeters lateral to MCL."

Retraction: If an apex impulse is seen, look just medially to see if slight retraction of the intercostal space occurs. This, too, is a normal phenomenon. It is not normal, however, to have actual retraction of rib. Rib retraction is commonly due to pericardial disease and occurs because the pericardium is bound firmly to the chest wall.

Lift or heave: When cardiac action is abnormally forceful, the sternum, or ribs, may be seen to lift with each heart beat. This is referred to as a lift or heave and should be confirmed by palpation. Both terms mean the same thing, but some authors refer to a slight movement as a lift and a more vigorous movement as a heave.

PALPATION:

Point of Maximum Intensity: If the apical impulse is not seen, try to locate the cardiac apex by locating a point of maximum intensity (PMI). The fingertips should be placed over the area where the apex is usually located and moved about to see if a pulsation can be felt. Having the patient lean forward may assist in identifying the apical impulse. If one is located, report the PMI as described earlier for apical impulse, i.e., by interspace and relationship to the MCL. Should it not be found easily, do not spend much time in searching since, as noted previously, the apex cannot be located in about half of the patients examined.

Lift or Heave: The precordium should be felt by placing the palm over the entire area to detect a movement of the chest wall with each systole. Heave due to increased pressure or enlargement of the right ventricle will usually be found in the sternum or near it, while overactivity or hypertrophy of the left ventricle will often produce motion of the chest wall near or lateral to the apex.

Thrill: A thrill is a palpable heart murmur or rub and is best described as a vibration. The sensation of a thrill may be reproduced by palpating the larynx while an "M" sound is being made. Thrill should be felt for across the entire precordium with the palm of the hand.

PERCUSSION:

The major objective of percussion of the heart is to detect the location of the left cardiac border (Fig. 13.4). Usually, the left border will be found at or medial to the MCL. If located outside this line, the lateral distance from the MCL should be measured and reported as for the PMI.

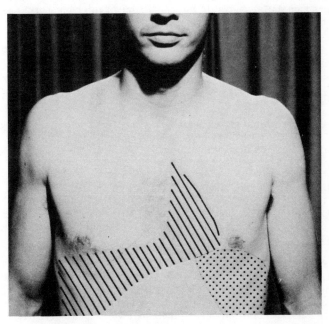

FIG. 13.4: Normal percussion areas. (Repeat of Fig. 11.13).
Hatched areas are dull and dotted area is tympanitic.

Since the heart is much more dense than the lung, percussion over the organ will produce dullness. This cardiac dullness is best detected by percussing in the fourth LICS from the anterior axillary line toward the mid-line.

Although it is more awkward to perform, percussion should be done, where possible, with the patient sitting or standing, rather than lying down. In the supine position, the patient's heart sinks away from the chest wall so that dullness is detected in a smaller area than it would be with the patient upright. The preferred technique is to percuss as lightly as possible, barely producing resonance over lung tissue, so that when the cardiac border is reached, the sound will disappear because of the dullness.

The left border of cardiac dullness (LBCD) should be percussed first in the fourth interspace, as suggested. Percussion should be repeated in the fifth and sixth interspaces to identify and report the location where the cardiac border is most lateral. Thus, "LBCD 2 cm. lateral to MCL in 5th LICS" means that this is the place where the cardiac border is furthest to the left.

The right cardiac border ordinarily cannot be percussed adequately. At the base (refer to Fig. 13.1), the heart lies too deep beneath lung to produce dullness, while the remainder of the right border is underneath the sternum. A brief percussion may be made about one centimeter to the right of the sternum to be sure that the heart does not project further than this, but this is not a mandatory portion of the examination, unless one fails to find a left border. (Congenital dextrocardia occurs in about one person in ten thousand so it is great "one-upmanship" to be the first to detect this rare abnormality in the patient.)

The student should try to see chest x-ray films of patients whom he has examined to see how close he has come to the actual border. The two methods of examination will not locate the border in exactly the same place, but they should not be far apart.

Enlargement or displacement of the left ventricle, which makes up most of the left border, will often produce the finding of the LBCD lateral to the MCL, and although such a finding suggests cardiac enlargement, it is not a reliable enough technique to be diagnostic by itself.

AUSCULTATION:

General: While the two heart sounds are heard all over the precordial area, there are locations where the sounds produced at each of the valves are transmitted best to the chest wall, and therefore heard loudest. Thus, the portion of the second sound produced by aortic valve closure is ordinarily heard best in the right second intercostal space near the sternal border. This is referred to as the aortic area. Similarly, the pulmonic area is in the left second interspace at the sternal border, the tricuspid area near the lower end of the sternum, and the mitral area at the cardiac apex (Fig. 13.5). The examiner should listen at these general locations, moving the stethoscope around to find the place where these sounds are loudest, on a particular patient's chest.

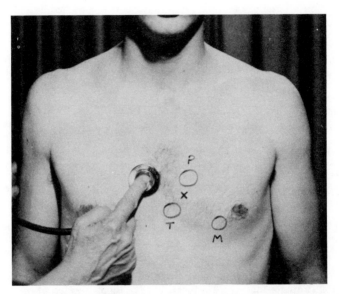

FIG. 13.5: Cardiac auscultation at the aortic area. Circles mark the valve areas. According to the old poem, "Aortic right, Pulmonic left, Tricuspid's 'neath the sternum, Mitral's at the apex beat, And that is how we learn 'em." Erb's point (see text page 189) is marked by an "X."

However, auscultation will not be limited to these four valve areas, but must include the entire precordium for an adequate examination. It is useful to vary the patient's position to see if sounds (and murmurs) can be better heard. Listening with the patient leaning forward while seated, and then again, when the patient is supine, may assist in the process of complete auscultation.

As indicated in the brief review of physiology, at the slow heart rate of sixty beats per minute, all of the events of a single cardiac cycle occur within a single second; at 120 per minute, within a half second. Thus, everything seems to be happening at once. In order to interpret what one hears, there must be a high degree of concentration, which the student must discipline himself to learn, and which he must practice to achieve.

The student must learn to "tune in" on specific events - to concentrate his full attention on one feature at a time. Since there are normally two sounds and two intervals, a logical method is to "tune in" on the first heart sound (S_1). Concentrate on this alone to the exclusion of all else, for enough cardiac cycles to be certain of its characteristics. Then shift attention to S_2 and listen to it alone. After this, listen to the systolic interval between S_1 and S_2. Try to hear nothing else. Lastly, fix on the interval between S_2 and the next S_1 - diastole.

Such concentration is not easily learned, but only by continued discipline will the examiner begin to develop competence in cardiac auscultation. Listening to recordings of heart sounds and murmurs is helpful in learning and practicing this technique of specific "tuning in." One must learn and train oneself to "listen for" sounds rather than just "listening at" heart sounds or murmurs.

It is important to keep in mind the facts relevant to heart sounds - that the first sound (S_1) is produced by closure of the A-V valves (mitral and tricuspid), that the second sound (S_2) arises with closure of the semi-lunar valves (aortic and pulmonic), and that these two sounds are heard over the entire precordium.

It is absolutely necessary to be able to identify the first sound and the second sound during all of cardiac auscultation. At heart rates of 90 or below, systole is distinctly shorter than diastole, so that identification of S_1 and S_2 is quite easy. However, as heart rates become more rapid, diastole begins to approach systole in duration, making timing a less certain technique for identification of the two sounds. At the aortic area both S_1 and S_2 are better heard than in other locations on the chest. Here, also, S_2 is distinctly louder than S_1, enabling the examiner to distinguish one from the other in almost all cases (Fig. 13.6). Confirmation may be obtained by palpating the apex beat (PMI) while listening. The apex beat is synchronous with S_1. If the apex beat is not palpable, the carotid pulse (but not the radial or femoral) may be palpated, as it rises just as S_1 ends.

By auscultation, S_1 is heard as a duller, lower-pitched and slightly longer sound than S_2. S_2 has a higher pitch and is snappier and shorter than the first sound. Fig. 13.6 is a sound recording (phonocardiogram) of normal heart sounds, which illustrates some of these features.

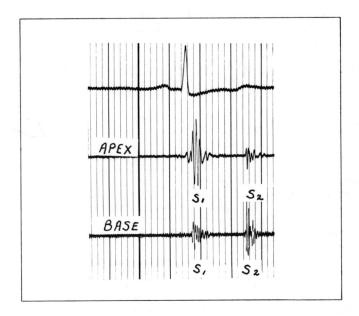

FIG. 13.6: Phonocardiogram of normal heart sounds. The upper
tracing is an electrocardiograph recorded for purposes
of timing. The middle line was recorded at the apex
(mitral area) and the lower tracing was taken at the pulmonic area. Note the fact that at the apex the first
sound is louder, while at the base, the second sound is
louder.

Technique: The examiner should place himself at the patient's right
side, routinely. This will assist him in developing a regular pattern
of examination and in keeping the earpieces of his stethoscope in
proper location in his auditory canals.

Certain sounds and murmurs are heard better with the patient upright
or leaning slightly forward, while others are brought out in the recumbent position. The student should, therefore, make a habit of
examining patients in at least two positions.

The clinician will listen to the characteristics of the heart sounds
first in his examination to determine if they are normal. Obviously,
such a judgment must be made on the basis of what one has heard in
many normal hearts. Intensity (loudness) is graded as normal,
louder or fainter than normal, or absent. Quality has to do with
the character of the sound, i.e., sharp, snapping, full, or booming.
Another feature of the character of a heart sound is whether it sounds

like a pure single sound or a "split" sound. This must be heard to be appreciated but it is a distinction which can be readily made once learned (see "Splitting," p. 185).

Remember that the diaphragm chestpiece amplifies sound and transmits higher-pitched sounds and that the bell transmits low-pitched sounds much better and is critical in certain portions of the examination.

CLINICAL AUSCULTATION

The examiner should be at the patient's right side and auscultation should begin at the aortic area, using the diaphragm of the stethoscope. Identify S_2, which is the louder sound here, and then begin the examination by concentrating your full attention on S_1. Listen to its loudness, pitch, and quality. Next, fix attention on S_2 and evaluate this sound. Only when the characteristics of S_1 and S_2 are determined and compared in your mind with the expected normal characteristics should you proceed.

Concentrate next on systole, the normally silent interval between S_1 and S_2. Any sounds heard in systole are to be described as accurately as possible. Then listen to the diastolic interval between S_2 and the next S_1. Here, too, there should be no sounds, normally.

Having completed this examination in the aortic area, shift the diaphragm of the chestpiece to the pulmonic area and repeat the entire sequence of auscultation: the S_1, then S_2, then to the systolic interval, and lastly to diastole. You will note that, as in the aortic area, the S_2 is louder than S_1 and that S_2 is a shorter, snappier, higher-pitched sound than S_1. Splitting of S_2 is often heard in this area, and may or may not be abnormal (see "Splitting," p. 185).

Before leaving the base of the heart, compare the loudness of S_2 in the aortic area to S_2 in the pulmonic area. You may need to shift the stethoscope rapidly between the aortic and pulmonic areas several times to make this comparison. S_2 is generally louder in the pulmonic area in children and young adults. By age 30, most adults will have an S_2 louder in the aortic area than in the pulmonic area. The loudness of S_2 (aortic) is roughly related to the arterial blood pressure in the systemic circulation, while loudness of S_2 heard in the pulmonic area is influenced by pulmonary artery pressure. Thus, for example, arterial hypertension will cause S_2 (aortic) to be even louder than normal. Factors which increase pulmonary pressures, such as chronic obstructive pulmonary disease, may lead to an increase of loudness in S_2 (pulmonic).

The finding of S_2 (pulmonic) louder than S_2 (aortic) in an adult over age 40 is abnormal. The relationship between S_2 (aortic) and S_2 (pulmonic) should always be established and recorded. Use of mathematical symbols is a convenient way to record this relationship. Thus, in the normal adult S_2 (aortic) is louder than S_2 (pulmonic) and would be symbolized as: S_2 (aortic) $>$ S_2 (pulmonic).

The examiner now "inches" his stethoscope down from the pulmonic area toward the lower end of the sternum. The first sound (S_1) at the tricuspid area may be normally louder than S_2 or both may be equal. Shift to the bell of the stethoscope to see if the lower pitched sounds are heard better than with the diaphragm. Once again, examine S_1, S_2, systole, and then diastole, evaluating the sounds and then the intervals for any abnormalities.

From this area, move the bell slowly toward the cardiac apex. The point at which sounds are loudest is called the mitral area, the cardiac apex. The examination of heart sounds and intervals is repeated at this location. Normally, S_1 will be louder than S_2 here, although the sounds may be of about equal intensity.

If there is significant emphysema present, with an increase in A-P diameter of the chest, either or both sounds may be difficult to hear at the tricuspid and mitral areas. Having the patient lean forward may help to bring these sounds out better.

Splitting: As noted earlier, the valves of the right and left sides of the heart snap shut almost simultaneously so that the sound produced is heard as a single sound. Should enough delay in the closures occur, the heart sound will be heard with two distinct components and it is said to be split (Fig. 13.7). Splitting is more often heard in first heart sounds at the apex, and in second sounds at the base.

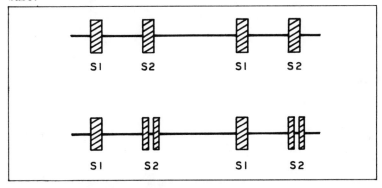

FIG. 13.7: Graphic representation of heart sounds. The upper line is normal. The lower represents a split second sound. Note the closeness of the two components of the split sound. Systole is the interval between S_1 and S_2; diastole occurs between S_2 and the next S_1.

It is important to be able to identify a split so as not to confuse it
with other sounds which may occur during cardiac auscultation.
This distinction will be made principally on quality and timing - the
split sound still has the same general quality (i.e., pitch, loudness,
and character) as the unsplit sound, but is made up of two distinct
components, one occurring immediately after the other. A crude
representation of this may be produced by saying aloud the sound,
"spit-spit-spit" to represent a single heart sound; then at the same
speed, pitch, and loudness, say "split-split-split." Pronouncing
the extra letter gives the word a split quality.

If a split sound is heard, the examiner should note and record variation in the split, with respiration. A split may occur in perfectly
normal hearts or under abnormal situations. The "physiological
split" of the pulmonic second sound will be heard to appear and
widen during inspiration and to disappear on expiration. Such a
split is a normal phenomenon. If the split does not vary with respiration, it is called a fixed split; if it becomes wider and more pronounced on expiration, it is called a paradoxical split since it varies
in an opposite way from the physiological split. Both the fixed split
and the paradoxical split have different causes and are generally
evidences of cardiac disease.

There are several other sounds which may be heard on cardiac auscultation, only two of which will be described here (Fig. 13.8).

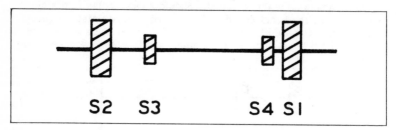

FIG. 13.8: Third and fourth heart sounds. Note that both occur during diastole.

Third Heart Sound (S3): In some normal patients, particularly in
those under thirty, a third heart sound (S3) may be heard. The
third sound has the following features:

    1. Heard best near the apex, not at the base of the heart
    2. May be accentuated by left lateral decubitus position
    3. Has a low-pitched sound (use bell of stethoscope)
    4. Occurs early in diastole
    5. May become louder with expiration
    6. May be more prominent with tachycardia

These features should suggest several maneuvers for the examiner to use to find or identify an S_3.

The exact cause of S_3 is not fully agreed upon by all authorities, but it is commonly accepted that while S_3 may be normal in young adults, it is to be considered abnormal in patients over 40, and should always be reported when found.

Fourth Heart Sound (S_4): A fourth sound may occur at the time of atrial contraction. It was noted, in the section on Physiology that, when the atria contract and fill the ventricles, ventricular contraction begins. Since this occurs prior to the beginning of the first heart sound, the fourth sound (S_4) will be heard at the end of the diastolic interval - or before systole begins (see Fig. 13.8). This is more often heard near the apex or left sternal border, but it may be heard in any location. However, since S_4 is a low-pitched sound, like S_3, it will be picked up more distinctly by the bell and can be distinguished from S_3 by the time of its appearance. S_4 is generally an abnormal finding.

Although other sounds do occur, their description will not be taken up in this text. When the student is sufficiently competent to be certain of the identification and characterization of these four heart sounds and of murmurs, he should then, by reference to other sources, expand his knowledge of sounds such as the opening snap, systolic ejection clicks, and pericardial knocks. He must, however, describe all sounds even if he is unclear about identification.

Triple Rhythm (Gallop): A triple rhythm refers to one consisting of three distinct heart sounds: S_1, S_2 and another of varied origin. This triple rhythm often resembles the sound of galloping hoof-beats, particularly when the heart rate is increased. There are several varieties of triple rhythm which are distinguished by the timing of the extra sound. It is very important to determine whether the extra sound occurs during systole (systolic gallop) or in diastole (diastolic gallop). Systolic gallops may be heard in normal hearts, whereas a diastolic gallop rhythm is almost certain to indicate heart disease.

Since, by definition, there will be three distinct sounds making up a gallop, the two normal heart sounds must be identified in order to know where the third component falls in the cardiac cycle. The major reference point for identification of the normal sounds is in the aortic area, where S_2 is loud, crisp, and distinct.

Triple rhythm is usually best heard with the patient supine, and most often is picked up at or near the cardiac apex. Once the examiner hears the triple rhythm of a gallop, he should begin to inch the chestpiece of his stethoscope toward the aortic area, using either the bell or diaphragm, depending on which allows him to hear all three sounds best.

As he approaches the base of the heart, the examiner will hear S_2 becoming louder and clearer. S_1 will also become more distinct and the extra sound will fade in intensity or actually disappear. This maneuver should identify which of the three sounds is "gallop-producing" and, therefore, in which phase of the cardiac cycle it appears.

There are, in fact, two types of diastolic gallop which are frequently referred to as "S_3 gallop" and "S_4 gallop" depending upon whether the extra sound occurs early in diastole where S_3 usually is heard (Fig. 13.9) or late in diastole, where S_4 is generally present. If this distinction can be made it should be reported, but this distinction is far less important than the determination that a gallop is systolic or diastolic.

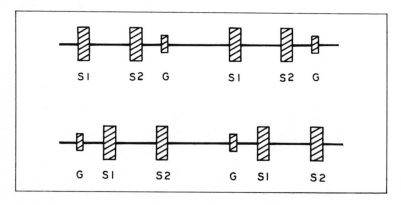

FIG. 13.9: Diastolic gallop sounds. The gallop-producing sound is labelled "G." The upper line shows an S_3 gallop rhythm sounding somewhat like the word "Ken-tuck-y." The lower line represents an S_4 (presystolic) gallop, with a "Ten-ne-see" rhythm.

As noted earlier, the presence of either an S_3 or an S_4, whether they produce a gallop rhythm or not, must be assumed to be abnormal and should be carefully described as to timing, location on the precordium, quality of sound, and change in respiration or patient's position. The distinction between an abnormal and a normal third or fourth sound should be left for the consultant.

Murmurs: Cardiac murmurs are the result of turbulent blood flow within the heart, produced at the valves, or through abnormal passages, such as openings between atria (atrial septal defect), ventricles (ventricular septal defect), or a patent ductus arteriosus. Ordinarily the term "bruit" is reserved for a similar sound heard over arteries distant from the heart. Murmurs have a greater duration than heart sounds.

Turbulence at a valve generally arises from narrowing of the valve opening (stenosis) or from blood flowing backward through a defective closed valve (insufficiency or regurgitation).

The timing of murmurs is based upon the time of the murmur in relation to the first and second heart sounds. The identification of the defect is not easy, for it is not always true that the murmur will be loudest at the named area on the chest identified earlier. Thus, aortic valve murmurs are generally transmitted toward the apex and may be at maximum intensity at the left sternal border or at the apex itself. Also, murmurs may be due to defects other than to damaged valves. The task of the examiner, therefore, is to establish the exact timing of the murmur, and then to describe carefully the location of maximum loudness, the quality, loudness, pitch, radiation, and change during exercise, respiration or movement of the patient.

It must be remembered, in cardiac auscultation, that all murmurs do not indicate heart disease and, conversely, that some cardiac defects do not produce murmurs. In general, all diastolic murmurs are to be considered pathological.

By definition, systolic murmurs occur between S_1 and S_2. If the murmur is loudest in mid-systole, it is referred to as an ejection murmur and is called "diamond-shaped" because of its appearance on the phonocardiograph (Fig. 13.10). The other common type of systolic murmur is one which is heard throughout systole and is more or less equal in loudness from beginning to end. This is called a pan-systolic or holosystolic murmur. Occasionally, a murmur is heard only in early or late systole and would be described in those terms.

Similarly, diastolic murmurs must be described in terms of onset, duration, and "shape." True pan-diastolic murmurs are less common than are pan-systolic. More often they are heard early or late in diastole. Early murmurs generally begin immediately after the second sound and fade out in late diastole (decrescendo); late murmurs begin near mid-diastole and become louder (crescendo) as they merge into the first sound. These are sometimes referred to as "pre-systolic" murmurs. Fig. 13.11 illustrates some characteristic forms or shapes of murmurs.

Murmurs must be described by the location of the point on the chest where they sound loudest. As noted earlier, these locations may or may not correspond to the valve sites due to transmission of the sounds. This is particularly true for murmurs of the aortic valve which are so frequently radiated to the third left interspace at the sternal border that this area is called the secondary aortic area, or Erb's point (see Fig. 13.5).

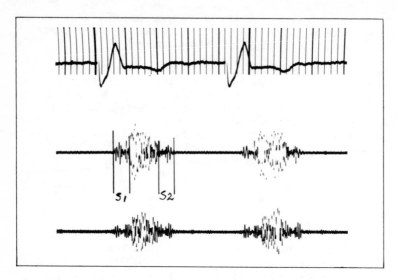

FIG. 13.10: Phonocardiograph of a systolic murmur. The upper
line is an electrocardiograph. The middle and lower
tracings were recorded with different electronic fil-
ters but both show the "diamond" shape of the systolic
murmur.

When listening for murmurs at the cardiac apex, it is a good practice to examine the area with the patient supine, and then to have
him move to a left lateral decubitus position, while listening. This
maneuver will occasionally exaggerate a faint diastolic murmur not
heard in any other position.

In addition to recording the point at which the murmur sounds loudest, the clinician should describe the radiation of the murmur. Such
radiation is often characteristic of a particular lesion and may be
quite helpful in diagnosis. Thus, the murmur of aortic stenosis can
often be tracked into the carotid arteries, that of mitral insufficiency
into the axilla, while that of mitral stenosis hardly radiates at all
from the apical area.

The pitch of a murmur is also an important feature to be described.
Low-pitched murmurs range from about 30-80 cps, medium-pitched
murmurs from about 90-150 cps, and high-pitched murmurs from
150 cps up to around 600 cps.

The examiner must also describe the quality of any murmur by descriptive terms. Commonly used words are blowing, rough, harsh,
rumbling, or musical. Other fanciful terms may be used if they

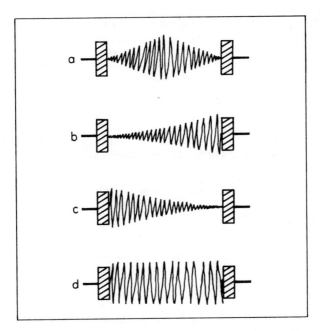

FIG. 13.11: Representation of several shapes of murmurs as seen
on phonocardiography. These may be either systolic
or diastolic in time:
a) Diamond-shaped
b) Crescendo
c) Decrescendo
d) Pan-systolic or Pan-diastolic

provide a good description. Thus, for example, the murmur of
aortic stenosis with calcification of the valve is often perceived and
described as a "sea-gull" murmur.

Thus, descriptions of murmurs require inclusion of many features:
timing, location, radiation, pitch, and quality. Additionally, the
loudness or intensity of a murmur must be described and recorded.
This is so subjective and so much related to the experience of the
observer that it is difficult to evaluate and to obtain agreement on.
Fortunately, it is not nearly so critical an item as timing or location for purposes of diagnosis or evaluation. Two systems are in
general use for grading the intensity of murmurs, one based on four
and one on six grades. The six grade system is as follows:

Grade 1 - the faintest murmur you can hear; often not heard at
first
Grade 2 - faint, but heard without difficulty

Grade 3 - soft, but louder than grade 2
Grade 4 - loud, but less loud than grade 5
Grade 5 - loud, but not heard if stethoscope is lifted just off
the chest (thrill will be present)
Grade 6 - maximum loudness; heard even if stethoscope is
lifted from chest

Obviously, the difference between Grades 3 and 4 is not exact, but the other criteria are rather easy to define. In recording the intensity by this system the observer must identify that he is grading on the basis of six, e.g., "Grade 4 (of 6) murmur," or "Grade 4/6 murmur." The four grade system is simpler and perfectly adequate. Here the criteria are:

Grade 1 - faintest murmur you can hear
Grade 2 - soft
Grade 3 - loud
Grade 4 - very loud

Reporting by this system would be identified as follows: "Grade 2 (of 4) murmur," or "Grade 2/4 murmur." If deep inspiration or deep expiration changes the intensity of a murmur, this should be noted.

If variations in heart sounds also occur, these should be noted to complete the description.

Table 13.1 is a condensed outline describing several common murmurs. Only a few descriptive terms are used and the student is cautioned to recognize that this is only a brief and incomplete starting point for interpretation of murmurs.

Friction Rub: In pericarditis, a friction rub may develop which can often be heard over the lower sternum. It is not usually related to systole or diastole, but may be heard during various parts of the cardiac cycle often beginning in late diastole and going through systole. Sounds may vary with respiration since the pleura may be involved where it attaches to the pericardium. The pericardial friction rub is typically transient and may change in character from time to time.

RECORDING

Heart

Insp. No heave. Apical impulse in 5th LICS medial to MCL
Perc. LBCD at MCL in 5th ICS
Palp. No heave, thrill or rib retraction
Ausc. Rate 80/min. regular,, sounds normal S_2 aortic $> S_2$
pulmonic, S_2 split at pulmonic on inspiration. No murmurs, gallop, rubs

TABLE 13.1

Area	Timing	Heart Sounds	Quality Of Murmur	Transmission Of Murmur	Probable Lesions
Aortic or Erb's pt.	Systole	S_2 normal or decreased, S_4 may be present	Medium pitch, harsh, ejection	Vessels of neck	Aortic stenosis
	Diastole	S_1 normal or decreased	High pitch, blowing, descrescendo	Left sternal border	Aortic insufficiency
Pulmonary	Systole	S_2 normal or decreased, S_2 split	Medium pitch, harsh, ejection	Little to none	Pulmonary stenosis
	Diastole	Generally normal	Medium pitch, blowing, descrescendo	Little to none	Pulmonary insufficiency
Mitral	Systole	S_1 normal or decreased, S_3 may be present	Medium pitch, blowing, pansystolic	Toward axilla	Mitral insufficiency
	Diastole	"Snapping" accentuated S_1, "opening snap"	Low pitch, rumble, crescendo	Little to none	Mitral stenosis
Left sternal border, 4th interspace	Systole	S_3 may be present	Medium pitch variable harsh, holosystolic	Variable	Ventricular septal defect
Left sternal border, 2nd interspace	Systole and Diastole	May not be heard	Variable pitch, harsh, crescendo-decrescendo	Precordium	Patent ductus arteriosus

TABLE 13.1: Typical characteristics of several common murmurs. The features listed are generally present, but vary according to the severity of valve damage and dynamic factors such as pressure. Also, where there is both stenosis and insufficiency of one valve, or damage to more than one valve, the characteristics of murmurs are modified.

PATIENT PROBLEM

Mrs. T.F., a 65-year-old widow with CC short of breath this a.m., felt "faint, weak."

Problem #1: Cardiac Murmur and Left Heart Failure

S: Good general health. No history of rheumatic fever. Had systolic murmur noted at age 38 but no symptoms until one year ago. Had episode of "feeling faint" upon exertion this a.m. Has never had ankle edema.

O: BP. L.A. 180/80 Pulse 100, vigorous beat. Pulses visible R.A. 170/80 sitting and lying

　　Insp.　Carotid pulse visible and pulsation noted in suprasternal notch. Apical impulse in 6th LICS, 2 cm. lateral to MCL.
　　Palp.　PMI forceful at location of apical impulse, slight lift at apex. Liver not enlarged.
　　Perc.　No pulmonary dullness. LBCD maximal in 6th LICS, 2 cm. lateral to MCL.
　　Ausc.　Few bilateral basal rales, posteriorly. S_2 accentuated. Blowing, high-pitched decrescendo Grade 2/6 murmur, heard best at Erb's point, radiating up to aortic area, carotid vessels, downward to apex. No gallop.

A: Probable aortic insufficiency with minimal early left heart failure.

P: Dx. ECG. Chest x-ray. Sed Rate. CBC.
　　Rx. Appointment with cardiologist for consultation, promptly.
　　Pt. Ed. Health status discussed regarding murmur, significance of S.O.B. Advised as to necessity for consultation and further tests, diet control, drugs and activity.

Problem #2: Anxiety

S: Has lived in same 8-room house for 35 years. Lost husband 3 years ago. Three sons married with families. Has not seen two sons since husband's funeral. One son visits monthly. Younger brother died of MI one month ago. Had been a teacher for 25 years. Retired - 6 months. Never had time for hobbies or outside groups. Complains of fatigue, yet does little. Went to senior citizens meeting, but uninterested in group.

A: Loneliness and depression as result of family loss and social isolation.

P: Consultation with Social Worker regarding appropriate expansion of social contacts.

Arrange return visit following medical evaluation for counseling.

_____
Signature

SUPPLEMENTAL EXERCISES

1. Describe completely, in problem oriented form, the symptoms (S) and physical findings (O) likely in a patient with severe mitral stenosis.

2. Which conditions are likely to produce sternal heave? Apical heave?

REFERENCES

1. Hurst, J.W. and Schlant, R.C.: Examination of the Heart, Part 3: Inspection and Palpation of the Anterior Chest. The American Heart Association, New York, 1967.

2. Leonard, J.J. and Kroetz, F.W.: Examination of the Heart, Part 4: Auscultation. The American Heart Association, New York, 1967.

3. Hurst, J.W. and Logue, R.B.: The Heart, Arteries and Veins, 3rd edition. McGraw-Hill Book Company, New York, 1974.

4. Lehmann, J.: Auscultation of Heart Sounds. Am.J. Nurs. 72:1242, July 1972.

5. Brown, M.S. and Alexander, M.M.: Physical Examination, Part 2: Examining the Heart. Nursing '74 4:41, December 1974.

6. Delancy, M. T.: Examining the Chest, Part 2: The Heart. Nursing '75 5:41, September 1975.

7. Sherman, J. L. Jr., and Fields, Sylvia K.: Examination of the Heart, Westinghouse Learning Systems. Multi-media Series.

CHAPTER 14

THE ABDOMEN

INTRODUCTION

The abdomen may be thought of as a shallow bowl containing the stomach, intestines, liver, spleen, kidneys, and other organs and blood vessels. The bowl is made up of the spine and muscles of the back and is covered by the anterior abdominal wall consisting of skin, fat, muscle, and connective tissue. Thus, the abdomen and its important contents are soft tissue structures. Palpation can, therefore, produce more information here than in the chest which is limited by its bony structures.

TOPOGRAPHICAL ANATOMY

As seen from the front, the anterior abdominal wall has the approximate outline of a hexagon with the xiphoid process at the top and the symphysis pubis at the bottom. The upper edges are formed by the costal margin and the lower edges by the inguinal ligaments which extend from the iliac crests to the symphysis pubis. The sides of this imaginary hexagon are simply the right and left sides of the patient (see Fig. 14.2). At first, it will be useful for the student to fix these points and lines by actual palpation before proceeding with the examination. It must be recalled that the abdominal contents extend up below the rib cage and down into the pelvis, outside this hexagon.

Due to variations in body build, the hexagon may be wide or narrow, long or short. In order to describe locations within the abdomen, the hexagon is divided into either four or nine segments. Since both systems or divisions are used, the student should be familiar with both. The simpler method is division into four quadrants made by a vertical line (the "mid-line"), from the xiphoid process to the symphysis pubis, and by a horizontal line across the umbilicus. The quadrants are simply named Right Upper Quadrant (RUQ), Left Upper Quadrant (LUQ), Right Lower Quadrant (RLQ), and Left Lower Quadrant (LLQ)(Fig. 14.1).

The second system (Fig. 14.2) marks off the abdominal wall by drawing vertical lines upward from the mid-point of both the right and left inguinal ligaments. Two horizontal lines are drawn - one across the lower rib margins and the other crossing the iliac crests. This produces nine areas and is a more convenient system for locating lesions or masses near the mid-line.

197

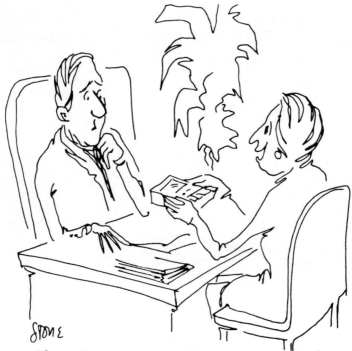

"I made a tape recording of my stomach
growling so you could listen."

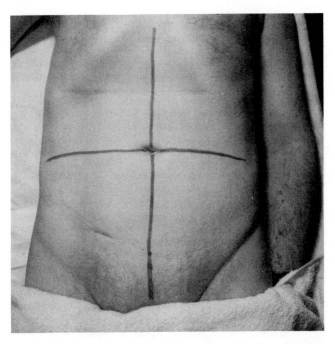

FIG. 14.1: The abdomen marked into quadrants. A surgical scar is
visible in the RLQ, and another crosses horizontally in
both upper quadrants.

The student must review the anatomical structures present in the
abdomen and their relationships before studying the physical examination. This knowledge is critical for an understanding of the techniques and results of the examination.

PHYSIOLOGY

The descent of the diaphragm on inhalation moves the liver, spleen,
kidneys, stomach, and intestines downward, producing outward motion of the upper abdominal wall. This motion is much more pronounced, on the average, in men than in women.

During the daytime, and particularly during eating, much air is swal-
lowed. This air, mixed with ingested fluids and intestinal juices, is
propelled through the stomach and intestines, producing bowel sounds
which, as might be expected, sound like gurgles and bubbles. Collections of air in the gastrointestinal tract produce the hollow note
on percussion called tympany.

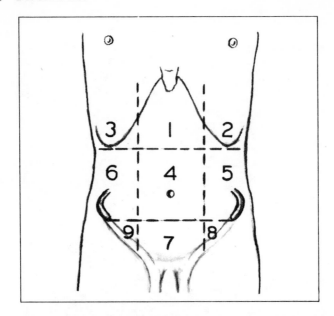

FIG. 14.2: Abdominal areas: (1) Epigastrium; (2,3) Left and right
hypochondrium; (4) Umbilical area; (5,6) Left and right
flanks; (7) Suprapubic area, or hypogastrium; (8,9) Left
and right iliac areas. Note the umbilicus below the center of the abdomen.

As the semi-solid feces are being formed in the colon, they are occasionally palpable. Urine, filling the bladder, may make it palpable and, if the full bladder is percussed, it produces a flat note.

The pregnant uterus rises out of the pelvis and, as it displaces intestine in the suprapubic area, can be appreciated as a solid mass
to palpation and percussion.

Late in pregnancy, the large volume of blood flow to the placental
circulation may produce a bruit - called the "funic souffle." Fetal
heart sounds may also be heard late in pregnancy.

EXAMINATION

For proper examination of the abdomen, the patient should be lying
comfortably in the supine position with his head supported by a pillow. He should have a narrow towel draped across the genital area
and, if the patient is a woman, the breasts should be draped also.
The patient's arms should not be raised since this position tends to
stretch the abdominal muscles, putting them under tension and making

the abdomen harder to examine. Generally, the arms should be at his side, and if they are in the way when the flanks are examined, they may be folded across the chest.

It is ordinarily not necessary to have the patient's knees drawn up unless the patient is uncomfortable with his lower extremities flat. Should the patient desire the knees-up position, careful questioning should be done about the location of pain if one or both lower extremities are extended, as this may produce valuable diagnostic information.

The examiner should inspect the abdomen from all angles but should develop the habit of performing most of the remainder of the examination from the right side of the patient. This positioning will help to reinforce a pattern of examination. It is often convenient to sit at the bedside for detailed inspection and for auscultation.

In the evaluation of the thorax, the sequence of examination is Inspection, Palpation, Percussion, and Auscultation. Here it is advisable to vary the order and to follow Inspection with Auscultation. The reason for this is that palpation may induce tenderness if there is a painful lesion in the abdomen, and this tenderness will interfere with the motility of the bowel - sometimes producing almost no motility for a period of time. This will change the frequency and character of the bowel sounds, whereas if the examiner had listened before palpating, his findings would have been quite different.

INSPECTION:

As for all other regions, inspection should begin with a general view of the region to detect significant variations from the normal. The examiner should keep in mind the anatomy of the area, and in his inspection should concentrate on the abdominal wall and then the abdominal contents.

It was pointed out earlier that the umbilicus is located slightly below the center of the abdomen. If it is observed to be distinctly higher than this, the examiner should be alerted to the possibility of a tumor in the suprapubic region (see diagram, Fig. 14.2) or of pregnancy which causes the uterus to rise into this region. The umbilicus may be lower than normal due to tumor underlying the epigastric region, or to ascites (see Fig. 14.4).

Contour: The normal abdomen should be flat and the lateral borders only slightly curved. If the abdominal wall is thin, the abdominal contents are reduced in size and the contour will be concave rather than flat. This is described as a scaphoid abdomen. On the other hand, the abdominal wall may protrude forward either in a localized area or throughout its entire extent. The flanks should be inspected to see if they are not generally straight but are bulging and rounded.

This is often an early finding when fluid is accumulating in the peritoneal cavity and is also commonly seen in simple obesity. Fig. 14.3 shows an example of severe bulging of the flanks.

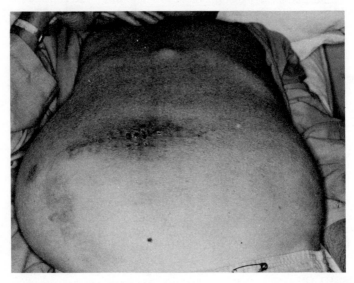

FIG. 14.3: Abdominal distention. This was due to excessive fluid (ascites). The umbilicus was removed following rupture of an umbilical hernia.

Skin: As elsewhere, the skin should be inspected for texture, color, lesions, scars, wounds, etc. which should be reported as described earlier.

Discoloration: The appearance of bluish discolorations or bruises in the abdominal wall should be viewed with great suspicion, for even though they may be due to trauma, they may also represent intra-abdominal bleeding. Such discolorations may be seen in cases of extra-uterine pregnancy, pancreatitis, metastatic tumors, etc.

Veins: The veins of the normal abdominal wall are usually not visible or are not prominent. A distinct increase in the number and the fullness of abdominal veins is probably abnormal and should always be reported. When prominent veins are seen (Fig. 14.4), the direction of flow in them should be recorded. In the normal situation, blood flows away from the umbilicus, i.e., upward above the umbilicus and downward below the umbilicus.

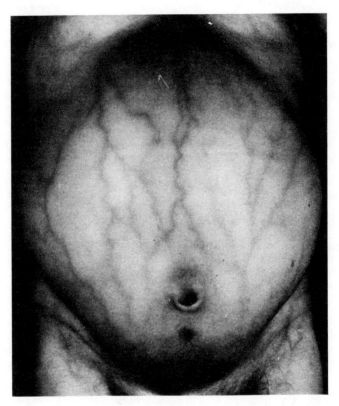

FIG. 14.4: Prominent abdominal veins and abdominal distention.
Photographed in infra-red light. Note here that the umbilicus is displaced downward.

Hernias: Inspection of the abdominal wall may also reveal the presence of a hernia, which is the protrusion of tissues or an organ
through an abnormal opening. There are several locations where
this is prone to occur in the abdominal wall: anywhere along the
midline including the umbilicus, in surgical scars, and above or below the inguinal ligament.

If small protrusions are noted, they may or may not be true hernias.
This may be checked by having the patient strain, increasing intra-
abdominal pressure. Most often, a hernia will bulge further out with
such a maneuver. Palpation will also assist in confirming the bulging of a hernia when intra-abdominal pressure is increased.

Respiratory Motion: The motion of the abdominal wall should be watched through several respiratory cycles. As noted earlier, most men are "abdominal breathers" in that they utilize the diaphragm more than women. What may possibly be abnormal is the absence of abdominal respiratory motion, particularly in a man. This may represent the first physical finding of peritonitis which causes the patient to hold the diaphragm still to reduce abdominal pain.

Pulsation: Portions of the abdominal wall may be seen to pulsate at the same rate as the heart. This is sometimes seen in patients with thin-walled scaphoid abdomens and occasionally with distended abdomens, particularly when the distention is due to fluid (ascites).

Peristalsis: Normal peristalsis is ordinarily not visible through the abdominal wall, but in cases of intestinal obstruction, waves may be seen to ripple across the abdomen. Whenever seen, peristaltic waves should be reported, since they are almost always abnormal in the adult.

AUSCULTATION:

There is much to be gained by careful attention to abdominal sounds and this portion of the examination should not be hurried. The clinician will listen for bowel sounds, arterial bruits, venous hums, and parietal friction rubs, particularly over-enlarged organs.

Bowel sounds: The mixing and moving forward of the liquid and air in the intestines produce brief bursts of gurgling, bubbling sounds. These peristaltic sounds are of medium to high pitch (200-1000 cps) and will therefore be heard best with the diaphragm of the stethoscope, which should be pressed lightly against the abdominal wall.

Peristaltic sounds are normally variable in frequency, pitch, and loudness. On the average, sounds will occur anywhere from two to three times per minute up to 10 to 15 times per minute depending upon the state of the digestive process at the time of examination.

The normal ranges in variability of bowel sounds must be learned by the examiner on the basis of listening to many hundreds of patients with normal intestinal function.

Examination of bowel sounds must be performed in each abdominal quadrant and for a long enough time to be certain that sounds are present in each area and are of normal quality.

The absence of bowel sounds in one area, when they are present and normal in other areas, is evidence of the fact that there is no intestine underlying the quiet area - that the intestine has been displaced from that location by tumor or by fluid.

When the gut is paralyzed, as in intestinal ileus, peristaltic activity is reduced so much that sounds are produced at a very slow rate - one per minute or even less. While the term "silent abdomen" is often used, total absence of peristaltic sounds for 5-10 minutes is quite rare. The examiner may wish to be seated at the bedside for the lengthy auscultation necessary for evaluation of a quiet abdomen.

Significantly increased peristalsis, with loud, rapidly produced bowel sounds (i.e., one every 2-3 seconds) is found in hypermotility of the gut. This condition may come from diarrhea or from bowel irritation due to gastroenteritis or to the presence of blood in the bowel (e.g., from bleeding duodenal ulcer).

Mechanical bowel obstruction is ordinarily associated with periods of "rushes" of sounds. During such periods of rushes, the sounds may be high-pitched (i.e., 1500-2000 cps), tinkling, or splashing in quality, and are frequently simultaneous with colicky pain perceived by the patient. This combination of rushes and colicky pain is diagnostic of obstruction. It must be understood, however, that the frequency and nature of the abnormal sounds will vary with the degree of obstruction and the duration of the process. For example, in nearly complete obstruction, after a period of time the bowel activity will weaken, the rushes become less frequent, and may finally disappear - producing a true "silent abdomen."

Arterial bruits: Since these are low-pitched sounds (i.e., under 100 cps), the bell should be employed. The examiner should routinely examine several areas where bruits are most commonly heard. These include the epigastrium - a few centimeters above the umbilicus - and the areas to the right and left of the umbilicus.

Most often, these sounds will be systolic in timing and will be heard a fraction of a second after the cardiac apical impulse or the carotid pulse is palpated.

Such bruits may be due to stenosis of the celiac artery, the renal artery, or to arteriosclerotic narrowing of the abdominal aorta. Renal artery stenosis may also produce a bruit lateral to the umbilicus.

It must be recalled that some cardiac murmurs may be transmitted quite well along the aorta, so that if the patient has a murmur and the student hears a vascular sound over the mid-line, it may be either a true bruit or the transmitted murmur. These are difficult to separate and the prudent student will seek help with this problem.

Venous hum: Another type of diagnostic sound which may be picked up is the venous hum. As the name suggests, the sound is generally less rough than an arterial bruit or murmur, is slightly higher-pitched than an arterial bruit (although the bell should still be used), and is commonly continuous through systole and diastole. Venous hums, if present, are most often found over the umbilical area, to the right of the umbilicus or over the liver region. While some venous hums may be normal sounds produced by the vena cava, any hum should be localized carefully and reported, as it may indicate the presence of cirrhosis of the liver with portal hypertension.

Friction rubs: These are similar in cause and quality to rubs heard over the pericardium or pleura. One should listen carefully over the liver (right upper quadrant) and over the spleen (left hypochondrium) while the patient takes several deep breaths.

A rub over the liver may be indicative of a hepatoma or of cholecystitis, while a rub over the spleen may be due to inflammation or to infarction of that organ.

PERCUSSION:

As noted earlier, the stomach and intestines contain varying amounts of air so that percussion over these organs will normally produce high-pitched tympanitic sounds. While the sounds may vary somewhat from one location to another, percussion over all four quadrants should produce a predominant tympanitic note within the abdominal hexagon. Any dullness should be investigated carefully.

In some individuals, the full urinary bladder may rise above the pubis enough to produce dullness but this is ordinarily limited to one or two centimeters into the suprapubic area. The disappearance of that dullness after the patient voids will confirm the cause. Pregnancy also will cause suprapubic dullness, generally in the latter trimesters.

Percussion will assist in confirming the findings on palpation of an enlarged organ or mass.

The presence of a collection of fluid in the abdomen (ascites) will modify the findings on percussion also. This is described in detail on p. 215.

PALPATION:

Considering the large number of organs in the abdomen and the ease with which the clinician may palpate the area, it is remarkable how little may be positively identified by this examination in the normal patient. The fingertips will sense differences in resistance but the examiner may sometimes complete a careful palpation without identifying clearly any intra-abdominal organ. It may be possible to palpate a few normal structures in a patient with a thin abdominal wall: the liver edge, the abdominal aorta, the lower pole of the right kidney, the 4th and 5th lumbar vertebrae, the uterus beyond the 3rd month of pregnancy, and the full urinary bladder (Fig. 14.5).

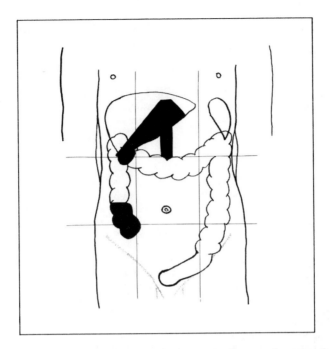

FIG. 14.5: Areas in black indicate portions of normal organs frequently palpable: liver in the epigastrium and right
hypochondrium, aorta deep in the epigastrium, lower
pole of right kidney deep in the right flank, cecum in the
right iliac and flank regions.

One word of caution is in order here. If the patient has identified an
area of pain in his medical history, this area should be left for last
in palpation. Premature palpation of a painful area may produce
spasm or rigidity of the abdominal wall so that the examiner is
robbed of the opportunity to evaluate the remainder of the abdomen.

There are several modes of palpation which the student must learn
in order to examine the abdomen thoroughly. These include ballottement, light palpation, and deep palpation.

Ballottement: A recommended technique is to begin in the lowest
portion of the abdomen and to bounce the fingertips upward at two to
three centimeter intervals roughly along each mid-inguinal line to
the costal margin. If this is done lightly and rapidly, the examiner
may be able to detect early rigidity of the abdominal muscles on one
or both sides (also called guarding), which is an early sign of underlying inflammation. Or he may be able to find evidence of a mass
beneath the abdominal wall.

If, for example, the liver is enlarged downward to the level of the umbilicus, ballottement will provide the examiner with a definite sense of resistance as he bounces his fingers from the RLQ to the RUQ. He will also note that the sense of resistance is quite different in the RUQ from that in the LUQ.

Since ballottement should be done very lightly with the fingertips, it will rarely produce severe tenderness even in an inflamed abdomen. In a patient with a painful abdomen it may be the only palpation which can be accomplished, and therefore, ballottement should be carefully practiced on every patient examined so that the student becomes skillful in this technique.

A more forceful type of ballottement is needed in situations where the abdomen is filled with fluid and the examiner is seeking to identify the lower edge of an enlarged organ such as the liver. As the fingers bounce upward from the lower portion of the abdomen, a distinct change of resistance will be felt as the liver is reached.

Light Palpation: This is performed by pressing the abdominal wall with the pads of the fingers lightly but firmly enough to indent the wall, but making no attempt to press deeply. All areas of the abdomen should be palpated and the sense of resistance of one side to the other should be compared. Light palpation should also be used to explore hernias identified earlier by inspection. A finger placed on a suspected hernia will pick up a thrust of the mass as the patient strains or coughs if it is, in fact, a hernia. Areas of tenderness should be felt as gently as possible to avoid muscle guarding.

Deep Palpation: When the entire abdomen has been adequately explored by light palpation, the examiner should press more firmly toward the back to identify tenderness or masses situated deep in the abdomen (Fig. 14.6). It is useful to use both hands to be able to palpate deeply and not numb the fingertips (see Fig. 5.1).

This examination must be done carefully but thoroughly and the examiner must learn to distinguish between normal discomfort produced by deep pressure and true tenderness.

The student will learn, with experience, the soft and rather elastic feel of normal abdominal contents, and the sensation of more firmness over the region of the cecum and sigmoid portions of the colon, the consistency of feces within the sigmoid colon, and the movement under his fingers as he displaces gas bubbles in the transverse colon. Once again it must be emphasized that until the student develops his own way of sensing what is normal by repeated examinations, he will fail to sense early abnormalities.

Abdominal Pulses: In many persons, the transmitted pulsation of the aorta may be normally palpable in the epigastrium and/or the upper

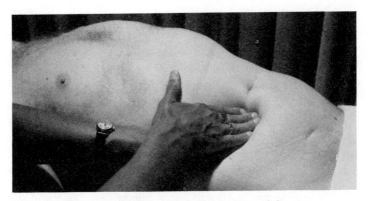

FIG. 14.6: Bimanual palpation of the abdomen.

umbilical region. With a thin abdominal wall, the aorta itself may
be palpable. It is important to distinguish a normally palpable aorta
from an aneurysm of the aorta. There are several points which may
help in this differentiation. The normal aorta is best felt in the
epigastrium, while an aortic aneurysm may be located here or in
the umbilical region. Attempt to palpate by pushing two fingers
deep enough to feel the sides of the structure. The normal pulsation
of the aorta will not push the two fingers apart, while a pulsating
aneurysm will often expand enough to move the fingers. Thirdly, an
aneurysm between the fingers will have a greater diameter. The
normal aorta should not be wider than 3 cm. in the epigastrium, or
more than 1.5 cm. at the level of the iliac crests where it bifurcates
into the iliac arteries. The presence of a pulsatile, expanding mass
in the mid-line of the abdomen is nearly diagnostic of an aortic aneurysm, and should be confirmed promptly.

Although outside the borders of the abdominal hexagon, the femoral
arteries are conveniently palpated while the patient is prone for the
abdominal examination. The femoral arteries can be found in the
upper portion of the thigh, just inferior to the mid-point of the inguinal ligament which forms the lower edges of the abdominal hexagon. They should be palpated simultaneously and are normally strong
and equal in intensity. Absence or significant weakness of one or
both pulses should be recorded, and auscultation performed for the
presence of bruit.

Palpation of the inguinal area for enlarged lymph nodes is also best
done at this time. One group of nodes is present along the inguinal
ligament and a second group extends downward along the course of
the femoral artery for a distance of 8-10 cm.

Lymphadenopathy is quite common in these areas due to frequent infections of lower extremities and a search for infection in the feet, legs, and groin will often turn up the source of the lymphadenopathy.

EXAMINATION OF THE LIVER

In most adults, the liver is completely tucked up under the thoracic cage, with its top under the dome of the right diaphragm and its lower edge at or above the right costal margin. However, the edge may also be found normally several centimeters below the costal margin. If the edge has not been detected in the abdomen by ballottement or light palpation, it should be sought for near the costal margin.

This is accomplished by making use of the knowledge that the liver moves during respiration - downward as the diaphragm moves down in inspiration. A successful technique is to place the right finger-tips lightly on the abdominal wall immediately below the costal margin at about the mid-clavicular line (Fig. 14.7). Tell the patient that you want him to take a deep breath, blow it out, and take in another deep breath. As he takes in the first deep breath, hold the fingertips lightly in place; as he exhales rapidly, push the fingertips upward under the costal margin and hold them as the patient takes in his second deep breath. Now, as the diaphragm and liver descend, the liver edge taps the examiner's fingers, and both the examiner and the patient will be aware of it. This is usually not painful but the liver edge is slightly tender. The clinician should be watching the patient's face during this maneuver as the patient may wince slightly when the liver taps the examiner's fingers. If there is more liver tenderness than is normal, or if the gallbladder is inflamed, the patient will suddenly stop the inspiratory movement when the examiner's fingers touch the liver edge. This "catching of breath" is highly suggestive of infection or inflammation of either or both of these organs.

This maneuver is often successful since it takes advantage of two other physiological facts - one, that the second deep breath a person takes is usually deeper than the first, and two, the transverse muscle fibers under the costal margin are relaxed by this breathing cycle.

The location of the upper border of the liver (dome) will have been identified during examination of the thorax (p. 142).

As the examiner percusses downward in the right mid-clavicular line, the upper border is marked by an abrupt change from lung resonance to hepatic dullness. As one continues percussion downward along the mid-clavicular line, there may be another abrupt change as hepatic dullness gives way to abdominal tympany at the lower border.

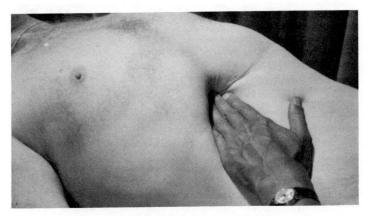

FIG. 14.7: Palpation for the liver edge.

However, this point is frequently not clearly defined, as the liver edge is often deeper in the abdomen than the body of the liver, giving rise to an indistinct change in percussion note.

Thus, the total span of the normal liver - about 10 to 15 cm. from dome to edge - is often best recorded by percussing the upper border and palpating the lower border in the mid-clavicular line.

It is critical to remember that the mere presence of a liver edge several centimeters below the costal margin does not define liver enlargement. Often in patients with pulmonary emphysema the diaphragms will be depressed, pushing the liver well downward into the abdominal hexagon. Only measurement of the liver span from upper to lower borders can be used as a dependable index of liver size. This measurement should routinely be taken (with the transparent ruler always in your pocket) and recorded.

Occasionally, the right lobe of the liver is congenitally elongated and may be readily palpated in the abdomen nearer the mid-line than the mid-inguinal line. If located, this long lobe (called Riedel's lobe) will move on respiration, will not be tender, but will lead to finding a liver measuring more than 15 centimeters from top to edge.

If there is reason to suspect liver disease - as, for example, in jaundice - blunt percussion may be of assistance in determining the presence of tenderness. This is performed by placing one palm flat over the right lateral chest and striking the back of the hand with the ulnar side of the fist (Fig. 14.8). The first blow should be gentle,

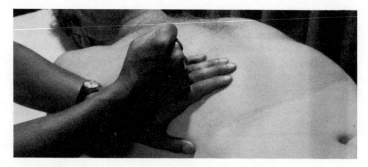

FIG. 14.8: Blunt percussion for liver tenderness.

and if no tenderness is produced, a second harder blow can be delivered. In acute hepatitis, the liver will often hurt when jarred and the pain will persist for a few seconds. Tenderness in the area may also be due to inflammation of the gallbladder.

In cases where the liver is definitely enlarged, auscultation for bruit or rub should be performed over the thoracic and abdominal portions of the liver.

EXAMINATION OF THE SPLEEN

The normal spleen is a soft, small organ located above the left costal margin centered under the tenth rib near the anterior axillary line and is, therefore, never palpable. It must enlarge to about three times normal size to be felt.

Examination for the spleen should take into account the fact that this organ enlarges downward and medially.

The spleen is searched for in the abdominal hexagon in the same general way as one explores for the liver, i.e., by ballottement up the left mid-inguinal line, then by light and deep palpation.

If the spleen is readily palpable, a distinct notch may be felt in the lower border which can confirm to the examiner that he has, indeed, felt this organ and not some other mass in the area. The spleen is a highly vascular organ, and if enlarged, should be palpated gently to avoid rupture.

When the spleen has not been located in the abdomen, it should then be sought under the costal margin. The examiner's fingers are pushed up under the left costal margin at about the mid-clavicular line and the patient should be asked to take deep breaths, exactly as in examination for the liver edge, described previously. Movement of the diaphragm downward in deep inspiration may push the moderately enlarged spleen onto the examiner's fingertips.

Further search may be done by bimanual examination. This is accomplished by having the patient lie on his right side, while the examiner's left hand compresses the posterior abdominal wall just below the palpable ribs. This maneuver moves the spleen anteriorly where, on deep inspiration, it may be felt by the right fingertips (Fig. 14.9).

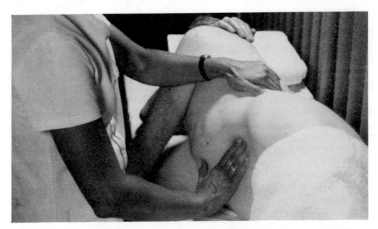

FIG. 14.9: Bimanual palpation for possibly enlarged spleen.

Remember that if the spleen is felt at all, it is significantly enlarged, whereas the palpable liver may or may not be enlarged.

Percussion is used also in this search. As noted earlier, the spleen is a small organ, normally centered under the 10th rib and the anterior axillary line. With the patient on his right side, as in Fig. 14.9, percuss downward along the anterior axillary line starting around the level of the nipple. One will pick up lung resonance down to about the level of the 9th rib and often will detect dullness, due to the underlying spleen, for a distance of 4-6 cm. before reaching an area of tympany in Traube's space, over the stomach bubble or gas-filled splenic flexure of the colon (see Fig. 13.4).

With significant splenomegaly, the area of dullness will extend to or below the costal margin. On deep inspiration, the area of splenic dullness may be quite pronounced and will fill much of the normally tympanitic area.

At best, percussion of the spleen is difficult to perform and interpret. The student must have a considerable amount of experience to be confident of his findings with this organ.

EXAMINATION OF THE KIDNEYS

The normal sized kidneys are not often palpable, except in the patient with a thin or scaphoid abdomen, since these organs lie deep in the abdomen on the posterior abdominal wall. The lower pole of the right kidney is ordinarily located about four centimeters above the level of the right iliac crest at the mid-inguinal line. The lower pole of the left kidney is often located about five centimeters above the left iliac crest near the mid-inguinal line. Like most of the abdominal contents, the kidneys descend on deep inspiration, although they move down less than the liver or spleen.

The lower pole of the right kidney is easier to locate than the left. It should be felt for bimanually, by having the left fingers press upward in the left costovertebral angle, and pushing the right fingertips deep at the point described above (Fig. 14.10), while having the patient taking deep breaths. The round lower pole may be felt as it moves downward under the left fingertips. The left kidney may be found with a similar technique - i.e., pushing upward in the left costovertebral angle with the left finger, downward with the right finger through the abdominal wall about five centimeters above the left iliac crest in the mid-inguinal line.

Because they lie so far posteriorly, percussion will not detect the presence of the kidneys.

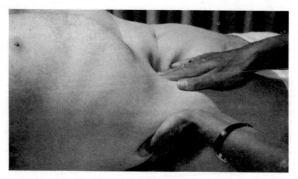

FIG. 14.10: Bimanual palpation for the right kidney.

ABDOMINAL TENDERNESS:

The basic aim of the clinician in examining the abdomen, where tenderness is present, is to locate the site and source of the pain as accurately as possible. This is frequently not too difficult when the patient has a localized area of pain on palpation. In order to locate the site of pain, whether the patient has local or generalized abdominal tenderness, one searches for the point of maximum tenderness. In the tender abdomen, deep palpation may produce a great deal of pain over a large area, so the examiner should try to find an area where the lightest touch produces tenderness. Gentle percussion will produce this lightest touch and may often pinpoint the area of maximum tenderness.

It sometimes happens that palpation in one area produces maximum pain in another area of the abdomen. Usually, this is due to transmission of the pressure by trapped gas in the intestines but, again, it is important to identify and describe the point of maximum tenderness, so the patient should be carefully questioned as to where he perceives the maximal pain when palpated.

When the peritoneum is inflamed, rebound tenderness may occur. This is induced by pressing over a tender area and quickly releasing the pressure. If the pain is suddenly worse when the examiner's hand is removed, rebound is said to be present and is a valuable sign of peritonitis.

Description of abdominal tenderness should include the precise location of the point of maximum tenderness, if one has been found, and the amount of pressure necessary to produce tenderness (i.e., by light palpation, moderate palpation, deep palpation or by rebound).

ASCITES:

Small amounts of abdominal fluid may not be detectable by any methods of examination but, as fluid increases, the first sign usually is a bulging of the flanks. Bulging of the flanks is also seen in obesity, however, and it is important to distinguish between the two. Simple pinching of the flank may help, since in distention due to fluid, the examiner may sense that he has primarily skin and muscle between his fingers rather than skin, muscle and fat. A specific test for the presence of larger amounts of abdominal fluid is the production of a fluid wave. This is done by placing a palm on one flank and striking the opposite flank briskly with the fingers of the other hand (Fig. 14.11). If the distention is due to fluid, a distinct transmission of the blow will be felt across the abdomen. To avoid feeling vibrations transmitted across the abdominal wall itself, a third hand is needed; an assistant or the patient presses the ulnar edge of his hand deep into the mid-line of the abdomen.

Another test is the examination for shifting dullness (Figs. 14.12, 14.13). With the patient supine, the abdomen is percussed toward one flank from the mid-line, and the point at which dullness appears is marked. The patient is then asked to roll onto the opposite

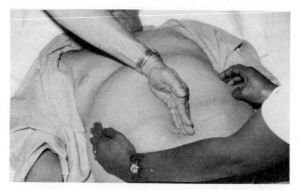

FIG. 14.11: Examination for fluid wave. Note the deep compression of the distended abdomen by the assistant's hand
to prevent vibrations from crossing along the abdominal wall.

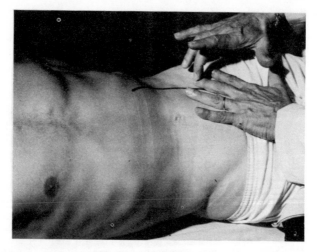

FIG. 14.12: Shifting dullness - supine position. Percussion lateral
to the mark produces dullness due to ascitic fluid in
the flank.

(unmarked) side and to lie in that position for about two to three minutes. This will allow fluid to drain away from the high portion of the
abdomen and for air-filled intestines to shift upward. Percussion
is now repeated toward the line marked earlier, and if the dullness
has shifted upward and has been replaced by abdominal tympany, the
clinician may be sure that there is fluid present in the abdomen.

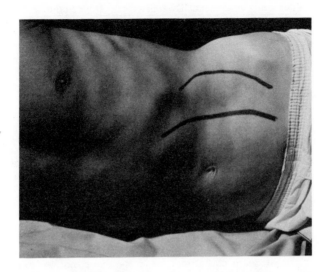

FIG. 14.13: Shifting dullness - right lateral position. Lower line is the one marked in Fig. 14.11. Fluid has drained from the flank, and dullness has shifted to the region lateral to the upper mark.

With severe degrees of distention due to ascites, the abdomen becomes tense and the umbilicus will be pushed outward and may even protrude above the wall. Palpation will help very little to detect anything in the abdomen causing the distention. Percussion will produce tympany, most pronounced in the umbilical and epigastric regions, with dullness elsewhere. This is due to the floating of air-filled gut toward the high point of the abdomen. Auscultation of bowel sounds will also demonstrate this central collection of intestinal gas.

RECORDING

Abdomen

Insp.	Abdomen flat, no skin lesions, no hernia, no pulsations.
Ausc.	Normal bowel sounds q. ten seconds. No bruits.
Palp.	No tenderness or masses; spleen, kidneys not palpated, liver edge at costal margin, non-tender.
Perc.	Normal abdominal tympany; liver 12 centimeters long.

PATIENT PROBLEM

Mr. A.L., 49-year-old male truck driver brought to primary care unit by neighbor because of abdominal distention and depression.

Problem: Abdominal Distention and Depression

S: Admits to at least one pint whiskey and several beers daily for past 10 years. In past month has been fatigued, developed abdominal distention. Has been attending alcohol clinic irregularly under court order because of multiple traffic violations and loss of driver's license. Separated from wife, lives in rooming house, has hot plate, eats poorly.

O: Insp. Abdomen is distended with bulging flanks; 98 centimeters girth at umbilicus; numerous spider angiomata over face, neck, arms; hair sparse on chest, genitals and in axillae; dilated veins over abdominal wall with flow   umbilicus from upper quadrants; umbilicus protruding.

   Ausc. Normal bowel sounds of three to four seconds heard best in epigastric, umbilical, and suprapubic regions; sounds are distant in flanks.

   Palp. Tense abdominal wall which can be indented by deep palpation to identify blunt liver edge eleven centimeters below right costal margin, non-tender, no other masses or organs palpable; no abdominal tenderness; fluid wave present.

   Perc. Dome of liver five centimeters above right costal margin; liver is 16 centimeters long; increased tympany in epigastric and umbilical segments, dullness over both flanks and diminished tympany in suprapubic segment; shifting dullness present.

A: Appears to be series of related problems - acute malnutrition superimposed on chronic alcohol abuse, depression over loss of family and job, and development of ascites, probably secondary to cirrhosis. Major problem is to relieve ascites and sort out serious socio-economic problems leading to current debilitated state.

P: Dx. 1. Recommend prompt hospitalization to physician.
      2. Per algorithm - order SMA-12, type and x-match 2 units blood.
      3. Record urine output.

   Rx. 1. Strict bed rest in unit holding bed until hospitalization can be arranged.
      2. Orange juice 120 cc. q. 1 hr.
      3. Call unit social worker to begin support program during admission and post hospital stay.

   Pt. Ed. 1. Discussed need for hospitalization due to probable liver disease; 2. Explained role of social worker and projected counseling with staff in hospital.

_____
                                    Signature

SUPPLEMENTAL EXERCISES

1. Make a list of the most common causes of acute abdominal pain. What are important elements of history and physical examination which will assist in distinguishing between some of these common problems?

2. Describe a method for identifying direction of blood flow when veins of the abdomen are prominent.

REFERENCES

1. Palmer, E.D.: Functional Gastrointestinal Disease. The Williams and Wilkins Co., Baltimore, 1967.

2. Cope, Z.: The Early Diagnosis of the Acute Abdomen, 14th edition. Oxford University Press, London, 1972.

3. Runyan, J.: Gastrointestinal Complaints. Primary Care Guide. Harper and Row, New York, 1975, pp. 29-33.

4. G.I. Series: Physical Examination of the Abdomen. A.H. Robins Co., Richmond.

5. Boyce, H.W. Jr. and Palmer, E.D.: Techniques of Clinical Gastroenterology. Charles C Thomas, Springfield, 1975.

CHAPTER 15

THE EXTREMITIES AND THE BACK

INTRODUCTION

The skeleton, joints, muscles, blood vessels, lymphatics, and nerves of the extremities and back do not make up a single defined system nor, strictly speaking, a region. For purposes of the physical examination, however, the extremities and the back should be looked upon as a whole and each of the component parts should be evaluated.

The skeleton consists of two parts: the central or axial portion and the attached or appended portion. The axial skeleton includes the skull, the spine, the ribs, and the sternum, while the appendicular skeleton includes the shoulder girdle and upper extremities plus the pelvic girdle and lower extremities. The functions of the axial skeleton are protection (skull and thorax) and maintenance of the upright position (spine) while the extremities provide for "fight and flight."

The great development of fine motion and sensation in the hand makes it unique as a tool and as a sense organ. It is a part of the legend of the Orient that the physician was limited in his examination of the harem women to inspection and palpation of the hand and wrist. Now that we are not so restricted we must not neglect the fact that careful examination of the skin, nails, joints, muscles, nerves, and pulses of the hands may detect signs of nearly 100 diseases, syndromes, or lesions! For instance, acrocyanosis, acrodermatitis, acromegaly, Addison's disease, albumin deficiency, alcoholism, amyotrophic lateral sclerosis, anemias, arteriovenous fistulae, arthritis, astereognosia, atrial fibrillation, and azotemia can begin the alphabetical list. In addition, cultural signs such as the shape and care of the nails, the wearing of rings, occupational marks and callouses, nicotine stains, etc., may aid the practitioner in an evaluation of the patient's personality and socio-economic status.

The recommended method of examination of the back and extremities is to perform a general inspection, then to evaluate posture, gait and balance, muscles, joints, the vascular system, and tendon reflexes. This sequence carries the examiner's focus from the general body, as a whole, down to specific tests.

GENERAL: An overall view of the head and neck, back, and extremities is made here, as elsewhere, for gross asymmetry of one side as compared to the other, for deformities, for skin temperature, for skin lesions, and for the presence of swellings or masses. Because of the large number of structures present here (bones, joints, muscles, ligaments, tendons, etc.); because of the high incidence of trauma to the extremities; and because of the relative ease of examination, many swellings, masses, or deformities can be found here. One type of swelling - edema - which occurs quite often in the extremities, particularly the lower extremity, deserves special mention here.

Edema is the infiltration of serum into the tissues, which may occur in a localized region such as an area of trauma, or may be more generalized. By far the commonest general type is dependent edema which pits upon pressure (Fig. 15.1). Since it is dependent, it will be found most often in the dorsum of the foot and the medial aspect of the ankle in patients who are not confined to bed. The dependent edema of bed-ridden patients will be located in the buttocks and the loose tissue over the sacrum and lower back. Distinction between pitting and nonpitting edema is an important point to establish and should always be recorded.

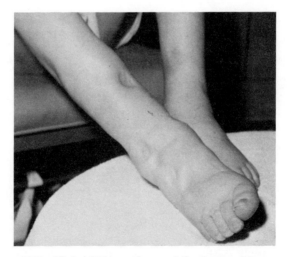

FIG. 15.1: Pitting edema of the foot and leg.

Dependent pitting edema is most often due to right heart failure, although there are many other causes such as venous or lymphatic obstruction, renal disease, nutritional deficiencies, etc. Non-pitting edema, such as myxedema, results from general thickening of the subcutaneous tissues rather than simple fluid accumulation.

POSTURE: In the upright position, the patient's head should be balanced over his shoulders, his hips and his ankles. When viewed from the side, the back should have three separate curves, each of which should be present but not exaggerated (Fig. 15.2): an anterior curve of the neck (cervical concavity), a posterior curve of the thorax (dorsal convexity), and an anterior curve of the low back (lumbar concavity). Viewed posteriorly, the mid-spinal line should be nearly perfectly straight and the shoulders should be level.

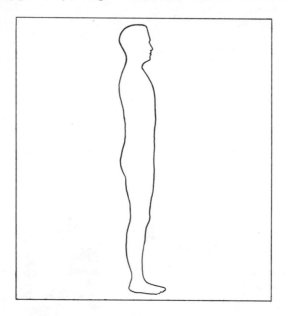

FIG. 15.2: Silhouette showing proper upright posture and normal curves of the cervical, thoracic, and lumbar spines.

As described earlier, an exaggerated anterior curve is called lordosis, an exaggerated posterior curve is kyphosis (see Fig. 11.8), and a lateral curvature is scoliosis (see Fig. 11.9). The presence of kyphosis or lordosis in one segment often produces a distortion of other curves so that a scoliosis is associated with a twisting or rotation of the spine and its attached ribs. These compensating abnormalities may be readily visible or may need to be confirmed by palpation. Abnormal curvature of the back may be due to spinal disorders, to muscle spasm, or to changes in the appendicular skeleton. For example, if one leg is shorter than the other, the pelvis will be tilted and the spine may have a scoliosis to maintain a nearly erect position.

Palpation should be performed to determine, if possible, the cause of abnormal posture. The spine and the paraspinal muscles should be examined for tenderness, swelling, or spasm.

PERCUSSION: Blunt percussion of the back with the ulnar aspect of the fist is used in two areas, over the vertebrae from the cervical spine down to the lumbo-sacral joint, and over the kidney. Jarring the vertebrae may induce tenderness in the presence of inflammation or destruction of the vertebrae or intra-vertebral discs. Locate the lower border of the ribs where they join the spine - the costovertebral angles (CVA) - and strike each angle with the ulnar side of the fist firmly, but not hard, over the kidneys (Fig. 15.3). Tenderness induced by this blunt percussion suggests kidney infection or inflammation.

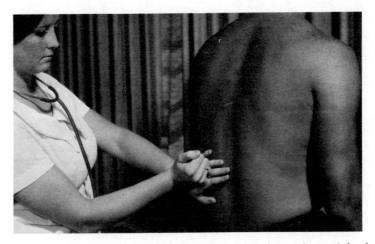

FIG. 15.3: Blunt percussion of the kidney over the costo-vertebral angle.

RANGE OF MOTION (ROM): Joints, of course, are designed to provide mobility, and they must be examined for this function. While the details of the ROM of each joint are very complex, the examiner must develop a pattern of evaluating at least the major joints through a portion of their active ROM. Observation of the whole patient, his gait, his behavior in undressing, in moving onto and off the examination table, etc., will give the alert clinician clues as to possible limitation of motion prior to specific examination (Fig. 15.4).

Active ROM of the back (spine) can be checked by having the patient bend from a standing position. The normal range is about 90º forward and about 25º to 30º backward.

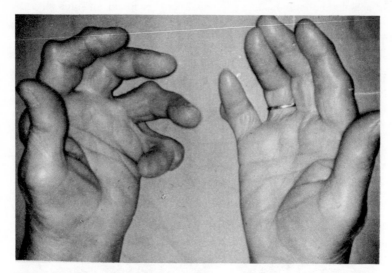

FIG. 15.4: Immobile deformed joints of the fingers and hand due to
severe rheumatoid arthritis.

ROM of the upper extremities may be examined briefly by comparing the patient's motion with your own (if you have no limitation).
Ask the patient to follow you in these calisthenics (moving from
fingers to shoulder): open and close the hands, flex and extend the
wrists, flex and extend the forearms, alternately turn the hands
palm up - palm down - palm up, raise arms to the sides, touch
hands overhead. This can all be done in about 10-20 seconds.

In younger individuals, the major joints of the lower extremities can
be tested as a group by simply having the patient perform a deep
knee bend. It is safer in older or weak patients to have the patient
seated on the examining table and to have the patient move individual
joints separately: flex feet up and down, bend and straighten the
knees, and raise the knees toward the chin.

Since the pattern suggested above is simply a brief screening of
ROM, it is to be considered adequate only if there has been no history of pain or limitation of motion, or if no limitation was detected
during the examination. If limitation has been found, closer examination by inspection and palpation is warranted. Further tests of
ROM are best left to the physiatrist, orthopedist, or physical
therapist.

GAIT AND BALANCE: Have the patient walk away from you and then
toward you. Watch for unusually short steps, a wide-based walk, or

restricted swinging of the arms, for evidence that the patient is watching the placement of his feet and, of course, for staggering or a tendency to fall (Table 15.1).

TABLE 15.1		
SOME ABNORMALITIES OF GAIT		
TYPE	CHARACTERISTICS	EXAMPLES
1. "Parkinsonian"	The body is held rigid, trunk and head bent forward. Short, mincing steps, sudden uncontrolled propulsive-like movements	Parkinson's disease
2. "Ataxic"	Staggering or reeling like an alcoholic	Cerebellar disease
3. "Slapping"	Feet wide apart, legs raised high and then feet slapped on the ground. Eyes fixed to the floor to help guide feet for placement	Disease of posterior column of spinal cord
4. "Spastic"	Jerking, uncoordinated movements	Cerebral palsy, multiple sclerosis
5. "Dragging"	Dragging of one leg around in a semicircle	Hemiplegia
6. "Scissors"	Thighs close together due to spasticity of adductor muscles	Spastic paraplegia

Balance is a complex function which depends upon sensation provided by the semicircular canals of the inner ear, upon "position sense" (proprioception) which informs the individual of the position of his body and limbs, and upon muscle coordination. These factors are examined by the Romberg test. Have the patient stand with feet together and eyes open to see if he maintains balance. Then have him close his eyes. Be sure that you are close to him to prevent a fall. Failure to maintain balance is called a positive Romberg's sign.

MUSCLE STRENGTH AND BULK: The examiner will already have a gross estimate of weakness or atrophy of major muscle groups by having done general inspection and by having watched the patient walk, arise from a seated position, undress, and perhaps step up to an examining table. In addition, a few major muscle groups of the neck, back, and extremities should be examined against resistance. With the patient facing forward, tell him to hold his head still while you attempt to turn his head by moderate pressure on first one and then the other side of the jaw. Unless there is gross weakness of the neck muscles, the patient should have no difficulty in holding his head still. Press down on the patient's shoulders and ask him to raise or shrug his shoulders. He should be able to do this easily. Biceps and triceps are quickly tested by having the patient hold his arm partly extended and asking him to keep that position while you push and then pull the arm (Fig. 15.5). Again, he should be able to resist these forces readily. Similarly, for the lower extremity, the patient should be able to resist both a pull and a push against the shin and the thigh.

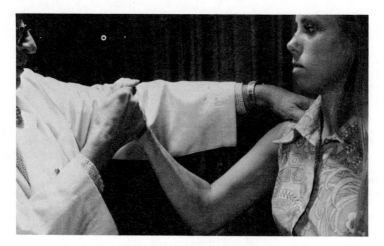

FIG. 15.5: Testing strength of the biceps muscle.

VASCULAR SYSTEM: Veins of the hand and forearm often appear dilated if the extremity is held below the level of the heart. These veins should collapse within a few seconds when the extremity is raised to about an angle of 30° above the horizontal. Failure to do so suggests increased venous pressure due to obstruction or to congestive heart failure. Veins of the lower extremities are often dilated in normal posture. Varicose veins are characterized not just by being dilated, but in being so dilated as to stand out from the underlying tissue and being tortuous (Fig. 15.6). If there is any question about the presence of true varicose veins, the patient should be referred for several other examinations which can determine the competency of the venous valves.

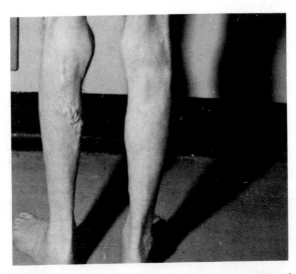

FIG. 15.6: Cluster of varicose veins of the left leg. Note also the reduction of muscle bulk evident in the gastrocnemius muscles.

When edema is found in the lower extremity, the examiner should be alerted to the possibility of venous thrombosis since this may be a life-threatening disorder. Early venous thrombosis usually produces no symptons, but when a vein is occluded by the thrombus there is usually pain, edema, and tenderness to palpation of the occluded portion of the vein. The extent of edema may not be readily evident so it is advisable to use a tape measure to compare the diameter of the involved extremity to that of the other side. A good practice is to measure the diameter of the limbs at ten centimeter intervals from a fixed point, such as the malleolus of the ankle or the patella, so that follow-up comparisons may be made accurately.

Examination of the radial pulse, which was performed earlier, is now repeated. Pulses are examined bilaterally simultaneously to compare their quality and the time of arrival at the examiner's fingertips. In the upper extremity, it is usually necessary to palpate only the radial pulses. If these are extremely weak or absent, the ulnar pulses should be examined, and if these too are weak or absent, the brachial arteries should then be located and examined. The brachial artery is most easily found a few centimeters below the axilla lying in the groove along the inner edge of the biceps muscle.

In the lower extremity, the femoral, dorsalis pedis, and posterior tibial arteries should be palpated routinely. The femoral arteries are readily located at about the mid-point of the inguinal ligament, i.e., midway between the anterior and superior iliac spine and the symphysis pubis, and should have been palpated with the patient supine during the abdominal examination (see p. 209). The dorsalis pedis artery follows a line which is drawn from the middle of the ankle into the groove between the great toe and the second toe (Fig. 15.7). It is best palpated on the instep of the foot. The posterior tibial artery is slightly more difficult to locate and is best searched for with two or three fingers. Place the fingers in the groove between the Achilles tendon and the tibia just above the medial malleolus, press deeply, and move the fingers toward the tibia (Fig. 15.8). These arteries are not palpable bilaterally in many normal persons, so do not spend too much time searching for them.

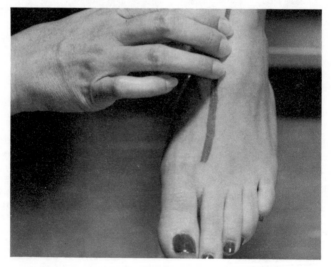

FIG. 15.7: Palpation of the dorsalis pedis artery.

If neither the dorsalis pedis nor the posterior tibial pulse can be detected on one side, the examiner should attempt to locate the popliteal artery. Although difficult to palpate, this artery can often be felt by having the patient flex the knee to relax the muscles (kneeling on a chair, if possible, is a satisfactory position). The examiner's fingertips are then pushed deep into the center of the popliteal space.

Absence of pulses in an extremity is highly suggestive of peripheral arterial disease, and the localization of obstructive phenomena may be determined generally by this type of physical examination (see Patient Problem at end of this chapter).

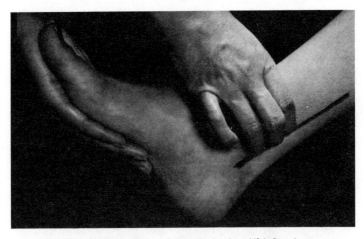

FIG. 15.8: Palpation of the posterior tibial artery.

LYMPH NODES: Palpation for lymph nodes in the groin has been described in the previous chapter, p. 209. As noted there, lymphadenopathy is frequently due to infections in the feet, legs, or genital area.

TENDON REFLEXES: The routine physical examination should include testing the biceps, triceps, patellar, and Achilles reflexes. These reflexes are tested by striking the tendon and watching for contraction of the appropriate muscle. It is not necessary for the muscle to contract forcefully enough to move the limb, but simply to contract. Therefore, the examiner should watch the muscle while striking the tendon. These reflexes will be difficult or impossible to elicit when the patient is tense and holding himself rigid, so relaxation is imperative for proper testing. Distracting the patient is often necessary. Reflexes on corresponding sides are compared with each other and against an arbitrary normal scale. Tradition has established a 5 point scale but it is our preference to ignore a 3+ score as being undefinable. In deference to tradition, we suggest the following scale:

0 = Reflex absent
+ = Reflex hypoactive
++ = Normal reflex
++++ = Reflex hyperactive

There is a wide range of normal and it is more important to compare reflexes from one side of the patient to the other than to strain one's imagination to fit an arbitrary scale.

The biceps reflex is obtained by supporting the patient's arm, placing the thumb firmly on the patient's biceps tendon (Fig. 15.9), and striking the thumbnail briskly with the reflex hammer. Watch the biceps muscle for contraction.

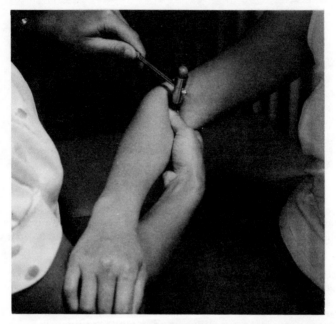

FIG. 15.9: Testing the biceps reflex. Note the way in which the examiner supports the patient's arm to afford relaxation.

In the same fashion, the patient's arm is supported to relax the muscles, and the triceps tendon is struck with the hammer just above the olecranon process (Fig. 15.10).

The patellar reflex is most easily obtained with the patient seated on the examining table with the legs dangling free. Tension may be relieved by having the patient swing his legs loosely for a moment before testing. The patellar tendon is struck just below the patella, and the quadriceps muscle group should be observed for contraction (Fig. 15.11).

With the patient seated on the table, the Achilles reflex is obtained by having the foot lightly supported by the examiner's free hand while the tendon is struck with the hammer. Sometimes, slight jiggling of the patient's foot prior to tapping the tendon will assist in obtaining relaxation (Fig. 15.12).

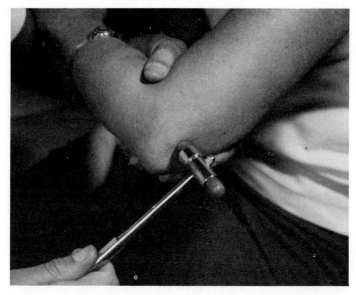

FIG. 15.10: Testing the triceps reflex. Again, the examiner is seen supporting the patient's arm.

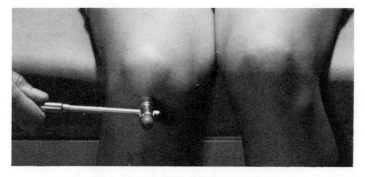

FIG. 15.11: The patellar reflex.

When patients are to be examined in bed, some variation of these positions is necessary but the principles to be followed are the same: get the patient and the limb as relaxed as possible and then strike the tendon briskly and with equal strength for all reflexes.

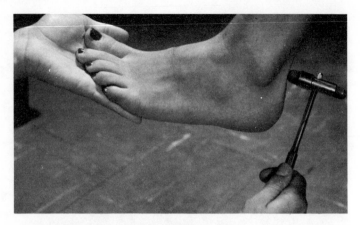

FIG. 15.12: Achilles reflex.

Plantar Reflex: The sole of the foot is stroked firmly with a hard, but not sharp, object such as a tongue blade, handle of a tuning fork, or a key. The normal response is plantar flexion of all of the toes, while an abnormal response (Babinski sign) consists of dorsiflexion of the great toe and spreading of the other toes (Fig. 15.13). An abnormal reflex should always be reported as Babinski positive.

RECORDING

The normal examination may be recorded as follows:

Back: Normal curvature, no spinal tenderness, no CVA tenderness.

Extremities: No skin, hair, or nail abnormalities. Full range of motion (ROM). Normal gait, Romberg negative. Muscle strength intact. No venous dilation. Radial, femoral, dorsalis pedis and posterior tibial pulses all palpable and equal. No lymphadenopathy. Biceps, triceps, patellar, and Achilles reflexes all 2+. Plantar reflex normal.

PATIENT PROBLEM

Mr. P.W., a 45-year-old diabetic man, presents himself at clinic because of leg pains.

Problem: Vascular Insufficiency

S: For past two years Mr. W. has had calf cramps which have definitely become worse over past two months. At first these were

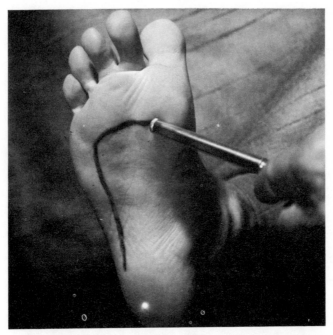

FIG. 15.13: Plantar reflex. The line drawn on the foot is the course of the instrument along the sole to elicit a plantar reflex. Here the reflex is abnormal and is called a Babinski positive.

noted only after several hours of exercise until the present time when he can no longer walk more than two blocks without needing to stop because of severe pains. Pain is crampy in type, involves calves of both lower extremities, is relieved by rest for three to four minutes. No medication ever tried for relief.

O: No asymmetry or swelling of lower extremities. Legs are pale, feet slightly mottled. Hair abruptly disappears from legs at about 15 centimeters above malleoli (Fig. 15.14). No hairs noted on toes. Skin below this level is cooler to touch than above. Femoral pulses present and equal. Dorsalis pedis and posterior tibials not palpable. Popliteals not felt. No bruits heard along femoral arteries.

A: The combination of abrupt loss of hair on legs, coolness of lower portion of leg, and absence of pulses of the foot is consistent with reduced arterial blood flow somewhere below the level of

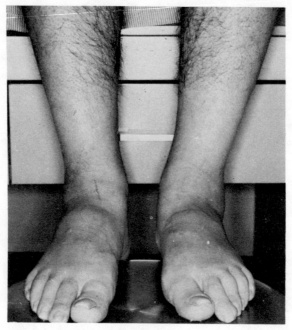

FIG. 15.14: Absence of leg hair due to arterial insufficiency. Note the sharp line of demarcation.

the femoral arteries. Because this is chronic (over 2 years) and the patient is a diabetic, this is most likely due to arteriosclerosis.

P: Dx. Refer to vascular clinic for further studies.
Rx. Patient advised to stop smoking, keep feet very clean.
Pt. Ed. Told that blood flow to feet is reduced, and that it is important to continue medical work-up.

_____
Signature

SUPPLEMENTAL EXERCISES

1. Obtain a set of charts or drawings showing the normal ROM of all major joints of the body.

2. Describe the abnormal features of the hand involved with rheumatoid arthritis and osteoarthritis.

REFERENCES

1. Fowler, N.O.: Examination of the Heart, Part 2: Inspection and Palpation of Venous and Arterial Pulses. The American Heart Association, New York, 1967.

2. Beethan, W.P. Jr. et al.: Physical Examination of the Joints. W.B. Saunders Co., Philadelphia, 1965.

3. Fairbairn, J.F.II et al.: Allen's Peripheral Vascular Diseases, 4th edition. J.B. Lippincott Co., Philadelphia, 1970.

4. Esch, D. and Lipley, M.: Evaluation of Joint Motion: Methods of Measurement and Recording. University of Minnesota Press, Minnesota, 1974.

5. Hoppenfeld, Stanley: Physical Examination of the Spine and Extremities, Appleton-Century-Crofts, New York, 1976.

CHAPTER 16

GENITAL AND RECTAL EXAMINATION (MALE)

INTRODUCTION

Cultural and sexual problems on the part of both patients and examiners often lead to a report of "deferred" and to a failure to examine these regions. This must be avoided by the development of a relaxed, yet composed, attitude on the part of the examiner who understands that disease of the genitalia and of the rectum is as important to detect as disease elsewhere. For example, all malignancies of the testes will be diagnosed - or suspected - on palpation, and approximately half of all rectal carcinomas are within reach of the examiner's index finger.

MALE GENITALIA

Anatomy: The skin of the penis is loose and free of hair except at the root. In the uncircumcised male it projects over the glans, forming the foreskin or prepuce. The urethral meatus is located near the center of the glans. Scrotal skin is loose and wrinkled by the dartos muscle.

The scrotal sac is made up of loose skin and the thin dartos fascia and muscle. Because of the looseness of the skin and the thin sheet of dartos muscle, the scrotum is normally wrinkled. The testes are ovoid, firm organs measuring roughly four centimeters in length, about 2.5 centimeters in the anteroposterior diameter and about two centimeters in width. The epididymis is a soft, cord-like structure which can be felt from the lower testicular pole, along the posterolateral aspect up to the posterior portion of the upper pole of the testicle where it enlarges. Arising from this enlargement, called the head of the epididymis, is the spermatic cord, which feels harder than the epididymis and somewhat like a strand of twine. The spermatic cord enters the inguinal canal at the external inguinal ring and, after three to four centimeters, enters the abdominal wall at the internal inguinal ring.

EXAMINATION

General: Because of the possibilities of infection, it is a reasonable practice to wear gloves in examining the genitalia. The genitalia are most easily examined with the patient standing and the examiner seated on a low stool.

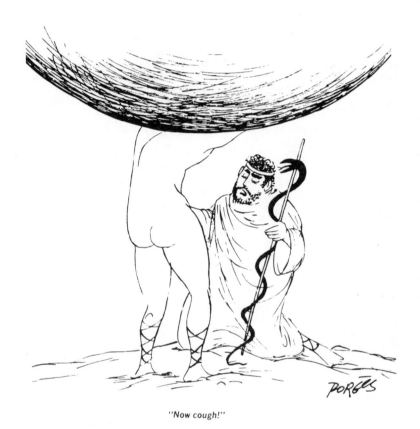

"Now cough!"

Pubic Hair: The distribution of so-called "male" or "female" patterns of the pubic hair is of little clinical importance since there are so many normal variations. Either absence or extreme sparseness of pubic hair, on the contrary, is usually significant and should be reported. This loss of pubic hair, along with loss or thinning of hair on the abdomen and in the axilla may be seen, for example, in advanced cirrhosis of the liver.

Penis: Because of variations in the size of the normal penis, only wide discrepancies are likely to be of significance. The penis should be inspected for edema, scars, and lesions. In the uncircumcised man, the foreskin should be retracted to expose the glans. The condition in which the prepuce is not able to be retracted is called phimosis. Gentle palpation for scarring or masses is carried out. Slight pressure near the tip of the glans should open the urethral meatus unless it is scarred. Observe the meatus for discharge.

Scrotum and Contents: Lesions of the scrotum are principally those of skin and should be reported as for skin elsewhere. Using the index and middle fingers of the right hand, in a scissors-like fashion, separate the two testes (Fig. 16.1). This will place the right testicle in the right hand and gentle pressure by the left fingertips will allow for careful bimanual palpation of the right testicle. The testicle should be evaluated for size, consistency, and masses. Holding the right testicle in place, palpate the epididymis between the fingers of the left hand from the lower testicular pole, along the posterolateral border, to the head, and then up the spermatic cord. Common lesions of the epididymis are scarring, generalized swelling, or tumors such as hydrocele. The spermatic cord is also subject to these same lesions. Any tumor found should be examined by transillumination in which a small light source (pen-light, flashlight) is placed behind the tumor in a darkened room to see if light passes through the tumor. Cysts generally transmit light, while solid tumors ordinarily do not.

The contents of the left scrotum are examined in the same manner, by separating the testes with the fingers of the left hand and with the right hand performing gentle palpation of the testis, epididymis, and cord.

Inguinal Canals: The inguinal canal, a curved three-to-four centimeter long tunnel, is the site of passage of an indirect inguinal hernia. The right canal is palpated most easily by the little finger or the index finger of the right hand which is pushed up through the scrotum with the fingernail lying against the spermatic cord (Fig. 16.2). The fingertip should not be able to enter the abdominal wall through the internal ring unless that ring is abnormally dilated. Weakness of the internal ring may signal a potential hernia and is tested for by holding the fingertip against the internal ring and having

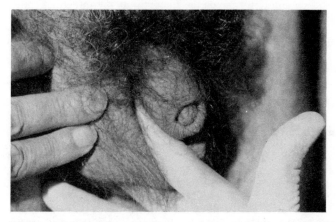

FIG. 16.1: Palpation of the scrotal contents. The right testis is
separated from the left by the first two fingers of the
gloved right hand and bimanual palpation is thereby
easily accomplished.

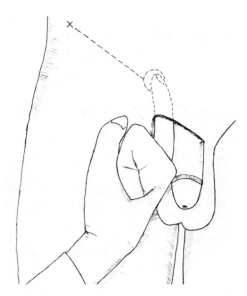

FIG. 16.2: Examination for indirect inguinal hernia. The circle
marks the location of the internal inguinal ring; x marks
the anterior superior iliac spine.

the patient cough or strain. Weakness or partial dilation of the ring
will produce a definite tap on the fingertip as the intestinal contents
are pressed downward.

An indirect hernia may already be present in the inguinal canal or
down into the scrotum. Such a finding warrants prompt referral.
The left canal is examined similarly, most conveniently with the
left index or little finger.

RECTAL EXAMINATION

Anatomy: The anal canal is a muscular sphincter, 2.5 to 4 mili-
meters in length, beginning at the anus where the perianal skin joins
the moist epithelium of the canal, and ending at the rectal ampulla,
a dilation which marks the end of the large intestine. The prostate
gland lies just anterior to the rectal ampulla and can be easily palpated through the thin rectal wall. It is a firm organ measuring
from three to four centimeters in width and about three centimeters
in length. On palpation, it seems to project less than two centimeters through the rectal wall. The normal prostate has readily palpable right and left lobes separated by a mid-line groove or fissure,
and a median lobe, lying below the groove, which cannot be felt.

EXAMINATION

The most convenient position for the routine rectal examination is for
the patient to stand with his feet apart, bent forward, resting his chest
on an examining table. The knee-chest position is also excellent.
For the bed-patient, a satisfactory position is achieved by having the
patient lying on one side with the superior thigh flexed, bringing the
knee as close to the chest as possible. Another position, suitable
for even sicker patients, is the lithotomy position.

Inspection: The buttocks should be spread widely to visualize the entire perianal region. Skin lesions, fistulas, external skin tags
(which are external hemorrhoids), or prolapsed rectal mucosa may
all be seen.

Palpation: There are several techniques which are helpful in accomplishing a successful rectal examination, all of which are based
upon the examiner's consideration for his patient. The more confidence and the less fear the patient has, the more likely is his cooperation. First, the examiner should tell the patient that this is an
uncomfortable examination, but that it should not be painful. Assure
the patient that you will stop if severe pain develops. Second, don't
surprise him. Tell the patient when you are about to begin palpation.
Remember that the lubricant, which should be spread liberally on the
gloved index finger, is at room temperature and is therefore much
cooler than the anus. Tell him that he will feel the coldness.

Third, and most important, never force the examining finger through the rectal sphincter. Place the lubricated pad of the finger against the anus and hold it there with light pressure. Wait for the sphincter to relax, and the finger will almost fall into the rectum without producing pain or sphincter spasm.

As the finger slides into the rectum, curve the finger so that it remains in contact with the anterior rectal wall, and the patient's prostate will be directly under the pad of the examiner's finger as it enters the ampulla. Examine one lobe at a time for hard masses within the lobe, and compare one lobe to the other for size (in three dimensions), consistency, and tenderness. Identify the mid-line fissure. Its absence is generally evidence of enlargement of the median lobe of the prostate, the one most likely to obstruct the urethra and cause urinary retention. Carcinoma is identified as a hard mass - often described as "stony hard" - while benign hypertrophy of the prostate often produces a firm rubbery enlargement In the aged male, the prostate may be atrophied, and therefore is soft and mushy or almost absent.

Tenderness of one or both lobes is generally evidence of infection - acute or chronic, recurrent prostatitis.

Next, examine the rectal wall by rotating the finger in first one direction, then the other, so that the finger pad has swept through an entire circle across the wall to identify a tumor or internal hemorrhoids. Carcinoma of the rectum or metastatic nodules are commonly palpable here. Feces will often be present and can be identified by their ability to be indented and moved. Being too soft, the seminal vesicles are not normally palpable but, if scarred, may be felt as thickened cords lateral to the prostate.

Evaluate the anal sphincter as you withdraw your finger. Of course, if the sphincter has a painful fissure, is strictured, or is obstructed, you may not have been able to go beyond this portion of the examination. On withdrawing the finger, note the presence of weakness of the sphincter muscles by pressing in several directions within the anal canal. Provision of toilet paper or tissue for the patient should be routine at the end of the examination.

Look at the examining fingertip for fresh blood, mucus, or stool. Record the color of the feces. It is good practice (if you are properly prepared) to smear the stool on a slide or porcelain plate and to test it for the presence of occult blood by the guaiac reagent.

RECORDING

Genitalia: Normal pubic hair. Penis circumsized, no lesions, no inflammation. Meatus patent. No discharge. Scrotum - testicles descended, symmetrical, no masses. No inguinal hernia.

Rectum: No external or internal hemorrhoids, no fissures or fistulae. Sphincter tone good. Prostate not enlarged, no masses or tenderness. Stool brown, no visible blood. Guaiac negative.

SUPPLEMENTAL EXERCISES

1. A common lesion of the scrotum is a varicocele. What is this and what is its appearance?

2. List common signs and symptoms of acute prostatitis.

3. Look up current morbidity and mortality statistics for carcinoma of the rectum. What percentage of rectal carcinoma is detectable by rectal examination?

CHAPTER 17

EXAMINATION OF THE FEMALE GENITAL ORGANS

INTRODUCTION

Despite an increasing openness regarding sexuality in this country, examination of sexual organs may evoke more psychological discomfort than an examiner can anticipate. There is often anxiety and apprehension regarding exposure, as well as the possible clinical findings and their implications. It is not unusual for women, both young and old, to avoid necessary examinations, often with serious results, because of previous unpleasant experiences during examination or communication from others of such discomfort.

Therefore, in order to foster relaxation, confidence, and mutual respect during this type of examination, the practitioner has a responsibility to provide a warm and interested atmosphere rather than one which may be interpreted as clinically detached.

It has been suggested that all practitioners, male and female, preparing to learn the procedures necessary to this examination, roleplay the part of patient, assuming the required position and experiencing the draping, exposure, and touch. The implications are obvious (see reference No. 3).

TOPOGRAPHICAL ANATOMY

The external genitalia (Fig. 17.1), collectively termed the pudendum or vulva, comprise the following structures: mons pubis (veneris), a rounded puff of fatty tissue over the symphysis pubis and covered by coarse, dark hair at puberty; the labia majora, two raised, rounded, longitudinal folds of skin, merging with the mons anteriorly and the perineal body posteriorly; labia minora, small, narrow, elongated folds between the labia major and the vaginal introitus with surfaces that are pink, moist, and resembling vaginal mucosa; clitoris, a slightly moist, glistening body of flesh projecting down toward the vagina; vestibule, the area between the labia minora from the clitoris to the urethral opening with soft, hairless skin containing sweat and sebaceous glands; Skene's glands and ducts, immediately within the urethra on its posterolateral aspect; Bartholin's glands and ducts, on either side of the lower vagina; hymen, circular or crescent-shaped membrane just inside entrance to the vagina; perineal body, including skin and underlying tissues between the vaginal entrance and the anal orifice supported by muscles; and the fourchette, a low ridge formed by the labia as they converge posteriorly above the perineum.

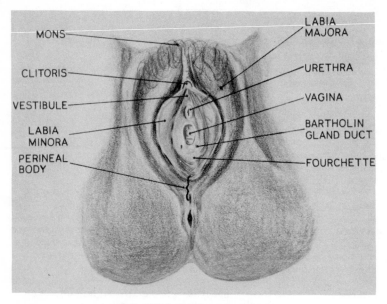

FIG. 17.1: External genitalia.

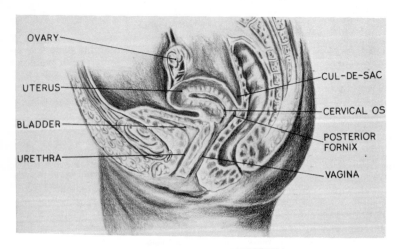

FIG. 17.2: Internal genitalia.

The internal genitalia (Fig. 17.2) comprise the vagina, a muscular, distensible canal with many folds or rugae and lined with pink mucosa about 7-8 cm. long, extending from the external genitalia to the lower neck of the uterus; the uterus, a pear-shaped organ about 8 cm. long, consisting of a body or fundus, a short, constricted isthmus, and a cervix 2-3 cm. in diameter lying in the midline of the vagina, pointed posteriorly and covered with pink, unbroken epithelium; two almond-shaped ovaries, about 4 cm. long, 2.5 cm. wide, located adjacent to the side wall of the pelvis; and two Fallopian tubes, or oviducts, about 11 cm. long, extending bilaterally between the folds of the broad ligament from the upper uterine fundus to an area beyond the ovary.

PHYSIOLOGY

The labia are normally close together in women who have never given birth, but then gape progressively with succeeding vaginal deliveries. They become thin with sparse hair in later years. In addition, the skin of the entire vulva becomes atrophic in the aged, often showing white plaques referred to as leukoplakia.

The size and development of the clitoris may be quite variable, but true enlargement usually represents some chromosomal or hormonal abnormality. Since it is analagous to the male penis, it is capable of engorgement and slight erection.

Bartholin's glands secrete into the vagina a clear, mucoid, lubricative fluid which assists the entrance of the penis during sexual intercourse. The hymen varies markedly; it may admit only one to two fingers or not be present at all.

The uterus is normally tilted slightly forward and is supported by ligaments (the round ligament to the fundus, the broad ligament to the pelvis, and the uterosacral ligament from the cervix to the sacrum). The uterine body can move with considerable freedom and can change to an abnormal position (excessively vertical or excessively horizontal). The cervical opening or os varies from being small and round to being a slit in parous women. A bluish appearance of the cervix and vagina is due to increased blood supply and is usually an early indication of pregnancy (Chadwick's sign), particularly in women who have never been pregnant before.

Ovulation may be accompanied by localized abdominal pain commonly referred to as "mittelschmerz" and, occasionally, by slight vaginal spotting.

Since the mucous membrane lining of the Fallopian tubes joins the peritoneum, infections from the vagina and uterus may spread into the peritoneal cavity causing inflammation (peritonitis).

Amenorrhea, or failure to menstruate, is most frequently due to pregnancy but may be caused by emotional disturbances, endocrine disorders, or the presence of disease. In women who are taking the "pill," the menstrual flow may be very scant and of brief duration, while women who have an IUD in place may experience heavy bleeding of up to 8 to 10 days. Dysmenorrhea, or painful menstruation, relatively common in young girls, may be due to a variety of conditions which require consultation.

EXAMINATION

Following a simple explanation of the necessary procedures, the patient is instructed to remove all her undergarments from the waist down and is clothed in an examination gown only. It will be necessary for her to void in order to empty the bladder prior to the examination. If cytologic examination is to be done, she should have been advised earlier to avoid douching for the previous twenty-four hours. Because the menstrual discharge may mask signs of discharge, lesions, or reddened mucosa, it is best to perform this examination before or after menstruation.

For the comfort of the patient, as well as for the legal protection of the male examiner, it may be advisable to have a woman in attendance during this part of the examination. The procedure includes:
 Examination of the breast (see Chapter 12)
 Examination of the abdomen (see Chapter 14)
 Examination of the external genitalia
 Cytologic smear
 Examination of the internal genitalia, and
 Rectal examination

It will be necessary to have available:

1. clean gloves
2. vaginal speculum
3. sterile cotton-tipped applicators
4. spatula
5. slides and test tubes
6. fixation solution
7. lubricating jelly
8. adjustable light
9. appropriate laboratory slips
10. microscope

The examination is conducted with the patient in the dorsolithotomy position on a table equipped with stirrups. A drape sheet is placed over the abdomen and legs to avoid unnecessary exposure. Once the drape is arranged, it is wise to elevate the head of the table about 30° or to provide a pillow, not only for comfort, but in order to maintain eye contact with the patient while the examiner sits. Depression of the center of the drape so that it falls flat on the abdomen will also maintain face-to-face contact.

The examiner stands or sits in front of the patient. Although the individual practitioner will have to find the position most comfortable, it seems advisable that the right-handed examiner use the right hand to separate the labia for inspection of the vulva, and to perform the digital part of the bimanual examination while the left hand is free for use of instruments and to perform the abdominal portion of the bimanual examination. This will, of course, vary from individual to individual. Gloves should be worn throughout the examination.

Throughout the examination, the practitioner should speak to the patient to inform her of what is going to happen, explaining what she is liable to feel and asking her to report any discomfort.

EXAMINATION OF THE EXTERNAL GENITALIA

Since the mons pubis is prone to skin lesions found elsewhere on the body, look for signs of dermatitis such as lesions, reddening or scratch marks. Edema may be a sign of vulvar varicosities or carcinomatous infiltration.

Retract the clitoral prepuce from its juncture with the clitoris and look for signs of inflammation, smegma, lesions and adhesions. The labia majora should be separated and the area inspected for the presence of adherence, laceration, or hematoma, as well as discharge, edema, varicosities, hernia, ulcers, or tumor masses. Sebaceous cysts also develop in these structures, but although annoying, are relatively insignificant unless they become infected and present a diagnostic question.

Examine the vestibule for swelling, inflammation, and prolapsed out-pouching of the urethral mucous membrane (caruncle) which is reddened and tender in infection. This area, as well as Skene's ducts and Bartholin's glands, is also a common site of cysts and venereal lesions, so that any discharge should be cultured.

While the lips of the labia majora are still separated, the fourchette and hymen can be inspected for old tears and scarring. The patient should be asked to strain or bear down, and the examiner alerted to any loss of urine from the urethra, or any protrusion which represents prolapse of the anterior or posterior vaginal wall or of the cervix itself.

EXAMINATION OF THE INTERNAL GENITALIA

This consists of the speculum examination and bimanual examination. Some practitioners prefer to do the bimanual examination first to locate the cervix and to facilitate proper insertion of the speculum. Others prefer the inspection provided by the speculum before performing palpation. Either sequence is acceptable.

Speculum Examination: Inspection of the cervix and the upper vagina can best be done by using a vaginal speculum. In addition, collection of vaginal and cervical scrapings for examination, culture and cytologic study may be readily accomplished when the vaginal walls are separated. Cytologic study should be done annually on all women over twenty-five years in order to identify precancerous lesions early enough to avoid invasive spread. Since the literature reports an increased incidence today of malignancies in even younger women, it may be advisable to carry out this examination routinely on all post-adolescent sexually active women, where possible. Unfortunately, thousands of women still die each year in the United States from cancer of the cervix. This is a serious tragedy when we realize that many of these women could have been cured, if their lesions had been identified early enough.

Select a warmed, but not hot, speculum of the appropriate size and use water alone as a lubricant to avoid contamination. Ask the patient to breathe slowly through her mouth in an effort to relax the pelvic muscles.

Separate the labia with one hand and move two fingers inside the vagina, retracting the vaginal wall by pressing posteriorly on the fourchette. Insert the speculum by holding it closed with the other hand so that the blades are nearly vertical, the handle pointed to the side (Fig. 17.3). Direct the tip of the speculum to the posterior part of the vaginal introitus to avoid possibly painful pressure on the external urethral meatus. Rotate the speculum back to the midline so that the blades are in a transverse position and the handle points downward (Fig. 17.4). Advance the speculum to full depth so the cervix can be exposed and, after opening the blades slowly, lock the speculum in its open position (Fig. 17.5). It may be important to mention here that the sight of a string or plastic tip coming out of the os is evidence that there is an intrauterine device (IUD) in place.

Once the cervix is adequately exposed, obtain specimens for Pap smear. Although there are several techniques employed, we suggest the use of a cotton-tipped applicator inserted gently into the cervical os to collect the first specimen (Fig. 17.6). A special spatula is used to scrape around the os (Fig. 17.7), and to obtain a collection from the vaginal pool in the posterior fornix. The material should be immediately transferred to the microscopic slide, promptly fixed with alcohol and ether or sprayed with a commercially prepared fixative to avoid distorting the cells by allowing them to dry, and sent to the laboratory.

In view of the increasing incidence of vaginal infections, it is recommended that cultures also be taken routinely during each examination.

With the speculum still in place, the cervix should be observed for color, laceration, discharge, erosions, ulcers, and new growths.

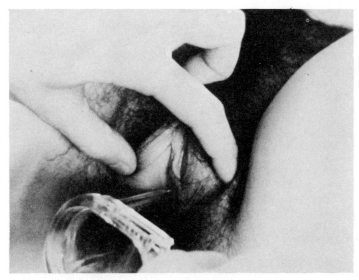

FIG. 17.3: Insertion of the speculum. Note the position of the handle to the right so that the blades are vertical for ease of entry.

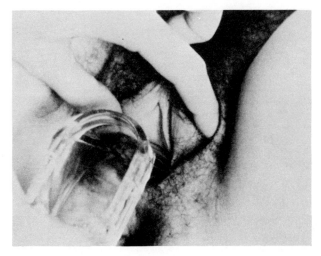

FIG. 17.4: Rotation of the speculum after insertion.

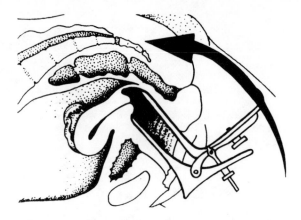

FIG. 17.5: Diagram of the speculum in position with blades opened.

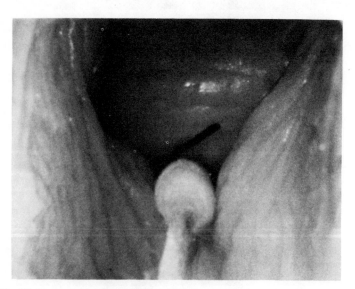

FIG. 17.6: Cotton-tipped applicator for collecting cells from the os.
Note the string of an IUD.

Inspect the cervical os for size, shape, color, polyps, and beefy
red appearance, as well as for bleeding spots. A marked change in
position may normally occur as a result of uterine retroversion, but
since any change in position may be indicative of uterine tumor, inflammation of the parametrium or malignant infiltration, this finding should be added to the problem list and consultation requested.

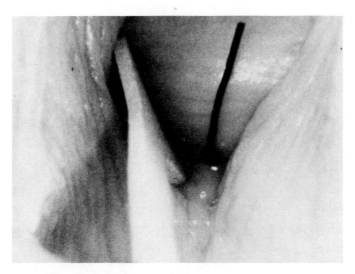

FIG. 17.7: Spatula scraping the cervix for cells.

The lateral walls of the vagina, visible between the blades of the speculum, should be inspected for texture, ulceration, abnormal redness or blueness, discharge, and evidence of bulging. As the speculum is unlocked and slid gently out of the vagina, the anterior and posterior walls may be inspected for cystic or solid tumors, ulcerations, and injury.

Frequently, a white vaginal discharge called leukorrhea may be found. It may occur at any age and affects almost all women at some time in their lives. Although it is not necessarily a sign of disease, but may be a manifestation of ovulation or normal desquamation of epithelial cells, leukorrhea may be a sign of a local or systemic disorder. Table 17.1 illustrates some of the typical findings in various types of vaginal discharge.

Bimanual examination: There are two parts to this procedure: abdominal-vaginal and abdominal-recto-vaginal. The examiner, again after carefully explaining the procedure, which may be slightly uncomfortable, stands before the patient who is still in dorsolithotomy position. The index and middle fingers of the examiner's gloved hand, held closely together, are lubricated and gently inserted into the vagina with slight pressure against the posterior vaginal wall (Fig. 17.8). The hand is then turned so that the back surface is parallel to the floor and the finger pads facing the anterior vaginal wall, in an attempt to avoid pressure on the sensitive urethra. Notation should be made of any firmness, induration,

				TABLE 17.1	

COLOR	CONSISTENCY	AMOUNT	ODOR	PROBABLE CAUSES
Clear	Mucoid	+ to ++	None	Ovulation, emotional stress, increased estrogen secretion
White	Thin with curd-like flecks attached to vaginal wall	+ to ++	None to musty depending on hygiene	Vaginal mycosis, Monilia albicans
Yellow-green	Frothy	+ to +++	Fetid	Trichomonas vaginalis vaginitis
Brown	Watery	+ to ++	Musty	Vaginitis, cervicitis, endometritis, neoplasm of cervix, endometrium or tube, post irradiation
Gray blood-streaked	Thin	+ to ++++	Foul	Vaginal, cervical endometrial, or tubal neoplasm

TABLE 17.1: Characteristics of vaginal discharge. Students are cautioned that these descriptions can serve only as a guide, and a great deal of variation may be expected.

tenderness, tumors, or cystic masses in the vaginal wall, as well as the amount of relaxation present. The examiner should be alerted to bulging of the posterior vaginal wall into the introitus, which is indicative of a rectocele, or bulging of the anterior wall, which occurs with cystocele.

Consideration should then be given to the consistency, tenderness on mobility, or fixation of the cervix. Normally the cervix feels like a button with a rounded face and a central depression; its consistency is similar to the tip of the nose. Feel for nodules and old lacerations.

Press downward with the abdominal hand while the pelvic structures are swept up against it with the vaginal fingers, and attempt to feel the uterus between the examining fingers and the abdominal hand (Fig. 17.9). With the vaginal hand palm up, separate the two fingers laterally so that one finger is on either side of the cervix, and attempt to outline the uterus. The five important characteristics which require attention include: size, mobility, position, consistency, and

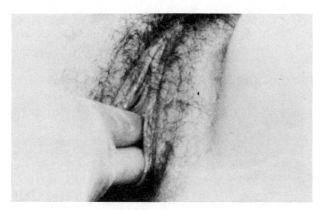

FIG. 17.8: Insertion of fingers into the vaginal vault. Note the vertical position of the fingers similar to the position of insertion of the speculum in Fig. 17.3.

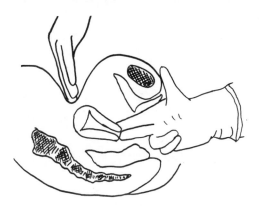

FIG. 17.9: Diagram of bimanual palpation of the uterus.

contour. Irregularity in surface such as in myomata can usually be identified easily. The cul-de-sac area should be examined for bulging, tenderness, and masses. Remember to explain your movements and the sensations she will have to your patient.

In order to locate the tube and ovary, place the vaginal fingers on one side of the cervix and push up and back. Place the abdominal fingers just medial to the anterior superior iliac spine and, by pushing downward so their tips approach the vaginal fingers, you should be able to locate the tube and ovary. (The right-handed practitioner may have to re-glove and change hands to feel for the left-sided organs with the left hand.)

The normal Fallopian tube can rarely be palpated. Once the ovary is located, it should be evaluated for size, shape, and mobility. It is important to remember that it is sensitive to pressure, so gentleness is imperative. The presence of unusual tenderness, enlargement over 5 cm., a fixed position from which it cannot be moved, or evidence of any irregularity in shape is noted.

RECTOVAGINAL EXAMINATION

This is another important part of the examination which can help to identify the presence of serious inflammation or tumor of the pelvis. Gently insert the index finger into the vagina and the second finger into the rectum. The presence of any inflammatory reaction, extensive malignant tumor, or granulomatous masses of the pelvic cellular tissue may be palpated in this manner.

Once the examination has been completed, the patient's vulva should be cleansed of examining lubricant, her legs removed from the stirrups, and she can be assisted from the table.

RECORDING: Normal Nulliparous Female

Genitalia

> External: Normal pubic hair, no labial swellings or lesions. Normal clitoris. Introitus admits two fingers. No urethral redness, swelling, or discharge. Skene's and Bartholin's not inflamed. Perineum intact, no scars.
> Internal:
>> Vagina - no bulging or masses, mucosa intact and pink.
>> Uterus - anterior, average size, regular shape, mobile, normal consistency.
>> Adnexa - tubes not palpated, ovaries not enlarged, slight tenderness.
>> Cul-de-sac - no bulging, tenderness or masses.
>> Discharge - clear, mucoid, 1+, no odor
>> Pap - to lab
>> Rectum - no external or internal hemorrhoids, no fissures or fistulae. Sphincter tone good. No masses or tenderness. Stool brown, no visible blood. Guaiac negative.

PATIENT PROBLEM

Mrs. S.D., a 22-year-old well-developed, white, married Grav. 0 Para 0 female, with CC "vaginal itch, burning on urination and vaginal discharge, one week duration."

Problem: Pruritis, Dysuria, Vaginal Discharge

S: Treated with erythromycin 4 weeks ago for RUL pneumonia. Was well until 7 days ago when she first noticed increased vaginal discharge with severe itch and burning on urination. Has taken Ovulen for birth control past two years, no untoward effects. Menses of 28 days x 3 days, no dysmenorrhea, no clots or spotting, uses 4 tampons q.d. No dyspareunia. Urine neg. for sugar in hospital. No family history diabetes.

O: Vestibule and urethra red and irritated.
Vagina - reddened mucosa, white curds clinging to wall.
Uterus, cervix and adnexa within normal limits.
Discharge - thin, watery 2+, no odor.
Pap - done - to lab.
Urine - neg. sugar.
Wet prep - no Trichimonads seen, cells typical of Monilia albicans

A: In view of recent Rx with erythromycin, increased susceptibility due to Ovulen, typical monilia cells seen on wet prep, suggest Monilia albicans vaginitis.

P: Dx. 2 hr. pc blood sugar.
Rx. Mycostatin suppositories BID one week.
Pt. Ed. Advise to avoid sexual intercourse, use of tampons and douching two weeks. If not cleared, return for consultation.

_____
Signature

SUPPLEMENTAL EXERCISES

1. Why should women be encouraged and instructed in visual and tactile examination of their external genitalia through the use of a mirror ?

REFERENCES

1. Novak, E.R., Jones, G.S., and Jones, H.W. Jr.: Novak's Textbook of Gynecology, 9th edition. The Williams and Wilkins Co., Baltimore, 1975.

2. Greenhill, J.P.: Office Gynecology, 9th edition. The Year Book Medical Publishers, Chicago, 1971.

3. Magee, J.: The Pelvic Examination: A View from the Other End of the Table. Ann Int Med 83:563, Oct. 1975.

4. Ulene, A.: OMNI OB/GYN Modular Instruction, "Pelvic Examination." Department of Educational Services, Ortho Pharmaceutical Corporation, Raritan, New Jersey, 1974.

CHAPTER 18

THE NEUROLOGICAL AND MENTAL EXAMINATION

INTRODUCTION

In performing the history and physical examination described to this point, the examiner has already performed almost every one of the elements of a screening neuropsychiatric examination. The purpose of this chapter is to arrange these elements into an organized whole, to recommend several additional tests which may be performed for a more complete neurologic evaluation, and to recommend a format for reporting the neurological evaluation of the patient, should it be desired separately.

GENERAL

The essential portions of this evaluation can be divided into the examination of cerebral function, the cranial nerves, the functioning of the cerebellum and motor and sensory systems, and the reflexes.

The examination summarized here is an adequate screening examination and is not a full, detailed evaluation of all psychiatric or neurologic functions, which must be left to the specialist.

CEREBRAL FUNCTIONS

The mental status of the patient is a critical portion of any evaluation and is properly recorded here. The entire medical interview, with appropriate questions, plus careful observation of the patient during the history-taking and the physical examination should provide the clinician with a sound basis for an evaluation of the patient's mental status.

Although there is some degree of overlapping in any classification, the cerebral functions may be placed in groups and reported according to the following outline:

1. State of consciousness: refers to the patient's functional level of responsiveness and may vary from alertness to drowsiness to stupor to coma.

2. Emotional state: reflected by his affect or mood which may be expressed by normal affect, hyperactivity (euphoria, hostility, or agitation) or hypoactivity (depression or flat, unresponsive affect).

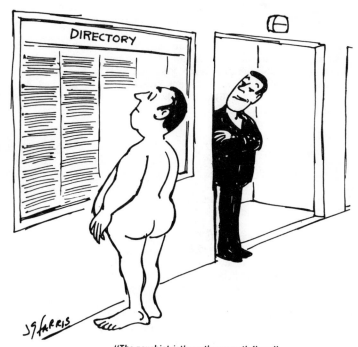

"The psychiatrist's on the seventh floor."

3. Intellect: may be considered to include high mental functions such as memory for recent and remote events, orientation to time, place and person, recognition of familiar objects or words, and ability to do simple calculations. Lack of any of these or abnormal thought content such as delusions, hallucinations, fixed ideas or bizarre expressions are reflections of a disturbed thought process.

4. Behavior: for purposes of this evaluation, refers to physical clues such as the patient's state of dress, appropriateness of gestures, facial expressions, and attentiveness to the examiner.

5. Speech: is a highly complex act which involves the cerebrum, the cerebellum, the cranial nerves, the mouth, palate, tongue, and larynx, and the respiratory system. It was suggested earlier that evaluation of speech should be recorded in the General Survey (Chapter 6) and it should also be included in this summary of cerebral functions.

CRANIAL NERVES

General: The function of each one of the cranial nerves will have been tested in the physical examination of the head and neck; therefore, the technique for examination of each will not be repeated here. The functions of the cranial nerve or group of nerves will be listed so that abnormalities can be related to the appropriate nerve.

The sense of taste (cranial nerves VII and IX) need not be routinely tested and is not included in the listing below. For cranial nerve VIII only the cochlear branch function is listed. The vestibular branch is concerned with balance but, routinely, this nerve function is not tested. Gait and balance are reported under the examination of the cerebellum in this summary. Similarly, nystagmus, which, if present, will have been identified and recorded during examination of the extraocular movements, should also be reported as a lesion of cranial nerves III, IV, and VI here, although, in fact, it may be due to a lesion elsewhere.

Specific Nerves:

   I. Olfactory - smell.
  II. Optic - visual acuity, visual fields, color vision.
 III. Oculomotor ⎫
  IV. Trochlear   ⎬   extraocular movement (EOM), nystag-
  VI. Abducens   ⎭   mus, elevation of upper lids, pupils.
   V. Trigeminal - sensation of forehead, face and jaw; closure of jaw.
 VII. Facial - movement of facial muscles, closure of eyes.
VIII. Acoustic - hearing, Weber test.
  IX. Glossopharyngeal ⎱ phonation, position of the uvula,
   X. Vagus   ⎰ swallowing, gag reflex

XI. Accessory - movement of head, shrugging of shoulders.
XII. Hypoglossal - protrusion of tongue, tremor of tongue.

CEREBELLAR FUNCTION

The cerebellum serves as the higher center for balance and muscle coordination. These functions should be tested separately. Only a few of the many possible tests are listed below, but these are adequate to identify cerebellar disorders.

1. Balance tests:

    a. Gait: Characteristic of a cerebellar disorder is a staggering, ataxic gait similar to that seen with alcohol intoxication. If the abnormality of gait is not due to an obvious physical abnormality such as paralysis of a lower extremity or muscle wasting, this abnormality should be reported here.

    b. Romberg: This is a test for sensory equilibrium leading to ataxia and has been described during the examination of extremities (p. 225, Chapter 15). Have the patient stand with his feet together and eyes open. If he does not begin to fall, have the patient close his eyes. With an impairment of station or posture, the patient may begin to fall - be prepared to catch him! Such a response would be recorded as a "positive Romberg" test.

2. Coordination tests:

    a. Finger-to-nose: Have the patient extend his arms fully to the sides and ask him to touch his nose rapidly, first with one fingertip and then the other. If this can be performed easily, have the patient repeat this with the eyes closed. An abnormal response would consist of "past-pointing" in which the fingertip will be brought beyond the nose, missing the target widely.

    b. Heel-to-shin: With the patient lying on the examining table, have him place one heel rapidly down the shin to the ankle. Ask him to repeat this using the other heel. Failure to do this smoothly and accurately will suggest a cerebellar disorder.

    c. Alternating motion: The normal individual should be able to coordinate alternating motions such as rapid pronation and supination of the hands or tapping the floor with his toes. These activities will be slow and inaccurate with cerebellar dysfunction.

MOTOR SYSTEM

Muscle Atrophy: In the examination of the neck as well as in the upper and lower extremities, the clinician should have observed and palpated atrophy of muscles and significant asymmetry of one muscle group from the corresponding group on the opposite side. Such atrophy should be recorded here to give a picture of the motor system as a whole in one place.

Muscle Strength: This testing was also performed in examination of the extremities (Chapter 15) and, if abnormal, should be recorded here also.

Involuntary Body Movements: A variety of involuntary movements may occur in either alert or comatose patients. These should be recorded here, although they may have been noted earlier in the region where observed (Table 18.1).

TABLE 18.1		
CHARACTERISTICS OF INVOLUNTARY MOVEMENTS		
TYPE	DESCRIPTION	CAUSES
1. Tics	tiny spasms of small muscles usually around eyes, face, and neck	Tenseness, nervousness
2. Twitches	same as tics, but may involve larger muscle and are more noticeable to the observer	Same origin
3. Tremors	fine or coarse trembling of large muscle or entire limb	Fatigue, alcoholic abuse, thyrotoxicosis, multiple sclerosis, Parkinson's disease
4. Convulsions	sustained contractions or intermittent contractions and relaxation of extremities; large, gross movements	Epilepsy, uremia, poisoning, tetanus, chorea

SENSORY SYSTEM

General: As for other portions of the detailed neurological examination, there are many sensory modalities which are capable of being tested. Routinely, light touch, superficial pain, and vibratory sense perception are tested in a few locations. Always start the examination first by testing opposite, corresponding parts of the body, asking the patient to compare the sensation on one side to that on the other. Do not pursue slight differences as they ordinarily are not significant. This examination should be done with the patient's eyes closed, although he should be told what is to be done and what responses are expected of him.

If a definite difference is reported by the patient between opposite sides, the abnormal area should be carefully outlined. Thus, if the patient notes diminished pain to pin-prick on the right forearm, testing should be done to determine at which level the abnormality is first noted, how low on the forearm it extends, and how far it extends on the flexor and extensor surfaces. A useful method for reporting the extent of such an area of abnormal sensation is to draw a diagram.

Light Touch: Using a wisp of cotton, touch the forehead, cheeks, arms, forearms, hands, chest, thighs, and legs. The abnormality will usually be in perception of diminished touch sensation.

Superficial Pain: Using a sharp pin, prick lightly on the above areas. Either decreased or increased sensation may be noted.

Vibratory Sense: Strike the tuning fork before touching it to each location to obtain roughly the same intensity of vibration. Place the base of the fork firmly against the skin pressing to make good contact with the underlying bone (Fig. 18.1). Test the shoulders, elbows, wrists, knees, shins, and ankles. Hold the fork on the part and note the patient's ability to feel when the fork stops vibrating. An abnormality here is either inability to feel vibrations at all, or, more often, stating that vibration has stopped while the fork is still vibrating briskly.

REFLEXES

In the examination of the extremities (Chapter 15), the tendon reflexes and the plantar reflex were described and recorded. The results should be reported here also.

RECORDING

Cerebral Function - alert and responsive, thought process, memory, and orientation intact. Appropriate behavior and speech.

Cranial Nerves:

    I. Identifies alcohol.

    II. Vision 20/20 O.D. 20/20 O.S. Color intact. Fields normal by gross confrontation. Fundi normal.

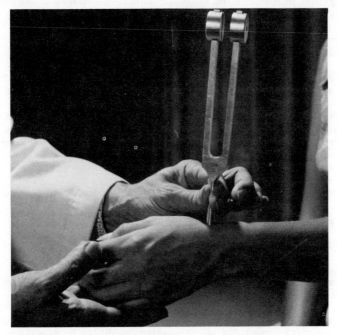

FIG. 18.1: Testing vibratory sense at the wrist.

III, IV, VI.   EOM intact. No ptosis. No nystagmus. **PERRLA.**

V.   Sensory intact, jaw closure normal.

VII.   Facial muscles symmetrical, no weakness.

VIII.   Hearing intact, Weber test normal.

IX, X.   Swallowing and gag reflex intact. Uvula rises in mid-line on phonation.

XI.   Head movement and shrug of shoulders normal.

XII.   Tongue protrudes in mid-line, no tremor.

Cerebellar function: finger to nose, heel to shin coordination intact. Gait normal, Romberg negative.

Motor system: No atrophy, weakness, or tremors.

Sensory: Intact to light touch, pin-prick, and vibration.

Reflexes: These are best illustrated either in chart form, or by use of a "stick-man" figure:

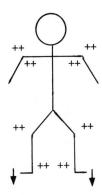

SUPPLEMENTAL EXERCISES

1. Describe in detail the typical physical findings of an established right-sided hemiplegia involving the upper and lower extremities.

2. Why are light touch, pin-prick and vibratory senses all examined in the screening neurological examination?

REFERENCES

1. De Jong, R.N.: The Neurological Examination, 3rd edition. Harper & Row, New York, 1967.

2. De Jong, R.N. et al.: Essentials of the Neurological Examination. Smith, Kline and French Laboratories, Philadelphia, 1974.

3. Patient Assessment: The Neurological Examination.

   Part I, Am. J. Nurs. 75:1511, Sept. 1975.

   Part II, Ibid 75:2037, Nov. 1975.

   Part III, Ibid 76:508, April 1976.

CHAPTER 19

THE SEQUENCE OF PHYSICAL EXAMINATION

INTRODUCTION

For purposes of clarity of teaching, the physical examination of each region or organ has been described as if each were a separate entity. Chapter 11 described inspection, palpation, percussion, and auscultation of the thorax and lungs from anterior, lateral, and posterior positions. Chapter 13 then described inspection, palpation, percussion, and auscultation of the heart, anteriorly. To actually perform a complete examination of a patient in this manner would require a repetition of examination of the same body region, resulting in much movement of the patient and the examiner, as well as a significant loss of valuable time for both. These repetitions must be eliminated by the development of a pattern of examination of the whole patient, which will not miss any portion of the examination and which will minimize wasted time. There is no single "right" order of examination which is used by all practitioners, or even by the same practitioner for all patients. The examination of a bedridden patient, of an ambulatory patient in the office or clinic, or of a seriously ill, feeble, or uncooperative patient will be varied according to circumstances. Additionally, if the patient presents a specific disturbing abnormality (e.g., abdominal pain, mass in the neck), this part may be examined first to reassure the patient that his major problem will receive priority, and not be relegated to the routine sequence of the examination.

It is strongly recommended, however, that the student develop a pattern for the complete basic physical examination and that he stay with this routine until it becomes a habit pattern. In this way, he will not skip around from one place to another wondering what to do next, and he will be less likely to miss a portion of the examination.

SUGGESTED SEQUENCE

The following is a suggested sequence for the routine examination of a fully cooperative ambulatory patient and is presented simply as one of several possible logical models:

1. Observe body movement and general status on entry.

2. Take history.

3. Record vital signs, test vision with Snellen chart.

4. Body as a whole:
    Inspect gait, balance, body build.

5. Head and neck:
    Inspect and palpate head, eyes, ears, nose, mouth,
    pharynx, and neck.
    Auscult cranium, carotids, and thyroid, if indicated.

6. Anterior thorax:
    Inspect anterior and lateral chest wall.
    Palpate shoulders, supra- and infra-clavicular spaces,
      axillae, breasts, ribs and sternum, precordium.
    Percuss lungs (anterior and lateral chest), heart.
    Auscult lungs (anterior and lateral chest), heart.

7. Posterior thorax:
    Inspect neck and back.
    Palpate lungs.
    Percuss lungs, diaphragm, costo-vertebral angles,
      spine.
    Auscult lungs.

8. Abdomen:
    Inspect anterior abdomen and flanks.
    Auscult bowel sounds and bruits.
    Palpate abdomen, flanks, and femoral arteries.
    Percuss abdomen and flanks.

9. Extremities (examine upper, then lower extremities):
    Inspect.
    Palpate joints, muscles, and arteries.
    Percuss tendon reflexes.
    Test touch, pin-prick, vibratory senses, and plantar
      reflex.

10. Genitalia:
    Inspect and palpate.

11. Rectal:
    Inspect and palpate.

It should be re-emphasized that this sequence is a suggested model
and that it is useful in developing a pattern of routine examination for
the clinician. More detailed examinations of a region, part, or organ will be added when abnormalities are detected. On the other
hand, no examination can be called complete which does not include
all of these elements of the work-up, no matter what the order of
examination.

CHAPTER 20

PRENATAL ASSESSMENT

INTRODUCTION

In this text we have presented a general guide for collection of information relating to history and physical examination which can be applied in almost all situations. There are occasions, however, where, in order to guarantee the thoroughness of the data base appropriate to that situation, additional information will be required.

During pregnancy, for example, it becomes important to know not only about the health history of the mother and her family, but to include information about the father as well. We know that certain genetic conditions which are transmitted from the father or his family may place the fetus in a high risk category.

We know that specific signs and symptoms accompany the physiological changes occurring in the mother's body as a result of the pregnancy. It is vital, however, to the delivery of health care, that signs and symptoms which may indicate real or potential problems be recognized early and reported appropriately so that proper therapeutic measures may be instituted rapidly. It is well-accepted knowledge that the sharp drop in maternal and infant mortality occuring in the 20th century is directly related to the quality of prenatal care received.

In attempting to provide, in this text, a guide for prenatal assessment and yet avoid redundancy, we have preferred to include only that information which would serve as a supplement to the general guide.

During the interview it is most important that the woman's response to the reality of the pregnancy and its implications be evaluated. Many women need time and guidance to help work through their feelings about pregnancy. It is important to stress that the emotional response of each pregnant woman to her pregnancy is unique. In this time when more women than ever before have the opportunity to decide for themselves whether or not to continue with a pregnancy, the speed with which problems can be identified and decisions made is crucially significant. The ability to elicit and identify these emotional problems relating to impending motherhood is a special skill worthy of development in those who deal with expectant parents; therefore, the guidelines presented earlier for development of a mutually beneficial relationship should be remembered during the initial encounter for prenatal evaluation and for subsequent continuing visits.

Since it will undoubtedly affect the woman's willingness to continue
and cooperate with the health supervision so vital to the well-being
of the mother and the fetus, the practitioner's ability to be concerned, supportive, and non-judgmental, even in the most unusual
situations, must be stressed.

HEALTH HISTORY

The health history should be as complete as one collected for any
other patient, with the following additional suggestions:

Chief Complaint: In most cases this will be simply, "My period is
three weeks late - I think I'm pregnant."

History of Present Illness: An introductory statement identifying
the age, marital status, gravida, and para is usually preliminary
to specific information which includes the date of the first day of
the last menstrual period and presumptive symptoms of pregnancy
experienced by the patient such as nausea and vomiting, fatigue,
tingling of breasts, and increased urinary frequency.

Past History

Medical conditions: Include questions about diabetes, hypertension,
rheumatic fever, tuberculosis, urinary diseases, venereal disease,
phlebitis, pulmonary embolus, as well as specific infections or environmental hazards which may have a bearing upon the health status
of the mother and/or fetus. A history of hematologic disorders as
well as any known allergies should be included. If anemia is present,
question the patient to find out what type it is to determine genetic
implications.

Surgical procedures: Should include those operations that may affect
or involve the reproductive system. Information gathered should include a summary of the events of hospitalization, types of intervention required, anesthesia, and any related problems or complications.

Immunizations (especially to rubella): An up-to-date record of immunizations should be noted.

Medications and drugs: Include all over-the-counter and medically
prescribed medications. Women with a history of drug addiction
should be carefully evaluated. The use of infertility drugs for conception must be noted.

Previous pregnancies: A record of previous pregnancies including
significant history about the mother, father, and baby, is necessary.

Obstetrical History:

> Age
> Year of delivery
> Week of gestation
> Weight gain during pregnancy
> Length of labor - type of delivery - forceps or spontaneous
> Presentation, e.g., vertex, breech
> Anesthesia, analgesia, or oxytocic drugs administered
> Premature rupture of membranes
> Episiotomy, bleeding or infection
> Puerperal problems
> Rhogam
> Significant health problems
> Genetic conditions or anomalies in family

Paternal History for Each Previous Pregnancy:

> Blood type
> Significant health problems
> Genetic conditions or anomalies in his family

Infant History:

> Sex
> Birthweight
> Weeks of gestation
> General condition at birth
> Apgar Score (if information available)
> Multiple births

Review of Systems: The usual review of systems should be obtained with special attention to the following areas:

> Breast: Changes noted such as tingling and fullness, color of areola; increase in size of areola, nipple and breast, secretion from nipples; monthly self-examination of breasts.

> Reproductive System: Include age of menarche, regularity of cycle, number of days and amount of flow, clots, intermenstrual bleeding, dysmenorrhea, premenstrual problems, frequency of coitus and post-coital pain or bleeding, methods of contraception used, history of infertility, date and findings of last Pap smear, and information about vaginal discharge such as odor, consistency, associated pain, and itching. Determine trimester of pregnancy by EDC (Estimated Date of Confinement), presence of Braxton-Hicks contractions, quickening, or lightening.

Family History: This should be as complete as that mentioned in Chapter 4 but should be certain to include the history of any genetic conditions or congenital anomalies as well as multiple births.

Personal-Social History: Gather data about adequacy of housing, ability to maintain a family unit, financial need in regard to prenatal care and hospitalization; assess ability of parenting; psychological status.

Patient Profile: The same guidelines mentioned earlier in the text should be followed.

PHYSICAL EXAMINATION

The physical examination, in addition to identifying the existence of any medical problems, will serve to reinforce the history in establishing the existence of pregnancy. It should include a general examination as outlined in this text with special attention given to palpation and auscultation of the abdomen for size and position of the fetus, and vaginal examination for additional data to support the diagnosis, as well as to evaluate the capacity of the birth canal. At this time, estimation of pelvic measurements may also be accomplished.

It may be of value for the student to review the normal changes which occur as a result of pregnancy and those which the examiner can expect to identify during the examination.

General Inspection and Skin: In general, the woman who is relatively healthy, well-developed and well-nourished, will not be adversely affected by pregnancy. Occasionally, there will be a loss of weight and dehydration early in the first trimester due to nausea and vomiting. If nausea becomes severe and persists, it may represent a serious problem which requires consultation for specific diagnostic treatment.

During pregnancy there is a general heightening of skin pigmentation so that the following become classic signs: chloasma (mask of pregnancy), linea nigra (darkening of vertical line from umbilicus to symphysis pubis), and striae gravidarum (silvery or reddish streaks on the abdomen and thighs due to stretching of tissue). In addition, there is an increased tendency to spider angiomas, which are not especially significant during pregnancy. Exposure to the sun may increase freckling during this period. Most of the signs disappear soon after delivery.

Head and Neck: It is most important to recognize that a generalized headache and blurred vision in the pregnant woman may be a sign of hypertension. These signs accompany a rise in both systolic and diastolic pressures. Edema of the face and eyelids should also be noted.

Palpation of the thyroid gland, which may occasionally become enlarged during this period, should be carefully conducted.

The Breast: The breast becomes generally enlarged during pregnancy but should still remain symmetrical in development. Tingling
and tenderness similar to that experienced premenstrually is an
early sign of pregnancy. The primary areola about the nipple becomes elevated, edematous, and pigmented during the second month
of pregnancy. It becomes soft and velvety to the touch and elevated
above the level of the surrounding skin. Colostrum may be expressed from the nipple by the end of the third month, while the
nipples themselves become larger and more sensitive. The secondary areola appears at the fifth month of pregnancy and is characterized by a series of washed-out spots surrounding the primary areola
due to the presence of non-pigmented sebaceous follicles. This sign
is of diagnostic value in the woman who has never been pregnant.

Heart and Lungs: Pregnancy may impose a risk for a woman who
has a history of rheumatic heart disease. The naturally occurring
increase in circulating blood volume often places an increased bur-
den on an already damaged heart. As the fetus grows, the pressure
on the diaphragm with subsequent limitation of the ability of the lungs
to expand may create an additional problem of dyspnea and orthopnea.

The existence of hypertension prior to, or occurring during pregnancy also creates problems for the expectant woman; a rising blood
pressure in the second half of the pregnancy should be considered a
possible sign of impending hypertensive disorder (toxemia). The
findings of blood pressure above 150/90 should always be considered
a danger signal and medical consultation should be sought.

The Abdomen: Enlargement of the abdomen is apparent after the
third month, when the uterus rises by its increased growth out of the
true pelvis. This enlargement is steady and progressive until the
last month of gestation. Early in pregnancy it is more pronounced
in multigravidas than in primigravidas because the abdominal walls
may have lost part of their tonicity and may be flaccid so that they
afford little support to the uterus, which then sags forward and downward. The fundal height is at the pubis by the third month, the umbilicus by the sixth month, and the lower part of the sternum by
eight and a half months. During the last two weeks of gestation in
primiparas the fetus usually starts descending. This descent, known
as "lightening," leads to easier breathing and to more frequent void-
ing due to the shift of the uterus away from the diaphragm and toward the bladder. Multigravidas may not experience this until the
onset of labor.

The linea nigra, which may be observed from the end of the second
month, although marked in brunettes, may be absent in blondes.
The pigmentation may remain after the pregnancy has terminated.
In brunettes, a dark circle appears about the umbilicus, and pigmented patches are observable over other parts of the abdomen. The
umbilicus itself should be observed for signs of hernia.

The abdominal signs of pregnancy on palpation are progressive increases in the size of the pregnant uterus. The fundus at the end of the third month is palpated in the plane of the pelvic brim, but is felt higher as each month passes. The pregnant uterus presents certain definite characteristics in shape. After the first two months, the uterus is egg-shaped, smooth, symmetrical, and soft. The fetal parts are detectable as early as the fifth month.

By placing the hand on the fundus, the examiner may detect painless intermittent uterine contractions as early as the fourth month. These contractions, known as the Braxton-Hicks sign, occur periodically through pregnancy, thereby preparing the uterus for labor.

Fetal movements detected by an experienced examiner may be considered a positive indication of pregnancy. They may be elicited by suddenly placing the hand upon the woman's abdomen, but are seldom elicited prior to the fifth month. During the fourth and fifth months the fetus is small in relation to the amount of amniotic fluid present, and a sudden tap on the uterus makes the fetus rise and rebound to its original position and tap the finger of the examiner. This is referred to as ballottement, which was described earlier in the chapter on examination of the abdomen.

The auscultation of fetal heart sounds is a positive indication of pregnancy. They are first heard by the eighteenth or twentieth week. Varying from 120 to 140 beats per minute, they are double sounds closely resembling the tick of a watch under a pillow. The rate should be compared with the maternal pulse. In the early months, the heart should be sought just over the symphysis pubis, but later it varies according to position and presentation of the fetus. In vertex presentations, fetal heart sounds are heard the loudest midway between the umbilicus and the anterosuperior spine of the ilium. In L.O.A. and L.O.P. positions sounds are generally heard best in the left lower quadrant. In R.O.P. the heart sounds are loudest in the flank toward the anterosuperior spine. Breech presentations are heard loudest at the level of the umbilicus. Later in pregnancy, other sounds auscultated include the funic souffle, uterine or placental souffle, and sounds due to movement of the fetus, as well as the gurgling of gas in the mother's abdomen. The funic or fetal souffle is a sharp, whistling sound synchronous with the fetal pulse, which is heard in about 15 percent of cases. It is inconstant in appearance due to the rush of blood through the umbilical arteries when they are subject to torsion, tension, or pressure, such as when the cord is around the baby's neck. The uterine souffle is a soft, blowing sound, synchronous with the maternal pulse and is usually heard distinctly upon auscultation in the lower portion of the uterus, because of the passage of blood through the dilated uterine vessels. It is not only characteristic of pregnancy, but may be

present in any condition where the blood supply to the internal genitalia is increased markedly, i.e., with large uterine tumors or enlarged ovaries.

Abdominal palpation for the determination of fetal position can be
accomplished by four Leopold maneuvers once the uterus rises out
of the pelvis. To perform this procedure, ask the patient to void,
then position her flat on her back with her knees flexed. The examiner should make sure the hands are warm before the examination to avoid contraction of the patient's abdominal muscles. In the
first maneuver, the practitioner faces the patient and places both
hands flat on the upper abdomen to ascertain which part of the fetus
is at the fundus of the uterus. Generally, the mass felt will be
either the head or the buttocks. The practitioner determines which
part of the fetus is felt by the consistency, shape and mobility of the
mass. The head is harder than the buttocks; the head is round and
hard and the transverse groove of the neck may be felt, whereas the
breech has no groove and feels more angular. The head moves in-
dependently of the trunk while the buttocks move with the trunk.

The second maneuver attempts to locate the back of the fetus in relation to the right and left sides of the woman. Facing the patient,
the practitioner places the palmar surfaces of both hands on either
side of the abdomen with deep but gentle pressure. The hand on the
right side of the abdomen remains fixed to steady the uterus while
the left fingers are used to slowly palpate the fetal outline. To palpate the opposite side, the functions of the right and left hand are reversed. During the procedure the examiner will note that on one
side of the abdomen the back is felt as a fairly firm, straight plane,
while the other side has numerous nodulations indicating the knees,
elbows and small parts of the fetus.

In the third maneuver, the practitioner attempts to find the head at
the pelvic inlet and determine its mobility. Using one hand, the examiner gently grasps the lower portion of the abdomen above the
symphysis pubis, using a thumb and fingers. If the presenting part
is not engaged, a movable mass will be felt.

The fourth maneuver determines if the fetal head is flexed, confirms
the location of the back, and aids in the determination of how far the
head has descended. It is performed by facing toward the feet of the
patient and using the fingers of both hands to palpate the lower abdomen around Poupart's ligament.

Pelvic Signs

There are changes in the appearance and character of the vagina and
uterus which occur quite early in pregnancy and which assist in the
diagnosis. The purple color of the cervix and vagina, referred to as
Chadwick's sign, is due to the marked congestion of pregnancy. This
sign may be observed in the cervix from the first month after

conception, but since it may remain in the vagina from previous pregnancies, it is not a specific diagnostic factor except in primigravidas.

Goodel's sign is a softening of the cervix. This sign can usually be determined in the primipara by vaginal examination as early as the sixth week. It begins at the lower border of the cervix and feels like a thin, velvety layer covering a firm body. As gestation progresses, the softening extends upward from below until it involves the entire cervix by the end of the eighth month. It is described as giving a sensation to the finger similar to that produced by palpating the lip.

In addition, there are changes in the shape, size, and consistency of the uterus itself. These changes, detected by bimanual examination at about the second month of gestation, are enlargement of the body of the uterus and change in shape to one which is irregular and globular and feels soft and elastic. Hegar's sign, in which the examiner can feel the softening of the lower uterine segment, appears at approximately the second month of gestation.

Internal ballottement of passive fetal movement is accomplished by placing two fingers in the vagina against the anterior uterine wall above the cervix, while the other hand steadies the fundus. With the two fingers toss the fetus upward in the amniotic sac; feel it fall back against the fingers. This ballottement indicates the presence of a movable solid content, and is usually detectable during the fifth and sixth months.

Since the ability of the pregnant woman to deliver her infant vaginally with minimal difficulty is affected by the capacity of her pelvis, it may be necessary to carry out an additional component of the examination measurement. Estimation of pelvic measurements to determine the existence and extent of pelvic contraction before the onset of labor requires special techniques which we believe are not germane to the objectives of this text. The student is, therefore, referred to obstetrical texts for specific descriptions of the techniques employed.

It may also be helpful to mention here, however, that there are specific laboratory data necessary to the complete data base during pregnancy. Initially, the urine should be examined for a complete analysis, but with subsequent visits, determination of the presence of sugar and albumin should be a regular procedure. In addition, blood should be drawn on the first visit for identification of type and the RH factor, and existence of syphilis, as well as a complete blood count. If there is indication of anemia, subsequent checks of hemoglobin and hematocrit will be necessary after therapy is initiated.

Carbohydrate metabolism is affected by the changes of pregnancy. Levels of fasting blood sugar are lower and the secretion of insulin is increased. Subclinical diabetes mellitus may be detected during the prenatal assessment.

Certainly, the method of thorough history and physical examination with supporting laboratory data which we have described is the first step in a program of guidance and health supervision for prospective parents which should promote a healthy mother and baby.

REFERENCES

1. Hellman, M. and Pritchard, A.: Williams' Obstetrics, 14th edition. Appleton-Century-Crofts, Inc., New York, 1971.

2. Page, W., Vilee, A. and Vilee, B.: Human Reproduction. W.B. Saunders Co., Philadelphia, 1972.

3. Blair, C.L. and Salerno, E.M.: The Expanding Family: Childbearing. Little, Brown and Co., Boston, 1976.

CHAPTER 21

ASSESSMENT OF THE NEWBORN

INTRODUCTION

The earlier chapters in this assessment guide have focused almost
exclusively upon the adult patient. Most of the information previously presented is transferrable to the evaluation of the infant and
child. However, the idea that the neonate and the child are but small
adults is an erroneous concept. It is important to recognize that
physiological, anatomical, and developmental considerations make
physical examination somewhat different. Some variations in examining techniques, in approach to the patient, and in interpretations
of findings are necessary. Birth events, patterns of growth, and
the accomplishments of developmental milestones are assessed in
the health status of infants and children. This chapter deals with
the differences between pediatric and adult physical evaluation.

When examining the newborn, you are primarily concerned with congenital deformities and metabolic disturbances. During the developing years, attention is given to signs of infection, endocrine disorder, malignancy and degenerative conditions, as well as impairment
of physiological functioning as a result of trauma. Throughout the
developing period you are also evaluating non-physical accomplishments: thought competency, interpersonal relationships, and development of self-concepts. All of these develop concurrently and
continuously interact and influence each other. There are specific
techniques to utilize, specific observations to make, and specific
questions to ask. The examiner must know what he is looking for.
Serendipity is not an asset in the examination.

We would like to point out that when you are examining the infant or
the child, you may also be dealing with the mother, or perhaps both
parents.

Careful explanation of each aspect of the examination and the findings to the parents who are standing by is a wise course to follow.
It serves to reassure them of competence and thoroughness in your
procedures, affords an opportunity for questions to be answered, and
helps to establish a relationship which may be extremely valuable if
referral or consultation for identified problems becomes necessary.
Every new parent is primarily concerned with the question, "Is my
child normal?" and when he is obviously ill, "What is the problem?"

THE NEWBORN

HISTORY: Prior to examination of the newborn, it is important to review the health history of the parents in terms of known medical conditions with hereditary characteristics which may influence the infant, such as diabetes and sickle cell anemia. The existence of genetically transmitted anomalies in the family will also give cues to observations which must be made. In addition, it is important to obtain information about the pregnancy and the delivery. Was there exposure to infections such as German measles, or teratogenic agents such as x-ray or drugs, early in the pregnancy? What were the results of RH typing and serology? Was there an elevation of the mother's blood pressure, indicating pre-eclampsia or bleeding due to placenta praevia with possible fetal anoxia? Was there use of analgesics and anesthetics throughout a long and difficult labor? Were forceps required or cesarean section performed because of cephalopelvic disproportion? Any of these factors might indicate potential problems with the infant and emphasize the necessity for close observation in the neonatal period.

EXAMINATION

The neonate is examined several times: immediately after birth, in the nursery, and once again prior to hospital discharge. This is usually about three days after delivery when the effects of maternal analgesia and anesthesia have passed and some adjustment to the new environment has occurred. He has, of course, been observed constantly by hospital staff while quiet, while active, and while feeding.

GENERAL: Cry, color, posture, size, respirations, body proportions, nutritional status, and movements of the head and extremities are evaluated.

The Apgar score at one minute and then at five minutes will give the examiner a beginning clue to the infant's general status (Table 21.1).

Obvious malformation such as anencephaly, missing limbs, and omphalocele will be recorded here, and then described in detail under the system involved. The weight and length of the infant are also noted. The neonate whose birthweight is under 2,500 grams is considered premature and will require special attention.

The newborn's temperature is taken first by rectum to determine rectal patency, but may be taken later by axilla or groin. It is not unusual to find a temperature of 34.5-36°C. (94-97°F.). Lower readings may occur as a result of birth trauma or a low environmental temperature. Elevated temperatures may mean dehydration after the third day, brain damage, or infection.

TABLE 21.1			
APGAR SCORE			
CRITERION		SCORE	
Heart rate	2 100-140	1 100	0 0
Breathing and cry	Immediate and strong	Fair	Apnea
Reflex irritability	Good	Fair	0
Muscle tone	Good	Fair or increased	Flaccid
Color	Pink	Fair	Blue
A score of 8-10 is excellent, 4-7 guarded, and 0-3 critical.			

Most examiners find it helpful to proceed as in the adult with the physical evaluation from head to toe in order to establish a systematic approach and ensure a thorough assessment. However, with infants, it may be a wise decision to auscultate the heart and the lungs first, for once the baby begins to cry as a result of turning and lifting, listening with the stethoscope becomes more difficult.

The Skin: The skin of the newborn should be observed as in the adult for color, hydration, texture, hemorrhages, and tumors.

Cyanosis, frequently present on the hands and feet, is referred to as acrocyanosis, and is due to sluggish capillary blood flow and cool surface temperature, but may be quite normal during the first 4 hours or even throughout the neonatal period. It will most likely diminish gradually, first from the hands and then from the feet, but if cyanosis remains beyond that time, a pathological cause may exist. Circumoral cyanosis in the neonate is definitely a danger signal. Since cyanosis is also influenced by the infant's crying, this phenomenon should be specifically recorded, if present.

In evaluation of pallor in the newborn, accompanying cardiac signs must be identified. For example, bradycardia usually accompanies the pallor of anoxia, while tachycardia usually accompanies anemia.

Although an erythematous flush over the body may be normal for 24 hours, a prolonged beefy red color over the entire body may indicate significant polycythemia, or possibly hypoglycemia. Vasomotor responses to temperature changes leading to "mottling" especially over the trunk and extremities are not unusual. The Harlequin sign, when one-half the body is red and the other half pale is usually temporary and not pathological.

Jaundice is usually a normal physiological finding after 48 hours of age, but its occurrence prior to this time is most often pathologic. It should be carefully looked for in the skin, sclera, mucous membranes, and nail beds of the newborn. For the most part, jaundice appearing within the first 48 hours may signify hemolytic disease, while jaundice which appears or persists for more than two weeks may indicate biliary obstruction.

Scratches, petechiae, and ecchymosis as a result of birth trauma are not unusual, particularly when forceps have been used; however, since they may also be indicative of infection or hemorrhagic diseases, they must be noted. A bluish pigmentation which may resemble an ecchymosis over the back or buttocks is called Mongolian spot and is of no clinical significance.

Telangiectases are quite common on the base of the neck, base of the nose, and the center of the forehead as well as on the eyelids, where they are known as nevus flammeus. Pigmented nevi and hemangiomas are birthmarks found any time during the first year of life, but the disfiguring permanent port-wine stain shows itself at birth.

Although local edema may be seen temporarily on the presenting part as well as on the genitalia of both sexes, generalized edema is characteristically seen in premature infants, infants of diabetic mothers, and in infants with severe RH incompatibility.

Additional normal characteristics of the newborn's skin include desquamation and milia, which are pinpoint white spots not surrounded by erythema, usually over the bridge of the nose, chin or cheeks.

The Head: Examination of the skull of the neonate is different because there are open sutures and anterior and posterior fontanelles. The fontanelles must be evaluated for their size and tension. The anterior fontanelle measures 4-6 cm. in its largest diameter at birth and normally closes between 5-18 months. The posterior fontanelle is 1-2 cm. at birth and usually closes by 2 months. Pulsations reflect the peripheral pulse. Bulging fontanelles are an indication of increased intracranial pressure, most commonly caused by hydrocephalus, meningitis, or intracranial hemorrhage. Depressed fontanelles are most commonly seen in dehydration and inanition. It will be necessary to measure the head circumference in order to have a base from which to observe skull growth which, in turn, indicates the development of the brain. At birth, the normal range for head circumference is 32 to 37.5 cm. for boys and 32 to 36 cm. for girls. We expect to find that the head circumference is 0.5 cm. or more, greater than the chest or abdomen. Tables are available indicating the norms for head circumference at various ages.

It is not unusual to observe asymmetry of the head because of intra-uterine molding, or to find masses such as cephalohematomas or caput succedaneum. Cephalohematoma is a soft and fluctuant, well-defined mass confined within the edges of the bone margin, not crossing the suture lines. Caput succedaneum is characterized by a soft, but ill-defined enlargement crossing suture lines, not fluc-tuant, and pitting on pressure. Although representing birth trauma, neither of these is cause for alarm in the absence of neurological signs.

Palpation of the newborn's head for craniotabes (Fig. 21.1) can best be accomplished by pressing the scalp firmly just behind and above the ears in the temporoparietal or parieto-occipital area. A crack-ling sound (crepitation) represents a softening of the outer table of the skull found in premature infants, some normal infants under six months of age, and a variety of conditions such as hydrocephalus, syphilis, osteogenesis imperfecta, etc.

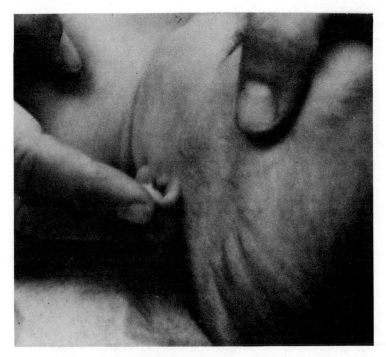

FIG. 21.1: Palpation of the head for craniotabes.

The Face: In general, the face is inspected for symmetry and paralysis. The distribution of facial hair is noted especially in the
premature baby. A small size chin referred to as micrognathia has
importance because the infant can experience breathing difficulties
due to the tongue falling backward and obstructing the nasopharynx.

The Ears: The height or positioning of the ears on the neonatal skull
is important to evaluate because there is a strong association between low-set ears and renal malformation or other chromosomal
aberrations such as Down's syndrome. Be careful, as you examine
the newborn's ears, to visualize the tympanic membrane. The largest speculum possible for the size of the canal should be used but
not passed deeply into it. Pull the pinna downward in infants. The
light reflex may be diffuse and not cone-shaped. Within a few days
of birth, deafness may be identified in the neonate, if he fails to respond to the snapping of fingers or a loud noise, with an eyelid twitch
or a complete Moro reflex. (The reflex is described later in the
section on Neurological Examination.)

The Eyes: The eyes of the neonate should be examined for structure
and function; however, since only peripheral vision is present during
the first few weeks, eye movements are normally uncoordinated.
Since the newborn's eyes are usually held tightly closed at rest, lift
him upright and turn him slowly to observe sclera, pupils, and extraocular movements. Discharges may be evident soon after birth,
primarily due to chemical irritation at first, ophthalmia neonatorum
(gonorrhea) within the first week, and viral infection later.

A Mongoloid slant in a Caucasian infant, represented by a lateral
upward slope with an inner epicanthal fold, may suggest chromosomal abnormality.

The newborn's eyes frequently demonstrate a searching nystagmus
and intermittent strabismus, but these conditions should disappear.
Ptosis of the eyelids is always a cause for concern. Drooping eyelids reduce the amount of light the retina receives and stunts its development. The assessment of vision is based on the presence of
visual reflexes, direct and consensual pupillary constriction in response to light, blinking in response to bright light and an object
quickly moved toward the eyes, as well as nystagmus produced by
rapid movement of vertical black lines across the visual fields.

Conjunctival or scleral hemorrhages are commonly found in the newborn and are rarely significant.

Although absence of the pupillary reflex is not uncommon during the
first three weeks of life, unilateral constrictions or dilation or continued absence of the reflex may represent pathology. It may be difficult to examine the fundus of the newborn because a strong orbicu-
laris muscle keeps the eyelid closed and retraction is almost

impossible. Examination will be facilitated in a slightly darkened room. Use of a cotton tip applicator placed adjacent to each row of lashes or an infant lid retractor may be necessary in order to observe for the red reflex and fundal landmarks with the ophthalmoscope.

The Nose: Patency of the nose may be tested immediately after birth with the attempt to insert a tiny suction catheter. A non-patent nasal passageway, represented by respiratory difficulties, may be associated with choanal atresia. Although sneezing of mucus is common, thick bloody discharge suggests congenital syphilis. Flaring of the nostrils is a positive finding which indicates respiratory distress.

The Mouth: The mouth should be inspected for hare lip (cleft lip) and cleft palate, as well as for the presence of tumors and cysts. The sucking, rooting, and gag reflexes should be tested. A nipple pressed to the side of the mouth should elicit a turning and sucking response by the newborn. After a day or two, absence of these reflexes may indicate brain damage. The presence of flat, white curds clinging to the mucous membranes of the newborn's mouth may represent thrush, a fungus infection which is a serious threat to the nutritional status of the infant because he is unable to suck without pain. Although spitting up and occasional vomiting are common in the newborn infant, persistent and projectile vomiting may indicate serious intestinal obstruction or neurological problems.

The pharynx can best be examined while the baby cries. Avoid the tongue blade as it may create a strong reflex elevation of the tongue and block the view. A shrill or high-pitched cry may be indicative of increased intracranial pressure. There should be very little saliva. Large amounts present in the newborn may indicate tracheo-esophageal fistula. Tonsillar tissue should not be present at birth.

The Neck: The neck is observed by placing one hand behind the upper back and allowing the head to fall gently into extension. The finding of a mass or deviated trachea may indicate any one of a variety of problems such as torticollis, fractured clavicle, or thyroglossal duct cyst.

The neck should be turned from side to side to elicit the normally-found tonic neck reflex. When the head is turned in one direction, with the infant on his back, the arm and leg on that side extend while the opposite arm and leg flex. This is the "fencer position." Absence of this reflex, which normally continues for 2 to 3 months, or prolonged maintenance to 4 or 5 months, may indicate central nervous system damage.

The Chest: The chest and abdomen of the newborn should be examined as a unit for their symmetry or fullness. Asymmetry may be due to a variety of pulmonary conditions as well as the presence of a diaphragmatic hernia with the intestine lodged on one side of the chest. Unequal excursion of the chest during respiration can point to atelectasis of a lung or a spontaneous pneumothorax, as in the adult. The AP diameter is usually equal to the transverse diameter at birth.

Enlargement of the breast, usually due to maternal hormones, may be seen in both sexes. Secretion of small amounts of milk from the newborn's nipple is rarely significant unless there is redness around the nipple. When this is apparent on only one side, a breast abscess is suspected. Extra nipples may be found. Wide-set nipples may be an indication of genetic disorder, i.e., Turner's syndrome.

The Lungs: Respiration in the newborn is chiefly abdominal, and from 30-50 per minute, irregular in rate and depth. Weak, grossly-slow or very rapid rates, and grunting are clues to pathological situations, but rales are normally heard in the newborn for the first few days. The breath sounds of the infant are broncho-vesicular, relatively louder than those of the adult, and may vary according to position. Breathing is usually alternatingly shallow and slow, then rapid and deep. The sound may be diminished on the side of the chest opposite the direction in which the head is turned. Intercostal, subcostal, and suprasternal retraction indicate labored breathing found in respiratory distress syndromes. Apnea may be found for short periods in normal newborns.

The Heart: Upon palpation, the apex of the newborn's heart may be found lateral to the midclavicular line and in the third or fourth interspace because it lies more horizontally than in the adult. The heart rate is regular but varies from 100 to 180 at birth. It soon regulates itself at 120-140 beats per minute. The first heart sound (S_1) is usually louder than the second heart sound (S_2) in infants at the apex. In the newborn, because of changing hemodynamics during the neonatal state, murmurs may become obvious only after the first several days, so that the need for repeated examinations becomes evident. It is often difficult to identify slight murmurs in infants because of their crying during the examination, so that it may become important to use a pacifier to quiet the baby. Murmurs are usually heard at the left sternal border in the third or fourth interspace or over the base of the heart, rather than at the apex. The most significant factor related to differentiation between innocent and organic murmurs are the findings of other significant cardiovascular signs, pulses, color, respiration, etc.

In the aortic area a thrill which radiates to the right side of the neck may indicate aortic stenosis, while in the pulmonic area a thrill radiating to the left side of the neck may indicate pulmonary stenosis (Fig. 21.2).

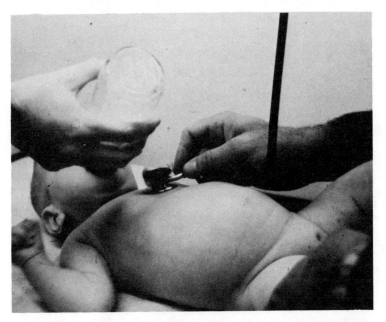

FIG. 21.2: Listening for heart sounds without interference with
crying.

The Abdomen: Examine the neonate's umbilical cord for the presence
of two umbilical arteries and one vein. A single umbilical artery
may be associated with other anomalies, especially of the heart and
kidney. In the newborn, the abdomen is protuberant because of   .
poorly developed musculature. It should be examined for distention,
scaphoid abdomen (depression due to dehydration or large diaphragmatic hernia), weakness or absence of abdominal muscles, dilated
veins, and visible peristaltic activity. Although the infant is an abdominal breather, excessive excursion may indicate pulmonary
disease.

Palpation of the abdomen for masses is especially important in the
newborn, but auscultation for bowel sounds should be done before
palpation because palpation may stimulate crying. Metallic tinkling
every 10-30 seconds can be heard normally. Usually the spleen tip
may be palpable under the left costal margin, and a liver edge can be
felt 2-3 cm. below the right costal margin. When examining the newborn, it is wise to begin the palpation in the lower quadrants and
move upward so as not to miss these organs. Hold the legs flexed at
the knees and hips with the left hand and palpate with the right.

In order to palpate the kidneys, the infant should be raised at a 45 degree angle with one hand supporting the occiput and neck and flexing the knees for relaxation, while the other hand palpates for the lower half of the right and the tip of the left kidney which can normally be felt in the newborn. Flank masses are usually of renal or adrenal origin, such as congenital hydronephrosis and Wilms' tumor.

The bladder may be percussed or palpated 1-4 cm. above the symphysis or at the level of the umbilicus. A markedly distended bladder may be difficult to palpate, so percussion is also necessary. Distention may indicate congenital urethral obstruction.

Genitalia: There are a variety of malformations which may affect the genitalia. Some are chromosomal in origin, while others may be due to the ingestion of hormonal drugs during the first trimester. An unusually large clitoris is found in pseudohermaphroditism, but since it may be a small penis, the urethral meatus should be identified. In the male, hypospadius, in which the urethral meatus is not on the glans, is common. Occasionally, there is an opening in the glans, but a secondary opening on the ventral surface of the penis is also present. The foreskin should be partially retracted, allowing inspection of the urethral meatus for patency and position. The testes should be palpated in the scrotum, which may appear enlarged, especially after breech delivery. The observation that one or both of the testes have not descended is significant. Although this is usually accomplished during the eighth lunar month of fetal development, it may take several months after birth or even years to occur and may require medical or surgical intervention. Look for hydroceles and hernias which are common findings in male infants.

In the female, a vaginal vault must be seen. The hymenal ring generally is protruding through the introitus and the labia are engorged due to the effect of maternal hormones. Fusion of the labia indicates a serious anomaly whereas simple adhesion may be due to inflammation. A slight bloody discharge may be quite normal in female infants for as long as a month and a thick white discharge may also be normally present.

Rectal temperatures should be taken judiciously, since imperforate anus may exist. It is imperative that consultation for rectal examination be made immediately in any suspicious case. If substantial amounts of normal meconium stool have been passed and there is no abdominal distention, there is no need to question the patency of the rectum.

Back and Extremities: The newborn should then be placed on his abdomen and the spine inspected and palpated for spina bifida, pilonidal sinus, and curvatures of the spine such as scoliosis. Tufts of hair over the spine and sacral areas may mask spina bifida or spina bifida occulta. The observation of symmetrical bilateral muscle movement of the hips and knees as the infant assumes intrauterine position

will give clues to possible problems. The extremities of the infant
are noted and fingers counted. Polydactyly (extra) and syndactyly
(fused fingers) are noted. Normally his elbows, hips, and knees
do not extend completely. The infant's hips must be examined for
dislocation by rotating the thighs with the knees flexed. Usually
they may be abducted and externally rotated so that the knees touch
the table top (Fig. 21.3). Unilateral subluxation will result in
limited abduction on the affected side. Flexion, external rotation,
and abduction of his hip can reveal limitation of motion or cause a
"pop" or sharp click of dislocation (Fig. 21.4). Although soft clicks
are common in the hips and knees, any suspicious finding such as
an uneven buttock and non-symmetrical thigh crease posteriorly
should warrant referral for hip x-ray of the infant (Fig. 21.5).

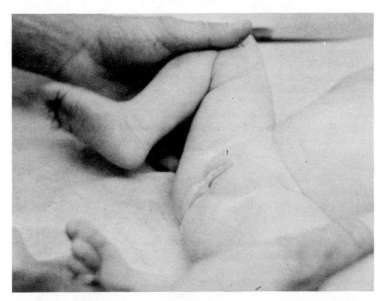

FIG. 21.3: Examination for hip dislocation.

The feet of the newborn may appear to be deformed as they retain
their intrauterine position. In examining the newborn's feet for anomalies, first scratch the outside, then the inside of the lower border
of the foot, which should make his foot assume a right angle with his
leg. If he has a clubfoot or metatarsus varus, it will not respond
appropriately, or may possibly respond only with forceful stretching.
True deformities do not allow manipulation to even the neutral position. Minor abnormalities may be evident, such as bowing of the
tibia. This is generally self-correcting. Metatarsus abductus, which
is a fixed angulation between the fore-foot and the hind-foot, generally

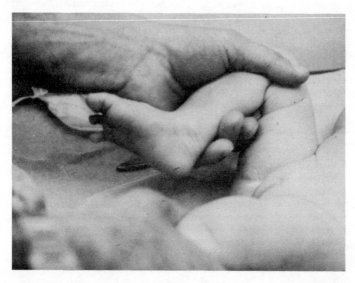

FIG. 21.4: Note position and action of examiner's hand as he checks for dislocation clicks.

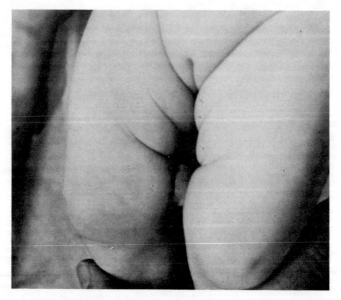

FIG. 21.5: Normally symmetrical thigh creases.

requires orthopedic care. Signs of congenital anomalies and chromosomal defects such as Down's syndrome include hyperextension of the phalanges and wrists, short, spadelike hands, simian crease (continuous crease across the palm), and a divergent great toe with a deep line on the sole between the first and second toes.

NEUROLOGICAL

Throughout the examination we have been evaluating the neurological function; observation of positioning, examination of muscle tone, reflex patterns, and listening to his cry. The normal lusty cry of the newborn can readily be distinguished from the weak, cat-like cry referred to as "cri-du-chat" of a neurological disorder. Since the nervous system is not completely developed, findings in the neonatal period will not coincide with those of the older infant or child.

A variety of responses which are present at birth, or appear shortly thereafter, including the grasp reflex (Fig. 21.6) will remain for only a short time or persist for a year or two. Several of these are mentioned here. In order to elicit the Moro reflex which should be present at birth, the infant's crib is jarred suddenly. The neonate should react by extending his arms, then flexing them with his hands clenched, and drawing his knees and hips up. This reflex should be present until about three to five months of age; its absence at birth or persistence after five months is indicative of severe central nervous system damage. In addition, if you observe him during his response for symmetry of movement of the arms and legs, you may observe signs of asymmetry due to fractured humerus, brachial nerve palsy, or recently fractured clavicle in the upper extremities; spinal cord injury, dislocated hip and myelomeningocele, which are identified by irregular reflex of one leg. Other examples are tonic neck reflex which also disappears after 4-5 months, as well as the sucking and rooting reflexes. The Babinski reflex is normal in the infant, but should not be present past the age of two (Fig. 21.7).

REFERENCES

1. Frakenburg, W.D.: Denver Developmental Screening Test Manual. University of Colorado Medical Center and Mead Johnson, Denver, 1968.

2. Barness, L.A.: Manual of Pediatric Physical Diagnosis. Year Book Medical Publishers, Chicago, 1969.

3. Graham, B.D.: Pediatric Examination in Physical Diagnosis. C.V. Mosby Co., St. Louis, 1969.

4. Vaughan, V.C and McKay, R.J. (eds.) Nelson's Textbook of Pediatrics, 10th edition. W.B. Saunders Co., Philadelphia, 1975.

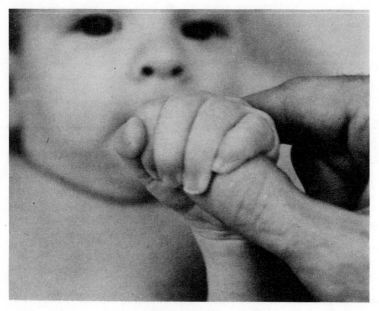

FIG. 21.6: Grasp reflex.

5. Barness, L.A.: Manual of Pediatric Physical Diagnosis, 4th edition. Year Book Medical Publishers, Chicago, 1972.

6. Chinn, P.L. and Leitch, C.: Child Health Maintenance: A Guide to Clinical Assessment. C.V. Mosby Co., St. Louis, 1974.

7. Barnett, H.L. (ed.): Pediatrics, 15th edition. Appleton-Century-Crofts, 1972.

8. Committee on Standards of Child Care, American Academy of Pediatrics, "Health Care of the Children and Youth." June, 1974.

9. Hoekelman, R.: The Pediatric Examination. In Bates, B.: A Guide to Physical Examination. J.B. Lippincott Co., Philadelphia, 1974.

10. Alexander, M.M. and Brown, M.S.: Pediatric Physical Diagnosis for Nurses. McGraw-Hill Book Co., New York, 1974.

11. Philip, A.: Neonatology - A Practical Guide. Medical Examination Publishing Co., Inc., New York, 1977.

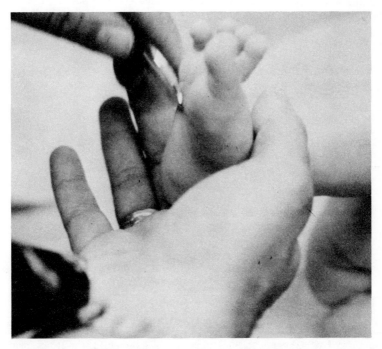

FIG. 21.7: Note the flaring and extension of toes characteristic of the Babinski reflex found in the infant.

CHAPTER 22

ASSESSMENT OF THE INFANT AND CHILD

INTRODUCTION

A regular schedule of examinations during the first year and continuing annually throughout childhood and adolescence sets a pattern for comprehensive health supervision that results in the early detection of health problems. For the most part, normal ranges of physiological development and behavioral abilities have been well-defined and are used as a comparison for the development and behavior observed in the child being evaluated.

The Recommendations for Preventive Health Care of Children and Youth* represents a guide for the care of well children who receive "competent parenting," who have not demonstrated any significant health problems, and who are growing and developing satisfactorily (Table 22.1). There are circumstances when additional visits or procedures may be recommended:

1. For first-born or adopted children, or those not with natural parents;
2. For parents with a particular need for education and guidance;
3. For children of a disadvantaged social or economic environment;
4. In the presence or possibility of perinatal disorders (such as congenital defects or familial disease);
5. For acquired illness or previously identified disease or problems.

HISTORY: The general guidelines for taking a history are adapted as necessary for the age of the child and the conditions surrounding the visit. Whenever possible, permit the older child to tell his own story first.

It will be necessary during an initial visit to gather data significant to the child's previous health. No matter what the age of the child, no assessment can be complete if the examiner is not aware of the antenatal, natal, and neonatal history. Significant factors relating to the health of the mother during pregnancy, parents' medical problems, infections during pregnancy, vomiting, toxemia, and bleeding

---

* Committee on Standards of Child Health Care of the American Academy of Pediatrics, June 1974.

TABLE 22.1: Recommendations for Preventive Health Care of Children and Youth

AGE[2]	2-4 Wks.	2-3 Mos.	4-5 Mos.	6-7 Mos.	9-10 Mos.	12-15 Mos.	16-19 Mos.	23-25 Mos.	35-37 Mos.	5-6 Yrs.	8-9 Yrs.	11-12 Yrs.	13-15 Yrs.	16-21 Yrs.
HISTORY														
Initial	·	·	·	·	·	·	·	At first visit	·	·	·	·	·	·
Interval	·	·	·	·	·	·	·	At each visit	·	·	·	·	·	·
MEASUREMENTS														
Height & Weight	·	·	·	·	·	·	·	At each visit	·	·	·	·	·	·
Head Circumference	▨	▨	▨	▨	▨	▨		▨						
Blood Pressure									▨	▨	▨	▨	▨	▨
SENSORY SCREENING														
Sight[3]	▨	▨	▨	▨	▨					▨ OR	▨	▨	▨	▨
Hearing[4]				▨	▨					▨ OR				
DEVELOPMENTAL APPRAISAL[5]	·	·	·	·	·	·	·	At each visit	·	·	·	·	·	·
PHYSICAL EXAM	·	·	·	·	·	·	·	At each visit	·	·	·	·	·	·
PROCEDURES[6]														
Immunization		▨	▨	▨		▨	▨			▨		▨		
Tuberculin Test[7]					▨					▨		▨		
Hematocrit or Hgb.					▨					▨ OR		▨		
Urinalysis[8]									▨					▨
Urine Culture (girls only)[9]										▨	▨	▨		
DISCUSSION & COUNSELING[10]	·	·	·	·	·	·	·	At each visit	·	·	·	·	·	·
DENTAL SCREENING[11]	·	·	·	·	·	·	·	At each visit	·	·	·	·	·	·
INIT. DENTIST'S EXAM[12]									▨					

1. Applicable in context of accompanying explanatory text and footnote references.

2. If a child comes under care for the first time at any point on the Schedule, or if any items are not accomplished at the suggested age, the Schedule should be brought up-to-date at the earliest possible time.

3. *Manual on Standards of Child Health Care*, 2nd Edition. Page 8 for details.

4. Ibid. Page 9, 127-130.

5. Ibid. Page 23-32, 120-126, 132-134, 140-144. Developmental appraisal is an integral part of each visit. Employ a standardized format at any time there is suspicion of developmental delay.

6. Ibid, page 131. *Report of the Committee on Infectious Diseases*, (Red Book) 17th Edition, 1973.

7. May be indicated yearly in certain areas and population.

8. At least 5-test dipstick.

9. Taken in morning, see Kunin, C.M., *Detection, Prevention and Management of Urinary Tract Infection*, Lea & Febiger, Philadelphia, 1972, Pages 60-69, for suggested methods.

10. *Manual on Standards of Child Health Care*, 2nd Edition, Pages 13-21. Discussion and counseling of child by the physician is of increasing importance at age 11 years and thereafter.

11. Ibid., Pages 11-13. Appendix 1, I. 135. Physician should inspect teeth and check on dental hygiene throughout childhood.

12. Subsequent exams as prescribed by dentist.

Key: ▨ to be performed.

complications are all pertinent. The examiner should know about the birth process: gestation, birthweight, duration of labor, type of delivery, sedation and anesthesia, state of infant at birth, etc. In addition, significant events occurring during the neonatal period, such as jaundice, cyanosis, convulsions, and feeding difficulties, should be reviewed.

The accomplishment of developmental milestones and nutrition must be evaluated. When did he first roll over, sit alone, walk, talk, and attain bladder and bowel control? How did he compare to his siblings? What of growth events and adjustments to school? Breast or bottle feeding, type of formula, solid foods, eating habits and allergies are relevant factors in the health history.

A review of all immunizations received, including response, should be clearly established and recorded.

No history is complete for the child without reference to personality factors, e.g., relations with siblings, other children, adjustments and achievement in school. The child's habits should be reviewed: eating, sleeping, exercise, urinary, bowel, and any evidence of disturbance clarified (e.g., excessive bedwetting, breath-holding, temper tantrums).

The relationship between parents and child can be observed throughout the interview and the examination and is of invaluable assistance in identifying potential or existing problems which require guidance and, perhaps, referral.

Use of the problem-oriented record helps to assure that no data are lost. The health record should be carefully maintained throughout the duration of the relationship between health professional and the family and made available whenever referral or consultation is necessary.

APPROACH TO EXAMINATION OF THE CHILD: The clinician will need to develop the skill, in approach to children, which is similar in objective to that cited earlier when relating to adults. Since each child is unique in his behavior and response to strangers, depending upon his age, relationship with parents, and emotional health, it is often difficult to anticipate the response he will make to the introductions and procedures necessary during the physical evaluation. When he is ill, it is even harder to accept the interference from the stranger examining him, who may remove him from the secure arms of his mother. Actually, much of the examination may be done while the child is sitting on his mother's lap or held over her shoulders. When the child sits on the high examining table, he is approached by the examiner at eye level, which may initiate an atmosphere of mutual respect. A friendly, kind, gentle, patient examiner with a soft voice will certainly have a better chance to accomplish his mission than one who rushes and quickly resorts to force and restraint.

Every attempt should be made to develop a trusting relationship by explaining what is being done, whether or not the child is old enough to understand every word. Even if the child is not old enough to fully understand what you are explaining, the words may be soothing and reassuring, if only to his mother standing nearby.

Although there may be differences of opinion on whether it is appropriate or wise to give the child advance notice of a potentially painful procedure, we find that most children, regardless of the age, prefer to be told the truth. Don't tell him it won't hurt if, in fact, it might.

The practitioner with imagination may dispel many of the fears a child may have of the variety of instruments used, by developing techniques of story stelling and games; but, of course, the ability to use these effectively or the assurance that the child will respond appropriately cannot be universally guaranteed. There may be times when no amount of creativity or playing will work, and some gentle restraint, preferably by the mother, will be necessary. If the need is explained in terms of safety and prevention of pain, a greater degree of cooperation may be elicited and may minimize any long-term negative effect.

The examiner should always wash his hands in warm water before touching the child. Undress the infant slowly to avoid drafts and chills. When appropriate, have the child himself, or his mother, do the undressing. Never assume that an infant is too young to roll off the table or a toddler reliable enough not to try to jump off. Watch that no sharp objects are left within the child's reach. The examination sequence may need alteration in order to deal with a restless child or prevent a painful or frightening task from stimulating a response in the child which will make continuation difficult. Some examiners prefer to reverse the order of adult examination and work from toes to head, while others begin with auscultation of the chest. This is usually painless and mystifying to the child and, if accompanied by an opportunity to hear his own heart (providing the age is suitable), it can be a fascinating experience which may make him more cooperative throughout the remainder of the procedure. In any event, you may have a few minutes of quiet before he responds with hysterical crying, making auscultation almost impossible. It is wise to leave the examination of the ears, nose, and mouth to the end, for these may certainly initiate negative responses.

It may also be necessary to skip some minor parts of the examination which have consistently been negative in findings during previous examinations in order to work quickly and not prolong the experience; however, never fail to examine the heart, throat, ears, lungs and abdomen.

An attempt to thoroughly describe here the procedure for examination of the child would result in a review of much of what has been said during the examination of the newborn, and what has been said during examination of the adult throughout the text. A few simple suggestions should suffice, in terms of modifications of the basic procedures to the examination of the growing child. Since it would be impossible to include in this text a complete survey of the range of normal findings during each stage of child development, the student is referred to any of the fine pediatric textbooks for further information regarding clinical data.

General Inspection: The examiner should look at the child and evaluate his general appearance. Does he look ill? Review general state of comfort, cooperation, nutrition, facial expression, consciousness, gait, posture, coordination, activity, and level of intelligence. What is his relationship with parents or guardians? How does he respond to the examination and the examinee?

It is appropriate to take the temperature, pulse rate, respiratory rate, blood pressure, weight, and height during each examination and compare these not only to the previous records, but to standard charts of normal values, remembering the wide variations in patterns. When there is a question regarding progress in height and weight, referral should be made to a pediatrician for evaluation. The mother can be instructed how to take the infant's temperature rectally in the office. This is then a much less frightening experience for both. A rectal temperature up to 37.8°C. (100° F.) is normal.

The Skin: The skin of the infant and young child should, of course, be observed for color, texture, turgor, and lesions. Pallor in the young child may be an indication of anemia, which requires laboratory evaluation. Taking a dietary history will help the clinician in evaluating an anemia when no cardiorespiratory causes are involved, and in outlining a plan for teaching, once therapy is indicated.

One or two patches of small, light brown non-elevated stains (café-au-lait spots) are within normal range; however, more than seven may be indicative of fibromas or neurofibromatoses. In children, turgor may be readily evaluated by feeling the calf of the leg, which should feel firm. Newborns, premature, and dehydrated infants may have loose, extra skin at the calf. Pitting edema is always a pathological sign, usually associated with long-term heart disease or kidney disease.

The most common skin disease of infancy is diaper rash. This may range from simple chafing to mild erythematous non-raised areas, to bright red, raised papules which form ulcers when they open, and may even become infected with organisms such as staphylococci, Candida albicans, or streptococci.

There is a variety of skin lesions which occur more often in children than in adults. The practitioner should take a careful history to identify possible causes and then describe the lesions specifically. With experience, characteristic data from history and description provide diagnostic clues which aid the examiner in problem solving. For example, eczema of infancy, occasionally associated with cow's milk sensitivity, reflects itself most often by scaliness on the cheeks, behind the ears, knees, and at the elbows. Flakiness on the head, especially over the fontanelles, is an indication of seborrhea, dermatitis, or cradle cap. Infectious conditions such as impetigo are frequently found in areas where children are living in close quarters, such as nursery schools or camps. The child usually demonstrates pustules filled with yellowish exudate, often crusted over, most frequently around the mouth and on the hands. Ringworm also occurs frequently in children. It can be identified by its characteristic scaliness. Erythematous lesions may be due to systemic disease. In rheumatoid arthritis, for example, painful, tender, reddened nodules 2-4 cm. in diameter along the fibula of the leg or ulnar surface of the arms are known as Erythema nodosum. Erythema marginatum is demonstrated by 1-2 cm. circular reddened areas with concrete borders and may be seen in children who have rheumatic fever.

The practitioner must also be aware of the significance of bruises. Ecchymoses and hematomas, especially on the extremities, are not unusual in healthy, active children. In fact, the absence of bruises in a pre-schooler is suspicious and may be indicative of a hypoactive child. However, when there is a history of weakness, fatigue, general malaise, and spontaneous bruises over the body, blood dyscrasias such as leukemia, platelet disorders, or hemophilia should be suspected. The abused or battered child will also appear with bruises over the body, but there is usually a history of unusual events and peculiar circumstances surrounding their occurrence. The practitioner should know that a few small pigmented nevi or spider nevi are commonly found in children.

The heads and hair of children should be examined carefully for signs of lice, mites, or ticks, especially when they live in the country or have animals who travel outdoors. Patches of unusual hair color may indicate pathology. In protein deficiency, the hair tips may have a reddish-rust color. The infant with a single patch of white hair may have a condition referred to as Waardenburg's syndrome, which may have an associated condition of congenital deafness.

The Head: During the first year the head is measured at its greatest circumference regularly and plotted on a growth curve scale to be compared to normal values (see Appendix III). Auscultation of the skull to detect a bruit is useless until the age of 6, because normal children have a bruit over the temporal area until that time. The head should be observed for control, positioning, and movements.

There should be no head lag past 3 months. In the event that the infant cannot control his head after that time, cerebral palsy may be suspected. If the infant sleeps on one side, flattening may occur.

The Face: The face should be evaluated for symmetry, paralysis, distribution of hair, size of mandible, swellings, and tenderness over sinuses.

The Ears: Examination of the ears assumes greater significance in childhood than it does in the adult because of the frequency of infections. Never fail to examine the child's ears. Gradually insert the largest speculum as possible to avoid discomfort. Rest one finger against the head so that any sudden movements will not result in injury. The child can be restrained by laying him on his abdomen. Pull the auricle back and down in infants, back and up in older children. Preschool children should have their hearing tested by the practitioner whispering simple commands at a distance of 8 feet. Tuning forks of pitches from 512 cps to over 2000 cps may also be used with this age group. A complete screening test with an audiometer should be done on all children before they start first grade. Evaluation of hearing on a regular basis should not be missed, since often even minor problems may result in inability to maintain scholastic activities in school, and false diagnosis of emotional mental disabilities may be made when, in fact, the problem is one of deafness.

The Eyes: The child's eyes should be examined as much as possible as described in Chapter 9 and the parents questioned about any difficulty they may have noticed, such as stumbling or complaints about double vision. A mild degree of strabismus may be present during the first 6 months, but is abnormal after that time. Most infants produce visible tears during the first few days of life.

In children over three years of age, a Snellen E chart can be used for testing visual acuity. Once the child knows his alphabet, a regular letter Snellen chart can be used for this testing. Visual acuity at three years is 20/40; at four to five years, 20/30; and at six years, 20/20. During the school years, the practitioner can distinguish between simple refractive error and organic ocular disease by asking the child to take his acuity test by looking through a pinhole in a card. When the pinhole card is used, acuity improves if refractive error is the causative factor, but does not when organic disease is present.

The Mouth: When you examine the mouth before the throat, you give the child an opportunity to become familiar with the light and tongue blade. Then have him stick out his tongue and say "Ah" louder and louder. Occasionally the tongue blade is unnecessary.

The teeth should be examined for their sequence of eruption, number, character, and position during infancy and childhood. Most misalignment of teeth in the young nursery school-age child is caused by thumb sucking. If this habit disappears by the time the child is 6 years old, the problem of misalignment tends to disappear with secondary teeth. Children have their full complement of 20 primary teeth by 2-3 years of age. Eruption of secondary teeth begins about the time the child begins elementary school and ends in late adolescence.

The Throat: The child's throat is carefully examined (Fig. 22.1) and the size of the tonsils evaluated. Enlarged tonsils may not be significant unless they are a focus of infection or interfere with swallowing and nutrition. The adenoids are generally not visualized unless they are extremely enlarged. Enlarged adenoids may interfere with the child's breathing and speech.

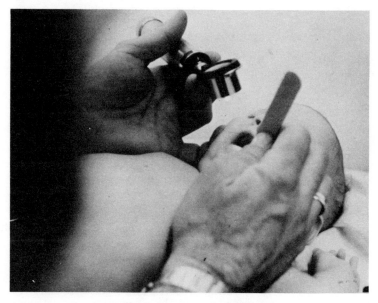

FIG. 22.1: Inspecting the pharynx.

The Neck: Neck mobility is an important assessment during childhood because of the possibility of central nervous system disease. Rigidity can be evaluated by placing the weight of the child's head in the examiner's hands while he is supine and flexing it. Resistance to movement may indicate meningitis. In the older child, the thyroid gland may be more easily defined with palpation from behind.

Lymphatic System: It is always necessary to evaluate the status of lymph glands in the child. Lymphadenopathy is usually a sign of infection but may be present with no other specific clinical complaints.

The anatomy of the drainage system should be reviewed to locate the infection site. For example, cervical adenitis usually indicates tonsilitis and pharyngitis, while submaxillary adenitis usually indicates stomatitis.

Thorax and Lungs: The thorax should be examined as in the adult for shape and symmetry, veins, retractions, and pulsations flaring of the ribs. Harrison's groove, pigeon breast, funnel shape, size and position of nipple, length of sternum, and intercostal or substernal retractions.

The thoracic wall, in infancy, is very thin so that ribs and sternum are readily seen. At about 1 year of age, the ratio of transverse diameter to anteroposterior diameter is 1:1.25. It changes little after age 6, when it is approximately 1:1.35 as in the normal adult.

Diaphragmatic breathing predominates with a simultaneous drawing-in of the lower thorax and protrusion of the abdomen on inspiration and the reverse on expiration. This is known as paradoxical respiration. Any unusual head movement with inspiration indicates severe respiratory disease. The percussion note heard throughout the infant's chest is normally hyperresonant. Any diminution may signify pathology.

It has been mentioned earlier that breath sounds in infants and children are normally louder and more bronchial in character, with expiration more prolonged than inspiration, than in adults. The clinician should use the bell or a small diaphragm stethoscope to listen to the infant's chest. This will provide for more specific location of sounds. Breath sounds are rarely absent in the infant or child even in the presence of disease because of the small size of the thorax and subsequent ease of transmission of sounds. The small size of the bronchial tube also allows for increased occurrence of rhonchi and rales. In order to distinguish between these, listen with the bell at the mouth and compare with what is heard at the chest, for while rhonchi can be heard orally, rales cannot.

Cardiovascular System: As the child grows older, it will become necessary to examine his blood pressure with a pediatric cuff. The blood pressure is normally 90/60 at about 6 years of age and about 110/65 at 10, when it begins to reach the normal adult reading.

Pulses should be examined, particularly the femorals, since the absence of a femoral pulse may indicate coarctation of the aorta. Normally, the newborn pulse of 120 per minute will drop to 80-90 by 7 to 9 years of age. In the child, because of the thin chest wall, the PMI is often visible between the 4th and 5th interspace. It is found left of the MCL before age 4, at MCL between 4 and 6 years of age, and right of the MCL after seven. The heart sounds are higher in pitch, shorter in duration. S_1 is louder than S_2 at the apex. Splitting of S_2 at the apex may produce an extra heart sound in one-fourth to one-third of all children. S_2 is louder than S_1 at the base and, although splitting here is rarely pathologic, referral may be indicated, especially when accompanied by other clinical findings.

Examine the heart with the child sitting up, lying down, and leaning to the left. Many children have sinus arrhythmias normally and premature ventricular contractions are not rare. Murmurs must be identified, and consultation should always take place when one is suspected. Physical signs related to cardiac disease such as inadequate weight gain, cyanosis, clubbing of fingers and toes, delayed development, tachypnea, tachycardia, heaving precordium, and edema, assist in the evaluation of significance of a murmur.

Any question or suspicion of cardiac disease requires early referral to a pediatric cardiologist. Final determination will require laboratory tests, chest x-rays, electrocardiograms, cardiac catheterizations, and other techniques. The clinician needs to assist the parents to understand why referral is indicated and to offer continued support. In order to encourage compliance with recommended regimens, counseling cannot be overemphasized.

The Abdomen: Protuberance of the abdomen may be seen throughout childhood when the child is standing on his feet. However, this should disappear when the child lies down. Infants often demonstrate umbilical hernias, ventral hernias, and diastasis recti, most often after two to three weeks of age. These are usually noted when the infant is crying. Most disappear within the first year. Because of the thin nature of the abdominal wall, superficial veins are often noted until puberty.

In children, light, superficial palpation of all quadrants should always precede deep palpation in order to prevent unsuspected discomfort. The area suspected as the site for pathology or pain should be examined last. If the child is particularly ticklish, try placing his hand partially under the examiner's. This should reduce sensitivity and permit relaxation. Verbal as well as non-verbal expressions such as facial grimaces will give clues to tenderness. Examine the spleen and liver, which are easily palpable in most children.

In young children, it may be difficult to localize intra-abdominal inflammation, for tenderness and spasm are rather diffuse. Pain in the right lower quadrant is frequently a sign of acute appendicitis, but is not necessarily specific. With the child lying supine, ask him to raise his head while you push down on the forehead. Extend the right leg at the hip as he lies on the left side, or flex and externally rotate the right leg at the hip with the knee flexed at 90 degrees. This should localize the pain in the RLQ. Examination for inguinal hernia is conducted as for the adult.

Extremities: The extremities should be checked for symmetry, mobility, unusual masses, infections, and joint pain. The wide range of joint motion of infancy diminishes during childhood until it reaches adult status.

Until about 18 months of age, there is a distinct bow-legged growth pattern. The appearance then becomes one of knock-knees until about 12 years. Twisting or torsion of the tibia inwardly or outwardly is common and usually corrects itself.

When the infant begins to walk, it appears as though he is flat-footed. Actually, this is because his legs are set wide apart and weight is borne on the inside of the feet. There is a degree of pronation of the feet and curving inward of the Achilles tendons. Since the longitudinal arch in infancy is hidden by adipose tissue, the foot appears flat. Watch the toddler and child in several positions, standing upright with the feet together, stooping and standing up to pick up something from the floor, and touching the toes. Have him shift his weight from one leg to the other to observe from behind signs of hip disease. The pelvis will tilt toward a diseased hip when weight-bearing occurs on the affected side, but will stay level with weight-bearing on the good side. Unequal limb signs can indicate blood vessel abnormalities or hip disease. Diminished mobility is generally caused by trauma. Masses such as ganglions of the tendon sheaths, and growths such as osteochondromas should be looked for. Joint pain can indicate trauma or neoplasms. When there is a question of possible growth disturbance, referral should be made to a pediatrician.

Neurological: We have already discussed much of the screening neurological examination conducted for the newborn and the infant. Examination during childhood is conducted quite similarly to that for the adult. In essence, throughout the history and physical examination, the clinician is gathering data significant for evaluation of the integrity of the central and peripheral nervous systems.

For review of all neurological findings, as in the adult, include evaluation of cerebral function, cranial nerves, cerebellar function, motor system, sensory system, and reflexes.

The Genitalia and Rectum: During the examination interview, consideration should be given to discussion of elimination habits and control. Many parents need assistance with problems which may exist or clarification of what is normal and what is not. Bedwetting is an anxiety-causing condition both for the child and the parents. It is advisable first to culture the urine to identify possible bladder or kidney infections which may be causing the problem and then explore with the parents other possible sources of stress. Since urinary infections are evidently more common than previously thought, particularly in young girls, urine cultures are recommended to be done annually in children between the ages of three and nine. When

symptoms present, more frequent examinations are necessary.
The size of the penis before puberty is not significant. In obese
boys the fat pad over the symphysis pubis may hide the penis.

To evaluate whether the testicles of the young boy have, in fact,
descended into the scrotum, have the child sit cross-legged on the
table. Palpation in this position will elminate reflexes which cause
apparent undescended testicle.

Examination of the female genitalia in young girls should be accompanied by explanations of organs, using a hand mirror. Vagino-
abdominal palpation to examine pelvic structures and direct visualization of the vagina and cervix are not considered part of the
screening physical examination at this age. If history or complaints
signify necessity for examination, referral should be made.

Rectal examination may be necessary when there is history of bleeding, pain, and severe constant constipation. The infant or child
should be in the supine position with knees and hips flexed upon the
abdomen with one hand while the examiner introduces the index finger of the other hand gently. Problems of this type are best dealt
with by a specialist.

Development (See Appendix II): Although we have mentioned the need
to evaluate growth and development several times in this chapter, it
is recommended again that the clinician become familiar with tests
such as the Denver Developmental Screening Test, a method used to
evaluate development and detect developmental delays in infancy and
preschool years, which is quite simple to administer. There are four
categories of testing: Gross Motor; Fine Motor - Adaptive; Language; and Personal-Social Development. This is not an intelligence
test, but is a screening instrument for use in clinical practice to determine whether a particular child is within the normal range. If
unexplained developmental delays are found, it is important to refer
him for further and more detailed diagnostic study.

We would like to emphasize that careful records of significant findings should be maintained, preferably in the problem-oriented method
we have described earlier in this text. This will serve as a method
of communicating the developmental changes which will occur, as well
as the record of preventive and therapeutic intervention.

SUPPLEMENTAL EXERCISES

1. Obtain copies of growth charts (see Appendix III for samples and
   details).

2. Describe how to elicit each of the following:
   Macewen's sign
   Chvostek's sign
   Transillumination of the skull

Setting sun sign
Doll's eye test
Brushfields' spots
Epstein's pearls

REFERENCES

1. Frakenburg, W.D.: Denver Developmental Screening Test Manual. University of Colorado Medical Center and Mead Johnson, Denver, 1968.

2. Graham, B.D.: Pediatric Examination in Physical Diagnosis. C.V. Mosby Co., St. Louis, 1969.

3. Vaughan, V.C. and McKay, P.J. (eds.): Nelson's Textbook of Pediatrics, 10th edition. W.B. Saunders Co., Philadelphia, 1975.

4. Barness, L.A.: Manual of Pediatric Physical Diagnosis, 4th edition. Year Book Medical Publishers, Chicago, 1972.

5. Chinn, P.L. and Leitch, C.: Child Health Maintenance: A Guide to Clinical Assessment. C.V. Mosby Co., St. Louis, 1974.

6. Committee on Standards of Child Care, American Academy of Pediatrics, "Health Care of the Children and Youth," June, 1974.

7. Hoekelman, R.: The Pediatric Examination. In Bates, B: A Guide to Physical Examination. J.B. Lippincott Co., Philadelphia, 1974.

8. Alexander, M.M. and Brown, M.S.: Pediatric Physical Diagnosis for Nurses. McGraw-Hill Book Co., New York, 1974.

9. DeAngelis, C.: Basic Pediatrics for the Primary Health Care Provider. Little Brown & Co., Boston, 1975.

10. Erickson, M.: Assessment and Management of Developmental Changes in Children. C.V. Mosby Co., St. Louis, 1976.

CHAPTER 23

ASSESSMENT DURING ADOLESCENCE

INTRODUCTION

Adolescence begins when secondary sex characteristics appear and ends when the individual completes somatic growth, is psychologically mature and becomes an independent functioning member of adult society. Essentially, we are dealing with youngsters between the ages of twelve and eighteen.

The clinician who relates to the adolescent must know and understand his special emotional needs, the developmental changes he has undergone, and the physiological differences true to his age group. When assessing the health status of the adolescent, the practitioner is not only concerned with his physical problems, but with family constitution and attitudes, culture of the group he belongs to, and the educational, recreational and vocational opportunities afforded him. General psychological status must be evaluated in terms of his self-acceptance, sense of identity, relationship with his family and his peers, and his adjustment to society as a whole.

In recent years, we have seen the development of Adolescent Clinics or Medical Practices devoted almost exclusively to care of the adolescent as a professional recognition that adolescents have special needs which require specially skilled practitioners.

The teenage years are ones when there is a great conflict in the individual's self-image between what he would like to be and what he is. It is not unusual for a student with a 93 school average to berate himself because he thought he could get a 95 average. Meanwhile, the pressures for accomplishment, for scholarship, for peer acceptance, and for financial advantages, are all around him.

APPROACH TO EVALUATION OF THE ADOLESCENT

The clinician needs to have skill in approaching the adolescent. He must be able to demonstrate interest in him as a total person. Initially, the practitioner must seek to establish a sense of trust and mutual respect. Accomplishing this can be a complex task, but it can be developed by demonstrating honest and genuine interest in what he has experienced in the past, what he is becoming and what he is hoping for in his life. Some young people may bring unpleasant memories of previous encounters with health care services and personnel to the present evaluation. These feelings may be so strong that the adolescent avoids seeking health care until it becomes a dire emergency. Inexperienced examiners often make the mistake of talking down to the young person as if he were a young child, which negates the establishment of a positive relationship and tends to "turn him off." It is unwise to turn to a parent accompanying the adolescent to explain procedures and plans for treatment before providing explanations directly to the youngster, before asking his opinions, and before listening to what he is saying or not saying.

Every adolescent should be knowledgeable about his own health status. He is able to understand explanations about treatments, procedures, illness, and health care preventive measures. The basic problem in many situations is that he is not informed and not educated. His right to knowledge has been ignored and denied. Adolescents are keenly interested in themselves, their bodies, and the changes occurring within. The wise clinician will recognize these needs and make an attempt to learn about the individual as a total person rather than focusing only on his expressed initial complaints. He will take every opportunity to provide the education he needs. Young people are becoming more interested in their health and they are seeking knowledge about the effects of drugs and alcohol, environmental hazards, and contraceptive devices. They are anxious to learn about natural foods and about non-traditional healing methods and respond to much of the scientific literature which is provided for them.

The adolescent often needs peers in order to relate to an adult. When someone his own age is present, interactions are more relaxed and spontaneous. Once he begins to know an adult in the presence of peers, establishing individual contact becomes more comfortable.

HISTORY

Chief Complaint: Not all adolescents seeking health care have an identifiable physical problem. Some young persons may use a vague minor discomfort such as occasional headaches or gastrointestinal upsets to obtain referrals for social or psychological counseling services. The real problem may be rather serious, or not quite as complicated as the individual believes. Common complaints include skin problems (especially acne), muscle pain, fatigue, and menstrual irregularity. Common disturbances often actually relate to drug use or abuse, alcoholism, sexual uncertainties or stress, unanticipated pregnancy, fear of or real signs of venereal disease, depression with or without suicidal tendencies, family adjustment difficulties, need for financial assistance programs, and school associated behavior problems. The practitioner should keep in mind that the three major causes of death in adolescence are accidents, cancer, and suicide. Whatever the problem expressed, it should be explored sufficiently to provide a thorough understanding of events leading up to, surrounding, and affecting the present situation. The important responsibility for the practitioner is to establish clearly the nature of the real problem and to plan with the adolescent for education, counseling, treatments, or appropriate referral based upon his total needs as an individual. We cannot overemphasize this principle. If the adolescent is disappointed with the relationship established during this health care contact, he may not follow through with referral, or accept the guidance necessary to help him cope with his physical, social, or psychological problems.

Evaluate the common complaint of fatigue in the adolescent completely, as for the adult. A careful history and physical examination may or may not reveal a physiological basis for this problem. More commonly, emotional and social factors are responsible. The pubescent often feels tired and appears to require an extra amount of sleep. Unfortunately, the early adolescent is also anxious to keep up with his older peers. He wants to watch late evening television when adult programs, perhaps previously restricted, are available. At the same time, the responsibilities of school work increase with a requirement for more reading and written assignments. All of this is occurring at a time when the need to join groups, social clubs, or particularly, competitive athletic teams, is at its peak.

The daily schedule for the adolescent is often a hectic one. Imagine a 14-year-old suburban boy who responds to the alarm at 5:30 a.m. in order to deliver the daily newspaper, arrives home in time to shower off the newsprint, grabs a breakfast pop-tart, runs for the 7:10 a.m. school bus, joins the football practice session immediately after school, takes the late bus home in time for 6:00 p.m. dinner and Star Trek, spends an hour for homework, 15 minutes of push-ups, walks the dog and then relaxes with Happy Days. We haven't even given him a chance for a group session at Carvel. No wonder he is tired!! The urban child may have just as many individual or group activities to keep him or her rushing.

The complaint of menstrual irregularity is a common one, especially during the first years of menstruation. Missed periods are not unusual. Dysmenorrhea is a particularly disturbing situation which should never be belittled. Although this may be a time of lessened fertility, the teenager must be aware that pregnancy can occur. Unfortunately, the fear that the missed period is not a normal physiological process, but rather a result of conception, is a particularly shattering one. There is no need to emphasize the emotional support needed and ability to counsel required on the part of the concerned clinician.

PAST MEDICAL HISTORY

Prior to the physical examination, review past health history with the adolescent and his accompanying parent. Whenever possible, time should be provided for interaction with the young patient alone. There may be significant information he will be unwilling to relate in the presence of his family. Guidelines to the history in the previous

chapter for infant and child, as well as for the adult, should be followed during the initial visit. A review of status of physiological
and sexual development is necessary. There may be concern about
delayed or precocious puberty which requires evaluation and referral. History of frequent accidents and injury may indicate emotional problems which are crying out for help. Obtain information
about past problems or situations which may influence the young
person's capacities. Devote special attention to information regarding adjustment with his family, peers of both sexes, school or
work situations.

PHYSICAL EXAMINATION

The examiner should be careful to allow the adolescent privacy during the physical assessment. Curtains should be drawn or the examining room door closed when the evaluation is being done. Young
people of both sexes usually want to disrobe in a private area away
from the view of the examiner. When it is necessary for the young
person to disrobe in the examining room, the practitioner may leave
the room and return when the patient is ready for the physical examination. Draping is done so that only the part being examined is
exposed at a time. Don't be surprised, however, if the adolescent
prefers not to be draped. We mentioned earlier that the young person may be more comfortable during interaction with adults when
one of his peers is present. This may or may not be the case during the physical examination. Ask the adolescent who brings along
a friend if she or he prefers to have the friend stay. Many practitioners make the mistake of insisting that friends leave the room.
Certainly we're not thinking of a group session in the examining
room, but having a friend stand by can be a very important source
of support. The examiner who permits this may be establishing a
reputation as a specially considerate and concerned human being, and
may gain an opportunity for additional health teaching. Of course, if the
adolescent feels comfortable enough with the friend in the waiting
room, his need for privacy may be a greater need than one for peer
support, so respect it. The following assessment guide is presented
to aid the practitioner in the assessment of the adolescent. Its focus is on the special adaptations of the physical examination for the
young person. Included in this outline are the common health problems of the adolescent. Procedures or techniques that are the same
as those for the adult patient are, for the most part, not included.

It is important to remember that the adolescent is interested in his
body, and the time of physical examination becomes an excellent opportunity for health teaching.

The examination may take longer than anticipated, but it is time well-
spent. The practitioner who explains the objectives for each component of the examination may find himself with a cooperative ally
who later comes for guidance at the earliest signs of a problem.

GROWTH AND DEVELOPMENT

During the year or two preceding puberty and throughout adolescence, rapid changes occur in the rate of growth and the physiology of the body as a result of maturation of the gonads and associated hormonal activities. Every individual grows at his own rate and there is a wide degree of normal range for body measurements. When body measurements such as height, weight, and head and chest circumference are recorded regularly and plotted on a growth graph, comparisons can be made with the growth identified on standard charts for the general population. The rate of growth and development depends on heredity, constitutional make-up, racial and national characteristics, sex, environment (including prenatal environment), socio-economic status of the family, nutrition, climate, illness and injury, exercise, position in family, intelligence, hormonal balance, and emotions.

Alterations in established growth patterns which cannot be attributed to physiological changes expected in this age group require further evaluation. The causes of uneven distribution in growth patterns, e.g., height remaining constant and weight continuing in upward direction, may indicate endocrine or metabolic disturbance or may eventually prove insignificant. The finding of a pigeon or barrel shape of the chest is a reason for referral for evaluation of the pulmonary system.

Weight and height records vary significantly in all children. As height increases take place due to the elongation of the long bones, so weight gain should also take place. There are frequently many emotional problems associated with the differences in rate of growth. The clinician must be alert to the adolescent's feelings about his size and shape. In early adolescence, the girls grow more rapidly than the boys, but later on the boys catch up and pass the girls. It is not unusual for boys to not reach full adult height until 21, while rapid growth ceases in girls at the onset of menses.

Boys are frequently disturbed by either a late start, with short stature, or a rapid start, with the skeletal system growing faster than supporting muscles, which tends to cause clumsiness and poor posture. Since large muscles may grow faster than small ones, the youth often lacks coordination. In addition, the hands and feet may grow out of proportion to the rest of his body, which causes more problems in coordination.

Preadolescent and adolescent girls (and boys as well) may experience a rapid increase in weight which is proportionally greater than the gain in height. The result is that obesity may occur and the individual appears stocky. Rarely is hypothyroidism, hypoadrenocorticism, or Cushing's syndrome a factor. Review of dietary habits should be done to evaluate whether the actual cause is overeating, with underlying emotional factors and/or lack of exercise.

Unfortunately, in our society, emphasis upon the desirability of a size 5 figure fostered by the mass media creates even more emotional problems in the obese adolescent girl.

Most of the symptoms of physical distress complained of by pubescents and adolescents are the manifestations of normal physiological changes occurring in their bodies and the inner emotional turmoil surrounding the expectations of them as they approach the responsibilities of adulthood.

Boys should be prepared well in advance for the normal changes in their bodies which generally occur in sequence:

1. Increase in size of genitalia
2. Swelling of the breasts
3. Growth of pubic, axillary, and facial hair
4. Voice changes
5. Production of spermatozoa
6. Rapid growth in shoulder breadth from about age 13 on
7. Occurrence of nocturnal emissions

Girls need preparation for the various changes which will be occurring in their bodies. Changes which occur in girls in the usual order of their appearance are:

1. Increase in transverse diameter of the pelvis
2. Development of the breasts
3. Change in vaginal secretions
4. Growth of pubic and axillary hair
5. Occurrence of menstruation sometime between the appearance of pubic hair and axillary hair

Parents should be advised to prepare their children for the various changes which will occur as well as the concepts of ovulation, fertilization, pregnancy, and birth. Young people need to know about menstruation as a normal physiological phenomenon well before it occurs. In our society, girls are experiencing the menarche earlier than in past years. Many have already begun to menstruate by the time they reach junior high school.

The clinician should be alert to these needs and concerned with facilitating appropriate discussions regarding feelings the adolescent may have about these changes. Adolescents often need an adult outside the family to relate to about problems they are experiencing, both the physiological changes and the many emotional problems they are faced with during this age.

GENERAL SURVEY

Vital Signs: During the age of adolescent development, the vital signs are affected by the various physiological changes occurring in the body. The body temperature may be slightly higher normally than in adults, with females higher than males. Temperatures up to 38.3°C. taken orally are considered within normal limits. The pulse rate varies significantly depending upon conditioning through physical activity, adaptation to psychological stress, and normal fluctuations within the age groups. For example, athletes in training have a slower heart rate than their peers. The mean pulse rate is higher in females than in males. Between the ages of 10 and 18 there is a normal drop in pulse rate and respiratory rate which probably reflects the slowing growth rate as the individual approaches full maturity.

The blood pressure, however, gradually increases to its normal adult level. While the mean blood pressure of the normal 10-year-old is 107/57, and 119/62 at 15, by the time he reaches 18 it is 122/64. The blood pressure reading is most significant if it varies markedly from these mean scores. A significant elevation correlated with protein in the urine and edema of the face, hands or feet, may signify glomerulonephritis. In girls, elevation associated with obesity, amenorrhea, and visual disturbances may signify pregnancy with early toxemia. Recently, through hypertension screening sessions, a rise in the detection of teen-age hypertension, especially in blacks, has been identified. Early recognition and management can prevent the multiple complications associated with hypertension.

A low blood pressure in the adolescent may be insignificant if there are no associated symptoms, or may reflect heredity, poor nutrition, drug or alcohol use, or other factors.

The practitioner should be particularly aware of the effects of drug use upon cardio-pulmonary function. Careful monitoring of vital signs along with observation for other drug-induced manifestations will help to identify the presence of this problem in individuals.

Skin: Skin problems in adolescents are so common that they are often considered normal manifestations of the process of growth and sexual development and age-related psychological stresses. Most adolescents have acne to some degree at one time or another during these years. Blackheads (comedones), followed by superficial and deep papules are commonly found on the forehead, chin, and cheeks, and may even extend to the back, shoulders, and chest. When pustules and cysts form, scars will result. It is imperative that referral be made when improvement does not occur as a result of diet and hygiene supervision.

Scars, needle tracks, and bruises are important clues which require detailed historical data in order to make a full and accurate evaluation. The implications in terms of possible physical abuse at home, drug abuse, or hematological disorders are all too complex to discuss fully here.

Pallor in adolescents, especially girls, is not uncommon. It usually is a reflection of a low hemoglobin level and poor nutritional habits. True anemias may exist so that full assessment through referral for laboratory studies should always be done. Since hepatitis and infectious mononucleosis are common in adolescents, any suspicion of jaundice must be investigated carefully as well.

Head, Face, and Neck: Examination of the head, face, and neck is quite similar to that done for children during early adolescence and for adults later on. Any history of head injury should encourage careful palpation for hemorrhagic masses. The scalp and neck often are the sites of sebaceous cysts so these should be looked for. The adolescent who scratches his head often may be communicating the presence of lice or seborrhea. In the presence of fever of unknown origin with or without rash, ticks should be looked for on the scalp.

Limitations in mobility of the neck often occur in adolescent athletes. When accompanied by fever and general malaise, the possibility of meningitis should be considered and investigated.

Lymph Glands: Adolescents develop infectious mononucleosis more often than any other age groups. Any individual with fever and generalized adenopathy should have full studies to determine the etiology.

Chest and Lungs: The chest and lungs must be examined as in the adults. Respiratory infection and asthma occur frequently in this age group. Adolescents seem more susceptible to tuberculosis. Abnormally slow respiratory rate may be the first sign of opiate poisoning or brain tumor.

Mouth: The adolescent in our country who has no caries is probably blessed with good heredity or is the child of a dentist who brushed his teeth for him and a mother who never gave pennies for the gum machine in the A&P. Otherwise, dental caries is a major problem in teenagers. They need frequent dental examinations and constant reminders about oral hygiene. Despite the fact that straight teeth and braces for teenagers are a sort of status symbol in our culture, underneath those braces plaque and decay may be forming. The mouth should therefore be carefully inspected.

Eyes: The adolescent requires frequent eye examinations. Myopia tends to increase during this age and school demands for increased reading and studying often result in eye strain. Evaluate visual acuity with glasses and refer for complete examination if deviations from normal are evident. The wearing of glasses fluctuates as an "in" or "out" vogue. In recent years, more and more teenagers have been fitted for contact lenses, usually without problems. Unfortunately, the cases of poor lens hygiene and overuse in this group are higher than necessary. Corneal abrasion is common. The practitioner should always refer such cases to an ophthalmologist in order to prevent permanent damage.

Nose: The teenager is especially conscious of his appearance. Often, minor deviations are interpreted as major defects and the self-image is destroyed. A deviated nasal septum may not only interfere with breathing ability but, in the adolescent, when accompanied by malformation and prominence, the shape of the nose becomes a major crisis. The interest in rhinoplasty today is so common among adolescents that it is almost considered a therapeutic, not merely a cosmetic, surgical procedure. Many surgeons and families alike report the occurrence of significant personality changes accompanying the repaired nose. When a prominent or distorted nose presents a serious problem to the teenager, the practitioner should not hesitate to refer the family for evaluation by a specialist.

Breast: The breast develops and matures during adolescence. Asymmetrical early development is not unusual. Some increase in breast tissue is expected and normal in early adolescent males. Patients with excessive and true tissue should be referred for evaluation. Now is the time to begin to teach girls to examine their breasts regularly. When adolescents are made aware of the importance of this procedure from puberty on, they will usually remember it throughout their lifetime. In this way, early lesions may be located and treated promptly. All other previously mentioned guidelines should be followed when examining the breast; however, the practitioner should be aware that young girls may be particularly sensitive about the examination.

Heart: The apex beat is usually found in the adolescent at the 5th left intercostal space at the MCL. No murmurs should be heard. In most cases, functional murmurs will have almost disappeared by the time of young adulthood, although in some instances they still persist. Any evidence of a murmur with or without accompanying cardiovascular signs is a cause for referral.

Abdomen: Examine the abdomen as in the adult. It should be soft and no pain should be expected with palpation. In the presence of a history of pain, it is appropriate to carefully elicit rebound tenderness. Appendicitis occurs more frequently in the adolescent period. Because teenage girls are dieting today, one week on and one week off, it is not unusual to identify striae over the abdomen due to rapid weight loss or gain.

Genitalia: It is essential to evaluate the presence of the testes in the scrotum in males. Undescended testicles at this age will most often be accompanied by sterility.

While the genital examination is usually limited to examination of the external genitalia, in young girls, if there is complaint of pain, discharge, or delayed menstruation, abdominal-pelvic examination should be performed. In view of the higher incidence of cervical cancer in younger girls today, Pap smears should be done annually on all sexually active females. When there is a history of the mother having taken stilbesterol during pregnancy, the adolescent should be examined for vaginal cancer. A few research studies have demonstrated the presence of urinary infections in girls supposedly without subjective or objective signs. It has, therefore, been recommended that urine cultures be taken at intervals during the years 15-18. A nitrite stick culture of a clean catch specimen along with routine urinalysis may be sufficient. The incidence of venereal disease has increased significantly in teenagers due to the lessened use of male prophylactics. Every case of increased vaginal discharge with a history of sexual activity should be evaluated.

Extremities and Back: As we mentioned earlier, the growth of long bones and large muscles during the adolescent period may create uncoordination and posture defects. However, by the end of this time span, the various childhood characteristics should have given way to more mature, adult stature. Knock-knees should have been straightened out and postural slumps corrected. The feet of the adolescent however, often show corns, calluses, and blisters. This is no small wonder when you evaluate the types of shoes in vogue for teenagers, or look at them on the street in bare feet. Their sizes have also changed rapidly, and with today's prices, they may often be wearing too small or ill-fitting shoes.

Any indication of asymmetry of the neuromuscular system requires early referral. Scoliosis is unfortunately common among adolescents, and during careful examination appears as alteration in symmetrical levels of shoulders or hips. If the teenager walks with a limp and there is no history of trauma, consider the possibility of slipped femoral epiphysis. In addition, any persistent severe pain or swelling in the long bones should also be immediately referred for evaluation in view of the possibility of osteosarcoma or Ewing's tumor which occur during this period. Muscle aches, pains, and tenderness are common in adolescents who are active sports participants. It is probably most unfortunate that our society places so much emphasis upon competitive sports in junior and senior high schools when muscle and bone growth is so significant. The Little League pitcher at 14 may have permanent injury with a lifetime of discomfort. Parents need counseling regarding the pressures placed upon young athletes in schools, and practitioners should not hesitate to assume responsibility for offering suggestions to individual students, teachers and school board members.

<u>Neurological and Mental Evaluation</u>: The clinician working with adolescents should evaluate carefully the past developmental history of this system. This evaluation should be as thorough and complete as described in Chapter 18 for adults. Complaints of frequent headaches, loss of consciousness, seizures, episodes of muscular weakness, numbness or loss of feeling in any part of the body, as well as visual disturbances among others, may indicate serious neurological problems.

Adolescents may experience a sudden insidious onset of epilepsy which is most frightening. Brain tumors may result in sudden symptoms with little previous neurological history. There may have been vague complaints such as headaches and fatigue for a period of time which were considered normal for the age group.

Evaluate the present mental status. The adolescent should be alert with responses appropriate to the situation, with judgment and insight into problems. Inappropriate behavior, delayed reflexes, lack of ability to think abstractly, and communicate intelligently in the presence of an otherwise unremarkable history may indicate use or abuse of alcohol or drugs. The adolescent must be encouraged to talk about how things are for him: Is he satisfied? What is his general mood or mental outlook? The practitioner must be able to put these signs together with the possible history presented of school work deficiencies, of poor parental relationships, of anxiety about personal abilities, and make an assessment which calls for consultation and counseling.

SUMMARY: It is quite obvious that the physical examination of the adolescent is much the same as for the adult. The guidelines presented throughout the text hold true for the young person with essentially the same basic principles we have been emphasizing throughout this text. Essentially, the unique problems are those of growth and development, and of adjustments to psychological and social stresses placed by family, peers and society. The skilled practitioner plans his professional activities in collaboration with his patient to help him to meet the needs that are his alone.

REFERENCES

1. Gallagher, J.R., Heald, F.P. and Garell, D.C.: <u>Medical Care of the Adolescent</u>. 3rd Edition, Appleton-Century-Crofts, New York, 1976.

2. Marlowe, D.: <u>Textbook of Pediatric Nursing</u>. 3rd edition. W.B. Saunders Co., Philadelphia, 1969.

3. Kagen, J. and Coles, R. (eds.): <u>Twelve to Sixteen: Early Adolescence</u>. W.W. Norton & Co., New York, 1972.

4. Brunswick, A. and Josephson, E.: Adolescent Health in Harlem. A.J. Public Health Supplement, October 1972.

5. Symposium on the Young Adult in Today's World, Part II. Nursing Clinics of North America, March 1973.

6. Kalafitch, A.: Approaches to the Care of Adolescents. Appleton-Century-Crofts, New York, 1975.

7. Daniel W.A.: The Adolescent Patient. C.V. Mosby Co., St. Louis, 1970.

8. Kugelmass, J. Newton: Adolescent Medicine. Charles C Thomas, Springfield, Mass., 1975.

CHAPTER 24

ASSESSMENT OF THE ELDERLY

INTRODUCTION

Lay persons and health professionals alike are well aware of the fact that the number of people in the "aged" population is increasing significantly. We are all also aware of the development of a much greater interest in the social and health problems of the elderly.

It is important for the health professional, however, to recognize that this increased interest in the elderly is of relatively recent origin in medical history. For example, in this country at the time of its birth, the average life span was about 35 years and the medical focus was largely on acute infectious disease and trauma in a young agricultural society. Diseases of the elderly were present, of course, but they made up only a small portion of the practitioner's daily activity.

Medicine made great advances in the nineteenth century which provided the basis for more treatment than had been possible before. Despite this, the elderly benefited much less than did children and younger adults.

Notable among these advances were the development of practical methods for vaccination against smallpox, the prevention of puerperal fever, the use of anesthesia, and the development of antiseptic techniques. Smallpox had always taken its greatest toll among children. For example, in the period before vaccination, about one-third of all children in England died of smallpox before they reached three years of age. Thus, the emphasis on vaccination was on protection of the children. Puerperal fever was a disease of younger women in their childbearing years.

Surgery was an ancient art and was extensively used in treatment of trauma - particularly for military casualties. The discovery of anesthesia and of antiseptic techniques led to a great extension of surgical treatment. However, since the elderly patients presented greater surgical risks, and since they had a shorter expected life span, the generally healthier and stronger young patients were the principal beneficiaries of the newer surgical procedures.

Thus, the treatment of the aged did not improve significantly. They remained in a less important category in the medical care process, since they were fewer in number and since their medical problems were often more complicated and less well understood. This attitude

315

toward the elderly is reflected in a story told by Dr. Paul Dudley White, the famous cardiologist. He pointed out that one of the case records of the Massachusetts General Hospital, about 100 years ago, listed the cause of death of a 45-year-old woman as "old age." (Dr. White died in 1973 at the age of 87.)

Out of this situation grew a number of concepts, habits, practices, school curricula, and prejudices which continued to emphasize the care of the young and the relative neglect of the aged.

Over the past 40 to 50 years, however, the situation has taken a distinct change. With better control of infectious diseases, better medications for cure or control of chronic illnesses, advances in clinical nutrition, and accelerated research into the problems of the aged, the life span of our population is now double that of 200 years ago. The decrease in infant and child mortality, coupled with better care for the aging person, has increased the numbers of the elderly population greatly. The expectations of our society now include adequate health care for all elements of our population, and this change is reflected in teaching, government support of research, and improved attitudes toward conservation of the health of the elderly.

While there are legal and social definitions of aging, there is no fixed medical criterion for this state. Aging is a highly relative condition. The professional athlete "ages" rapidly in his career and may be forced to change his occupation at 30 or 35. At the other extreme, persons may be active and highly productive for 8 or 9 decades in literature, the arts, and other intellectual pursuits. For example, Goethe completed "Faust" when he was 82, Titian painted his last masterpiece, "Christ Crowned With Thorns," at 95, Verdi composed the opera "Falstaff" at age 87, and Stradivarius was still at work making violins when he died at 93.

There are numerous examples from many fields similar to the above, indicating that creativity does not cease with the achievement of an arbitrary birthday. As health professionals, we must not assume that any person is senile, incompetent, or of little importance simply because of age.

Most important for us, as clinicians, is our attitude in the evaluation of the elderly patient. If we feel that anyone over 60 (or any fixed age) is "on his last legs" physically and mentally simply because of his age, the examination and assessment are likely to be skimpy and, therefore, inadequate. The elderly patient requires the same courteous, competent evaluation as does his younger counterpart. In addition, he needs a sensitive examiner who will use all available personal skills and understanding in appraising the patient. A smile, a gentle manner, a slower pace in speaking, patience in eliciting the history, a steadying hand on or off the examining table - all communicate the special caring so supportive to the older patient.

THE AGING PROCESS

GENERAL: There are many anatomical and physiological changes which are clearly associated with aging. What is not so clear is just which changes are directly due to chronological aging itself, and which are related to factors such as heredity, diet, previous illnesses, occupation, "wear-and-tear," environment, etc. Current research and review of older data will undoubtedly assist in clarifying the roles of many of the features of the process which we call aging.

We do know from many studies that aging is not a uniform process, in that there are great variations in aging from individual to individual. It is also known that, in a single person, aging will involve certain organs, systems, or functions and will spare others. Thus, aging does not follow a fixed pattern directly related to the length of life.

With this important feature of variability in mind, one can properly consider certain general characteristics of the aging process.

ANATOMICAL CHANGES: Some examples of the changes in body cells, tissues, and organs which are often seen are the following:

> reduced body weight
> shortened stature due to atrophy of intervertebral discs
> reduced bone mineral content
> loss of tissue water (e.g., skin, muscle)
> reduced number of taste buds
> impaired elasticity of the lens of the eye
> increased AP chest diameter
> reduced arterial elasticity
> progressive arteriosclerosis
> fewer kidney glomeruli
> reduced brain weight and number of cortical cells
> reduced number of fibers in nerve trunks

As a rule, when these changes do occur, they are more distinct and severe in the seventh decade and beyond.

PHYSIOLOGICAL CHANGES: In the general "slowing down" process of aging, a number of individual organ functions become less competent. These include:

> lowered visual acuity
> hearing loss, particularly for high frequency tones
> reduced vital capacity of the lungs

    reduced pulmonary ventilation on exertion
    lowered oxygen uptake during exercise
    reduced cardiac output
    reduced secretion of gastric acid and gastric hormones
    decreased renal function
    less mobile joints
    reduced strength of muscles
    reduced blood flow to the brain
    slower nerve conduction
    slower reaction time
    reduced basal metabolic rate
    lowered glucose tolerance
    less effective immune protective mechanisms
    decreased pain perception

The presence of a number of these reductions, particularly if some are severe, limits an individual's ability to respond to stresses of various types. He can no longer meet demands for prolonged physical exertion and cannot tolerate the effects of disease, injury, or emotional upheaval as well as he could several decades earlier.

In general, therefore, as a person ages, he adapts less well to changes from his basal resting state and must live within a narrower range of activities.

MENTAL FUNCTIONS: Some general features of change in these functions are:

    lowered scores on intelligence tests
    fixed habits which are harder to change
    slower rate of learning
    slowed speed of mental activity (e.g., arithmetic)
    poorer memory of recent events
    retention of memory for distant events, but less reliability of
      content
    lack of attention to surroundings
    more disinterest in current events

It has been pointed out that some of these features may not be due to actual lack of intellectual capacity but, rather, to reduced motivation. Elderly persons also attach less importance to some of these items than do the young.

Several studies have shown that when people remain in stimulating environments through their later years, they seem to retain mental capacity better than those whose environment is dull and uninteresting. This has important implications for prevention and treatment of reduced mental functions in elderly persons.

EXAMINATION

GENERAL: In order to assess the health care needs of the geri-atric patient, the clinician will not need to learn any new methods for interviewing or physical examination. Basically, the techniques for obtaining a health history and a physical examination are no different from those described for the adult in Chapters 2 - 19. The assessment of the problems of the elderly should be as complete as that for younger persons. However, the actual conduct of both the history and physical examination will differ somewhat and the examiner needs to know and understand the changes of the aging process described in this chapter.

Depending on the actual anatomic, physiologic, and psychologic aspects of the individual patient, certain modifications may be in order. If the patient is fully alert mentally and in good physical condition, there will be little difference in the examination. On the other hand, for a patient who is impatient or inattentive, the history must be abbreviated at the first visit.

Similarly, for a patient who seems to tire easily or to be physically weak, the physical examination may need to be curtailed.

In either case, the clinician must be prepared to focus the examination on critical matters first and to aim toward completion at subsequent visits. Knowing how to modify either the history or physical examination is a matter of judgment which will come with knowledge and experience. There are a few guidelines, however, which may be of assistance in changing the pattern of the initial evaluation where indicated by the patient's mental and/or physical status.

First of all, the clinician must make a rapid, general assessment of the patient in order to judge how alert, attentive, and strong the patient is. This will give the examiner a basis for judging how much of the history and physical he may be able to accomplish at the first visit.

The next chapter, on the comatose patient, presents the concept of "shifting gears" as needed. In the examination of the elderly patient, the clinician must frequently resort to such a modification of the routine pattern.

THE HEALTH HISTORY: Several suggestions may guide the interviewer in obtaining the health history:

1. Keep the questions simple, clear, and pertinent.
2. Use language that the patient can understand.
3. Speak distinctly and directly to the patient and wait for the response.
4. Avoid extensive writing during the interview.

5. Pace the questioning to the ability of the patient to respond.
6. Avoid the appearance of rushing.

Chief Complaint and Present Illness: These remain the most vital
portions of the history and, without question, have the first priority. Verification of information through family members or records, where available, is highly desirable.

A most important consideration is that pain perception is often reduced, as noted earlier. This reduction may be minimal or may be
nearly total, particularly with visceral pain. Thus, disorders which
are ordinarily associated with severe pain (e.g., obstruction of the
ureter, perforation of the intestine) may possibly produce only minor
symptoms.

Past History: As noted in Chapter 3, this element should consist of
diagnosed illnesses which are considered medically important. For
the aged patient, medical diseases and surgical procedures, likely
to be of long-term significance, are to be asked about. Certainly,
diabetes, hypertension, myocardial infarctions, renal or liver disorders, for example, will be of importance. Surgical removal of
organs or tumors and repair of heart valves are key subjects to
explore.

Of lesser consequence are illnesses or minor surgical procedures
of the distant past which are unlikely to influence the patient's current status. Examples are the usual childhood diseases, extremity
fractures, removal of non-malignant skin lesions, single bouts of
pneumonia, or passing of a renal stone, etc.

Information about immunizations is of little consequence except, perhaps, for data about tetanus boosters in a patient whose current
problem is related to trauma.

Drug allergies and a record of current medications are of distinct
importance in the history and should not be neglected at this
interview.

Thus, the past history may be reviewed in briefer format, if it is
felt necessary, but the examiner should be aware of any pertinent
items left out for exploration at a later date.

Review of Systems: Guidelines for a modified review are difficult to
provide since the circumstances of the patient's present illness will
determine the requirements for questioning. For example, if the
chief complaint consists of a generalized, poorly defined problem
such as fever, malaise and weight loss, it is likely that a major diagnostic problem exists and therefore, a nearly complete review
of systems is indicated. Even here, some items relating to problems

of the distant past may be eliminated such as skin problems, use of
eye glasses, hearing loss, menstrual history (in a woman well past
menopause) or pregnancies (unless complicated).

Any current or recent problems, however, must be explored in detail no matter what the problem may be. If time presents difficulty,
the ROS may be broken into two or more sessions. Since the most
common medical problems among the elderly relate to pulmonary,
cardiac, gastrointestinal disease, and neuro-psychiatric disorders, review of these systems should take priority.

Particular attention must be paid to the patient's dietary habits, for
disorders of nutrition become far more prominent in older persons.
Dental problems such as loss of many teeth or ill-fitting dentures
often interfere with eating an adequate diet.

Since complaints about improper bowel function are almost univer-
sal, special attention should be given, in the ROS, to this problem.
Care must be taken to distinguish abnormalities, such as alternating diarrhea and constipation and tarry or bloody stools, from simple constipation. The patient with the latter should be assured that
a bowel movement once a day is not necessary, and that proper diet
and fluid intake are much to be preferred to constant use of
laxatives.

Family History: As indicated in the description of this element
(p. 45), questioning about first-order relatives will generally be
adequate. Almost all of the familial disorders will have become
manifest well before the sixth or seventh decade, so detailed questioning in this area can be safely deferred for a patient in this age
group or beyond.

Personal and Social History: Items of particular concern to the clinician relate to the daily living pattern, the social environment, economic status, the physical environment, and self-image of the aged
person.

Activities of Daily Living: Particular attention must be paid to the
patient's dietary habits, for disorders of nutrition become far more
prominent in older persons. The listing of a 24-hour intake often reveals gross inadequacies, especially in protein foods. Lack of knowledge about foods, misconceptions, dyspepsia, and limited income
are factors which also may contribute to the development of
malnutrition.

Complaints of inability to sleep at night are often heard from aging
patients, especially when they have limited exercise or when they
nap during the day. It is important for the clinician to know, however, that the normal sleep pattern in the elderly person consists of
frequent intervals of awakening and sleeping.

Occupational exposure to dusts or toxins in the past may produce disorders such as pulmonary fibrosis or carcinoma of the lung many years later. Thus, an occupational history is required, even for the retired person, as is a history of tobacco or alcohol use even in the person who has quit such habits.

Certainly, the present socio-economic status of the patient is of great importance for an adequate evaluation of the current state. As is well known, poverty and loneliness are potent influences on any patient's health status, and this is particularly true of the aged.

The physical conditions of the patient's home including space, utilities, stairs, etc., should be determined. In addition, information about the patient's community and its resources is of vital importance. Although discharge planning for hospitalized patients should begin at the time of admission, realistic planning is seldom done unless someone interviewing the patient upon admission is alert to questioning in this area. Some homes and communities where the aged live, especially where they live alone, are not able to provide for their special needs when families are unable to help. With adequate time to plan, temporary (or permanent) alternate arrangements can often be made, and unnecessarily long hospitalizations or nursing home stays may be prevented.

It is in the areas of interpersonal functioning and environment that multiple hidden problems may directly affect not only the mental status but the physical health and well-being of the patient as well.

THE PHYSICAL EXAMINATION: The actual technique of performance of the examination is not essentially different for the aged patient than for the younger adult. Each element of the examination remains important for the proper evaluation of the patient; none may be safely eliminated.

Since the examination itself does not differ from the routine described in previous chapters, the sections below, on each region, will indicate the pertinent earlier chapter, so that the student can refer to it readily as he reviews this material.

One may expect to find some of the features described in the section on the Aging Process in the examination. It is also valuable to look closely for signs of malignancy, cardiovascular disease, arthritis, and malnutrition - all more frequently present in the elderly.

Basic Data (Chapter 6): As noted earlier, there is a tendency in late age for stature to shorten and for body weight to be somewhat reduced. There are no precise tables to indicate the normally expected changes. However, if the changes are due simply to aging, they should be of small degree and should occur slowly.

Blood pressure should <u>not</u> increase with age. It is now well known that the adage that "systolic pressure should be 100 plus the patient's age" is grossly incorrect. The standards for normal blood pressures in the aged are no different from those of the fully matured young adult. Elevated pressure is the result of disease - not of aging.

<u>Integument</u> (Chapter 7): Since the water content, the elasticity, and the subcutaneous fat are all reduced, it is to be expected that the skin will be drier, more lax, and that it will appear thinner. The natural defenses of aging skin are less competent, so more fungal infections may be present and eczema is more common.

Most skin lesions have the same appearance as in younger patients. There are several which are much more common in the elderly, particularly senile keratoses and seborrheic keratoses. The latter are plaques made up of the outer (keratin) layer of skin, raised slightly above the skin surface. They are of varying size and range in color from tan to black. These seborrheic keratoses are often seen on the face and neck and are unimportant lesions.

Senile keratoses are nodular in shape, quite firm to the touch and scaly on the surface. They occur most often on areas of the skin exposed to the sun. Since they occasionally undergo malignant change, they should be described carefully and reported.

Thickening of nails, particularly of toe nails, is generally not a direct result of aging. If present, this is generally due to fungal infection.

<u>Head, face, and neck</u> (Chapter 8): While the examination does not differ from that of the adult, signs arising from strokes and occlusion of the carotid arteries should be searched for carefully because of their increased incidence. The examination of all cranial nerves should be complete, and palpation plus auscultation of the carotid arteries will aid in detection of possible occlusions. Surgery to correct such occlusion may be life-saving.

<u>Eyes</u> (Chapter 9): As noted in the section on the process of aging, a frequent change is loss of elasticity in the lens. This leads to inability to focus on near objects, referred to as "farsightedness" or presbyopia.

Distant vision is tested by use of the Snellen chart, but since presbyopia is almost universally present in the older patient, near vision should also be evaluated. This is simply done by having the patient read from a newspaper, magazine, or book. If the patient wears reading glasses, have him use them for this test. A person with normal near vision, or one with properly refracted reading glasses, should be able to read newsprint at a distance of 15 to 30 cm. (6 to 12 inches). Failure to do this warrants referral for further examination.

A change associated with age is arcus senilis (Fig. 24.1). While this does appear more often in older persons, it is not pathological, nor is it associated specifically with arteriosclerosis, as was formerly thought.

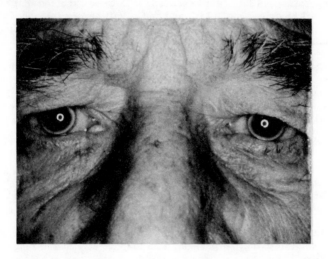

FIG. 24.1: Arcus senilis. Here the rings around the limbus are complete.

Cataracts are also frequently found and can be identified by dark areas in the examination of the red reflex with the ophthalmoscope. In extensive cataract formation, the red reflex may be totally absent. Since these are present in the lens (see Fig. 9.1), they will come into sharp focus with the ophthalmoscope lens set from +15 to +10.

Any suggestion of increased firmness of the eyeball is enough to indicate referral for tonometry testing for glaucoma. Many clinicians advocate routine tonometry for all persons over 50 years of age.

The Ear, Nose, Mouth, and Pharynx (Chapter 10): Hearing loss is commonly a problem for the elderly person, particularly if it involves a loss in the normal conversational range (i.e., 80 to 2000 cps.). Since the tuning fork tests hearing only at a single frequency, it is preferable to test the patient by the whispered voice test. Any indication of hearing difficulty is cause to refer the patient, since such loss can interfere significantly with the patient's ability to keep in good contact with his environment.

Evaluation of teeth or dentures must be careful enough to determine the patient's ability to bite or chew properly - functions which are important for his overall state of nutrition.

Cancers of the mouth, tongue, and pharynx increase in frequency with age, so careful inspection and palpation are indicated.

Thorax and Lungs (Chapter 11): The aging process has direct effects on the chest cage and on the process of ventilation of the lungs. The A-P diameter of the thorax is increased, dorsal kyphosis often develops (see Fig. 11.9, p. 145), and there is a reduction in chest expansion. These changes are secondary to degeneration of the intervertebral discs, stiffening of ligaments and joints, and weakened musculature. Arthritis of the spine, a common disorder of the elderly patient, may also interfere with adequate chest expansion. These changes in the chest wall lead to the common findings of hyperresonance on percussion and reduction of the loudness of breath sounds even in healthy lungs.

Chronic bronchitis, emphysema, or a mixed entity called chronic obstructive pulmonary disease are all frequently found in the aged, particularly in smokers and those who have been exposed to dust or fumes in their occupation.

These disorders produce somewhat different physical findings but all have the effect of increasing the air content of the lungs and making expiration more difficult. Thus, the hyperresonance and diminished breath sounds, noted earlier as a result of aging, are exaggerated. In addition, auscultation often reveals prolonged expiratory breath sounds and rhonchi in one or both phases of respiration.

Carcinoma of the lung increases in frequency up to the 7th decade of life and should be searched for diligently. Often, there are no physical findings unless a bronchus becomes partially or completely obstructed. Although signs are variable, partial obstruction will often cause a localized, unilateral wheeze (sibilant rhonchi), while complete obstruction of a bronchus leads to collapse of the lung peripheral to the obstruction. In this situation, depending upon the size and location of the collapsed (atelectatic) lung, there may be diminished expansion of the chest on the side of the lesion, an area of dullness, diminished breath sounds, and reduced voice transmission.

Breast (Chapter 12): There is a change in the texture of the female breast arising from involution of the milk glands and ducts. There will be a reduction in breast size, and the ducts will become stringy and fibrous to palpation.

The examination of the breast, however, will not differ from that described, and the search for masses must be as detailed in the elderly as in the younger woman.

Heart (Chapter 13): The heart may be expected to be of normal size, or smaller, due to some degree of muscle atrophy secondary to the aging process. With changes in the AP diameter of the thorax and some emphysema which often occurs, percussion of the left border of cardiac dullness becomes less accurate, and the PMI frequently cannot be palpated.

Heart valves become thicker and more rigid, due to fibrosis, and often do not shut completely, leading to the production of murmurs. The heart sounds themselves are not as loud, and they are sometimes difficult or nearly impossible to hear if emphysema is present.

Atrial fibrillation is much more common in the elderly, so careful attention should be paid to cardiac rate and rhythm, presence of pulse deficit, and varying intensity of S_1.

Abdomen (Chapter 14): Physical examination of the abdomen must take into account the fact that the diaphragm is frequently low in the thorax, being flattened by aging changes or by emphysema, as noted earlier in this chapter. Because it is low, the diaphragm can move only a short distance between inspiration and expiration.

This depression of the diaphragm will push the liver downward so that it is frequently palpable in the abdomen. The student has been cautioned, previously, not to assume that a palpable liver is an enlarged liver, and special caution must be observed in the elderly in whom the liver is frequently palpable. Percussion of the upper border of the liver under the ribs and palpation of the lower border in the abdomen will give the clinician a measure of the span of the organ, and that span is the most reliable index of liver size on physical examination.

There are no other important differences in the physical findings on abdominal examination of the elderly. However, special attention should be given to the search for masses, since neoplasms increase in frequency with advancing age. Duodenal and gastric ulcers, diseases of the gallbladder and biliary system, hiatus hernia and diverticulosis of the colon are all commonly present also, but more often their presence is suspected by symptoms rather than physical signs.

Aneurysms are more frequent in the aged and should be searched for here as well as in other palpable arteries. In the abdomen, aneurysm of the aorta may be detected on physical examination if careful deep palpation is done along the midline from the epigastrium down to the inferior portion of the umbilical region.

The femoral arteries are most conveniently palpated while the patient is supine for the abdominal examination. It is recommended that auscultation of these arteries be routinely performed in the elderly patient since aneurysms or occlusion of the vessels may be present.

Extremities and Back (Chapter 15): With the degeneration of inter-vertebral discs, the frequent presence of arthritis of the spine, and the dominance of flexor muscles over extensors, there is a change in posture of aging patients. The head is thrust forward, kyphosis of the dorsal spine is exaggerated, the arms are carried in slight flexion, and there is some flexion of the leg on the thigh. The ideal posture (see Fig. 15.1) is infrequently maintained.

Gait may be influenced by any of the disorders noted in Table 15.1 but, in addition, poor vision, arthritis, and the characteristic flexed posture may also cause a loss of the easy, "loose-jointed" gait of the younger adult.

Loss of balance, however, is not a consequence of the aging process, but follows disorders of the semicircular canals, loss of proprio-ceptive sense, or cerebellar disease.

Lack of regular exercise, as well as the aging process, leads to re-duction in muscle bulk often seen in the elderly patient. Muscle strength is often found to be fairly well preserved despite the reduc-tion in bulk.

Decreased range of motion (ROM) of the neck, back, and extremities is to be anticipated. This limitation is due to stiffening of ligaments and joints arising from the aging process as well as to the develop-ment of arthritis.

It is important to determine whether any limitation in ROM is pri-marily due to painful joints or to mechanical difficulties in motion, since the pain of arthritis is often more readily treated. A useful technique is to palpate joints for pain before testing the ROM by movement.

Osteoarthritis is commonly found in the spine and in peripheral weight-bearing joints such as hips, knees, and ankles.

Examination of veins and arteries is carried out in the same detail as for the adult. Since peripheral arterial disease is more commonly present, it may be expected that weaker pulses will be found. Of par-ticular importance is the determination of differences in pulse strength from one side to the other, for this may identify localized areas of partial arterial occlusion. Such findings warrant referral, for ap-propriate therapy may prevent the development of gangrene.

Deep tendon reflexes are likely to be hypoactive but should not be ab-sent. Comparison of reflexes from right and left sides is most im-portant for proper interpretation of this examination. The plantar reflex may be absent without signifying an abnormality but, as with younger patients, dorsiflexion of the great toe and spreading of the toes is distinctly abnormal.

Male Genital and Rectal Examination (Chapter 16): While tumors of the testes are more frequently seen in young men, they are not to be overlooked in the elderly, so bimanual palpation of the scrotal contents is to be done routinely. Often the testes will be soft, small, and somewhat atrophic in older males.

The knee-chest position may be quite uncomfortable for patients with arthritis of the spine, shoulders, hips, or knees, so the less stressful lateral or lithotomy positions are preferred for the rectal examination.

Benign prostatic hypertrophy, carcinoma of the prostate, and carcinoma of the rectum, are all lesions more commonly found in the aged and should be searched for diligently.

Female Genital Examination (Chapter 17): With loss of estrogen production there are several changes in the genitalia which are to be expected. The external genitalia will show a loss of vulval hair, subcutaneous fat is reduced, producing flattened labial folds, and the introitus is smaller.

In the vagina, the epithelium thins, the wall becomes less elastic, and secretions are much reduced, producing a smooth, shiny and dry vaginal canal. The cervix becomes small, as does the entire uterus.

The position for speculum examination, most often performed with the patient in the dorsolithotomy position in stirrups, may need to be modified if arthritis is present. The simple lithotomy position or lateral Sims' position will allow for a thorough examination without stressing the patient unduly. Due to the narrowing of the introitus and vagina referred to above, it is desirable to use a pediatric speculum to avoid pain or the induction of bleeding which may follow use of the standard adult instrument.

While uterine myomas are less frequent in postmenopausal women, the incidence of uterine cancer remains high, so careful inspection and regular Pap smears are always in order.

Because the uterus is significantly smaller and more mobile in elderly women, bimanual examination is often more difficult to interpret, but the critical characteristics of size, mobility, position, consistency, and contour should all be identified and reported. Unless an ovary is enlarged due to disease, it is rarely palpable, since it too is smaller than in the young woman.

Neurological and Mental Status Examination (Chapter 18): Keeping in mind the differences to be found in the elderly patient, the clinician will proceed in the manner used for the adult examination.

However, great care must be taken in this evaluation of the aged patient so that the events associated with aging are not misinterpreted as evidence of psychologic or organic disorders.

Since, for example, the incidence of stroke and peripheral neuropathy increases with aging, and since both may produce weakness of specific muscle groups and loss of reflexes and/or sensory perception, the examiner must accurately describe and record these abnormal neurological findings to allow the cause to be identified.

REFERENCES

1. Galton, L.: Don't Give Up On An Aging Parent, Crown Publishing Co., Boston, 1975.

2. Miller, M.H.: If the Patient Is You, Chapters 3, 4 and 5, Chas. Scribner's Sons, New York, 1977.

3. Chinn, A.B.: Working With Older People, IV, Clinical Aspects of Aging, DHEW, Public Health Service Publication No. 1459, Washington, 1971.

4. Cowdry, E.V. and Steinberg, F.W.: The Care of the Geriatric Patient, 4th Ed., C.V. Mosby Co., St. Louis, 1971.

5. Burnside, I.M.: Psychosocial Nursing Care of the Aged, McGraw-Hill Book Co., New York, 1973.

6. Busse, E. and Pfeiffer, E.: Behavior & Adaptation in Late Life. Little, Brown & Co., Boston, Mass., 1969.

CHAPTER 25

EXAMINATION OF THE COMATOSE PATIENT

INTRODUCTION

The major emphasis of the textbook has been on the examination under optimum conditions, i.e., adequate time for the examiner and a fully cooperative patient. There will be many situations in which these ideal circumstances will not pertain, where it will be necessary for the practitioner to "shift gears" - to increase his speed and/or to eliminate certain portions of the examination. Situations such as the evaluation of an uncooperative patient, an acutely ill, or severely injured patient, obviously demand modifications of the history-taking process and the physical examination. An extreme example of such a situation is the evaluation of an unconscious person.

PATIENT STATUS

The first, and by far the most important, step in the evaluation of the comatose patient is the requirement to judge rapidly the adequacy of the patient's respiratory and circulatory systems to sustain life and integrity of the brain. The essential ingredients are a patent airway and adequate ventilation to provide oxygen, enough blood glucose to avoid permanent metabolic brain damage, and a pulse rate and systolic blood pressure sufficient to provide circulation of the oxygen and glucose to the brain.

Priority, therefore, must be given to examination of the pharynx, to the vital signs, and to the level of blood glucose. A significant abnormality of any of these calls for deferment of further examination until emergency treatment is initiated. A team is urgently required under these circumstances, for the work-up must be continued while treatment is in progress.

APPROACH

While there are many conditions which may produce coma, there are far fewer than the total list of conditions which cause illness in general. Familiarity with common causes of coma narrows the list of possibilities and thereby makes certain parts of the "routine" examination more important and others unnecessary. One classification of the causes of coma is the following:

Exogenous Intoxication: alcohol, barbiturates, opiates, carbon monoxide or other gas poisoning, lead or other heavy metal poisoning, insecticides, etc.

Metabolic Disorders: uremia, diabetic ketoacidosis, hypoglycemia, hepatic failure, etc.

Trauma: concussion, subdural hematoma, extradural hemorrhage, heat stroke, electrical shock, etc.

Infection: meningitis, encephalitis, malaria, rabies, etc.

Syncope: circulatory shock secondary to blood loss, myocardial infarction, arrhythmias, pulmonary embolism, anaphylaxis, ruptured viscus, etc.

Neuro-psychiatric: epilepsy, hysteria, basilar artery thrombosis, intracranial hemorrhage or embolus, etc.

Review of this classification, and of some of the specific causes, will help the examiner to concentrate his attention on certain elements of the history and the physical examination.

Despite the urgency of the situation, jumping to conclusions is no more warranted in the evaluation of the comatose patient than in any other situation. The history and physical examination must be abbreviated but not carelessly performed.

HISTORY

Since the comatose patient cannot give a history, this element of evaluation is often totally neglected to the detriment of the patient. Questioning people who brought the patient in, or relatives and friends who can be reached quickly, may be life-saving. Examination of the patient's clothing and purse or wallet may reveal important clues such as a diabetic identification card, a bottle (full or empty) of medication, or a suicide note. Information from previous medical records should be obtained if available promptly.

PHYSICAL EXAMINATION

In the immediate assessment of the patient's status, the respiratory and cardiovascular systems took first priority, but that examination was performed quickly to evaluate the viability of the patient. These systems should now be re-evaluated in more detail when searching for clues as to the etiology of the coma. Since coma is a manifestation of a serious neurological disorder, the neurological system must be carefully examined. A suggested order for this type of physical examination is:

Vital Signs: Nearly continuous monitoring of pulse, respiration, blood pressure, rectal temperature, and urine output is obviously mandatory.

Head: Inspect and palpate for skull trauma. If blood is detected in the hair, the scalp should be shaved rapidly to allow for careful examination.

Face: Inspect for symmetry of facial muscles.

Eyes: Inspect for pupillary size, equality, and reaction to light, nystagmus, or "wandering" of the eyeballs. A funduscopic examination should be done for evidence of papilledema.

Ears: Inspect for blood or spinal fluid in the canals or behind the eardrum. Inspect for bulging or rupture of the drum.

Nose: Inspect for leakage of spinal fluid or blood.

Mouth: Smell the breath for odor of alcohol, acetone or hepatic fetor. Inspect the tongue for bite-marks and the palate for bleeding.

Neck: Flex the head to detect resistance or rigidity.

Chest: Inspect for rate, rhythm, and depth of respiration. Percuss and auscult for signs of consolidation or lung collapse.

Heart: Recheck rate and rhythm. Auscult for murmurs.

Abdomen: Inspect for bruising. Auscult for bowel sounds.

Extremities: Inspect for evidence of trauma, for needle tracks on the forearm, and for puncture marks on the thighs. Assess for muscle tone. (This may be done by raising and dropping both arms, or legs, at the same time.) Attempt to obtain reactive movement by jabbing a pin into each hand and foot. Examine tendon and plantar reflexes. These evaluations are done to detect inequality of response from one side to the other.

Level of Consciousness: This is evaluated by the patient's responsiveness to stimuli. The more vigorous the stimulus needed to obtain a response, the deeper is the coma. Thus, spoken words, shouted words, mild pain stimuli (slapping or pin-prick), deep pain stimuli (pressure over the eyeballs at the medial portion of the upper orbital ridge, squeezing the testicle or the Achilles tendon) are progressively severe stimuli. The patient's level of consciousness should be re-evaluated regularly during the comatose state based on responses to such stimuli.

It is not expected that the student or practitioner will memorize this sequence of examination, but it is given as a guide to the areas of the examination most likely to produce information related to the etiology of coma. The full evaluation of the comatose patient, of course, requires the selection of appropriate laboratory studies, a review of which is beyond the scope of this text.

As stated at the beginning of this chapter, the evaluation of a comatose patient is reviewed not so much as a pattern for this examination, but as an illustration of the variation from the routine when circumstances are not optimal.

Thus, for the comatose patient discussed above, the history is condensed, therapy is begun, and the physical examination is limited to those areas of immediate concern for the patient's survival. On the other hand, with a patient who demonstrates an urgent need to talk, the entire time of a visit may need to be spent discussing a chief complaint and a psycho-social history.

The principle should be clear - that the clinician's judgment must be used to set priorities in the patient assessment process based on the immediate needs of the patient. Subsequent visits are often necessary to piece together a complete history and physical examination.

REFERENCE

1. Plum, F. and Posner, J.A.: Diagnosis of Stupor and Coma, 2nd Edition, F.A. Davis Co., Philadelphia, 1972.

CHAPTER 26

PUTTING IT ALL TOGETHER

Within this text we have been trying to express a philosophy which we believe must serve as a guide to the practitioner throughout his professional life. The best modality for the total assessment and management of the patient is a competent, caring clinician who looks upon his patient as a person and who diagnoses and treats that person's illness - not a disease.

Since the phenomenon of <u>illness</u> is the process of interaction of one or more <u>problems</u> in a <u>specific host</u>, assessment of any person's health status requires the synthesis of knowledge about the individual, his problems, and the illness. Absence of adequate information about any of these elements leads, inevitably, to less than optimum patient care.

Information about the host is primarily dependent upon obtaining an adequate health history with accurate data about past medical history, family history, and personal and social history. The careful review of current symptoms, a thorough physical examination, and selected laboratory information form the data base for evaluation of the host's response to the <u>disease</u> - i.e., the patient's <u>illness</u>.

An important step in total assessment is the establishment of a diagnosis, or, in terms of the problem-oriented record, the refinement or resolution of the problem.

The establishment of a correct diagnosis depends upon two major processes - the collection of data from the patient and the analysis of the data. This textbook is principally a guide for the collection of data from the medical history and the physical examination. No proper or complete analysis of data can be made if the data base is inadequate or in error. Failure to elicit the fact that there have been several deaths from coronary heart disease in the patient's immediate family will interfere with the clinician's interpretation of the anxiety state in a middle-aged man with mild chest pain. Failure to pick up the diastolic murmur and to see the splinter hemorrhages in the nail beds will not allow the diagnostic process to consider that the patient may have subacute bacterial endocarditis. Failure to perform a rectal examination, thereby missing the presence of a carcinoma, will lead to improper analysis of the patient's symptoms and to an incomplete diagnostic process. It is obvious that a careful, thorough, and accurate data base must be constructed prior to the process of data analysis. The practitioner must be able to perform this accurate type of examination by a lifetime of improvement through practice.

The second phase of the diagnostic process - the analysis of data - is a logical evaluation of the facts accumulated in the initial data base. The practitioner selects those abnormalities in the data base which seem most important and then tries to associate these abnormalities with various disease entities. His ability to do this well is based upon his knowledge of basic sciences and of clinical medicine, i.e., of the disease process.

If the examiner does not know that certain drugs can damage the liver and thereby produce jaundice, his analysis of the causes of jaundice in a patient will be faulty. If the practitioner is unaware that there is disease known as osteogenesis imperfecta, he certainly cannot make this diagnosis, and his assessment of the patient's medical status will be incomplete. Knowing one's limitations and knowing when referral is in order are normal expected parts of the process of evaluation and management of illness.

As indicated in Chapter 2, the establishment of rapport with the patient is a major goal in the work-up process. It should be clear by now that adequate assessment of the host and of his symptoms and signs depends upon good interchange between the clinician and his patient.

This rapport is also a significant factor in the management of the patient's illness. It must never be forgotten that the taking of a history and the performance of a careful physical examination are parts of the therapeutic process as well as of diagnosis. Every health professional who comes in contact with the patient has a role to play in reducing the patient's anxiety and uncertainty, but the clinician who initiates the evaluation of the patient can provide the best therapeutic support for the patient in his anxious state by a careful, thoughtful assessment of the whole person.

" . . . for the secret of the care of the patient is in caring for the patient."

APPENDIX I: SAMPLE CASE REPORT

This is presented as a sample of a complete writeup of a patient's history and physical examination. It incorporates all of the elements of the data base expected from our students in a suggested order and format. As recommended throughout, the recording makes minimal use of the terms "negative" or "normal" but emphasizes, by use of specific entries, what information was sought on history, and what was observed or tested in the examination.

The patient's history in this example incorporates several problems. The physical findings, however, have been extracted from the sections entitled "Recording" in the chapters on physical examination and are, therefore, all within normal limits. The order of the reporting varies slightly from that of the text and is presented here in a more convenient order:

BASIC DATA: Mrs. J.H.A.   Date of Examination
1234 Middleville Road
Stony Brook, N.Y
Date of Birth: 9/24/1930, Washington, D.C.
Source: Patient. History seems reliable

HISTORY: CC: "Headache for 20 years."

PI: Mrs. A had only infrequent headaches through childhood and adolescence, but beginning at about age 25 (two years after her marriage) she noted the beginning of a right-sided temporal headache which at first seemed to be present once or twice a year, particularly in hot weather. For the past 4 years she has had these headaches at 2-3 month intervals, but for the past week has had nearly daily bouts which have become much more severe, accounting for her visit to the office today.

Characteristically, the headache begins as a spot of pain on her right temple, becomes penetrating and seems to bore right into her skull. Within a 2-3 minute period the pain spreads to the whole right side of her face and neck. The headaches vary in severity from moderate to so severe that Mrs. A. must stop what she is doing to lie down. Has vertigo with severe headache only. Usually they last from 2-3 hours. She knows of nothing that will bring on or relieve an attack although she is aware of the fact that they usually occur after 2 or 3 o'clock in the afternoon and do not awaken her at night. She has had anorexia and nausea with severe sttacks but has never vomited. She has seen no "flashes" or "sparks" prior to or during these attacks.

A brother, age 40, has had a similar problem which is under treatment as migraine. Her case was considered by her brother's doctor (J.P.M____, M.D.) not to be migraine and she was given some tablets (type unknown) last year which did no good since her attacks were generally over within 3 hours whether she took the tablets or not. Now takes 3 aspirin tablets at onset of headache. She had an EEG as part of her work-up which was said to be normal.

PAST HISTORY

Medical: Pneumonia, right 1956. Duodenal ulcer 1970. No difficulty in past 5 years.

Surgical: Appendectomy 1951. No sequelae.

Injuries: None.

Allergies: Penicillin, manifested by drug fever and urticaria - 1956. None known to foods, other drugs, pollens or contact materials.

Immunizations: Smallpox, typhoid and one other (type unknown) before going abroad in 1969.

Current medication: None other than in PI.

REVIEW OF SYSTEMS

General: Overall state of health is good. No major weight changes. Can carry out normal ADL except when headache is severe.

Integument: No eruptions, rashes except for urticaria (see PH). No disorders of hair or nails.

Head: See PI. No history of trauma.

Eyes: No vision problems. Wears glasses past 5 years only for reading. No diplopia. No eye exam for past 5 years.

Ears: Normal hearing, no tinnitus, no infections.

Nose: No epistaxis, discharge, or sinusitis.

Mouth, teeth, gums: Visits dentist 2x/yr. No major problems.

Throat and neck: Infrequent sore throat, no neck stiffness or pain, no hoarseness.

Breasts: No masses, discharge, bleeding.

Resp.: No wheeze, cough, SOB. Has colds about 3x/yr. No Rx other than aspirin. Last x-ray 1 yr. ago - neg.

<u>CV</u>: No chest pain, palpitation, hypertension, or vascular problems.

<u>GI</u>: Appetite good. One BM every day. No jaundice. Ulcer (see <u>PH</u>) requires no Rx. No nausea - except as in PI.

<u>GU</u>: No dysuria, hematuria, nocturia, VD.

<u>GYN</u>: Grav 0 Para 0. No contraception. No reason known for lack of conception. Onset menses age 12, q. 25-28 days. LMP 5 days ago. No dysmenorrhea. Pap smear done 6 mo. ago at routine check-up - negative.

<u>Musc.</u>: No weakness, joint pains, cramps.

<u>NP</u>: No syncope, vertigo (except with severe headache - see PI), dizziness. Intelligent and well-oriented in 3 spheres. Sensorium intact. No paresthesias. Affect seems good but there is a sense of rigidity and "perfection-seeking" about her responses which seems inconsistent with her attempt to be friendly and helpful. No apparent depression.

<u>Lymph-Hemat</u>: No adenopathy, bleeding disorders.

<u>Endocrine</u>: Prefers cold weather, but is tolerant of heat. No glycosuria, polydipsia, excessive sweating.

FAMILY HISTORY

M. died at age 67 - heart attack.
F. died at age 70 - pulmonary embolism.
1 sister d. age 3 mo. of congenital heart dis.
1 brother in good health except for headache (see PI).
No history of diabetes, cancer, hypertension, or other familial
  disease.

PERS/SOC HISTORY

<u>Activities of Daily Living:</u>

<u>Diet</u>: (See table on following page)

<u>Sleep</u>: 6 hours, sometimes wakes to urinate but generally falls back to sleep unless worrying about something.

<u>Exercise</u>: Rarely. Little physical activity except swimming in summer.

<u>Occupation</u>: Real estate salesperson - 15 years. Hours vary so has little time for recreation. Combined family income adequate.

Diet:

Time	Food/Fluid	Approx. Amount
8 A.M.	Juice	4 ounces
	Toast	1 Slice
	Coffee (Milk & Sugar)	1 Cup
11 A.M.	Coffee (Milk & Sugar)	1 Cup
1 P.M.	Roast Beef Sandwich	
	Vegetable Soup	1 Cup
	Tea	1 Cup
4 P.M.	Fruit Salad	1 Cup
7 P.M.	Pork Chops	2
	Mixed Vegetables	1 Cup
	Baked Potato	1
	Tossed Green Salad	Small bowl
	Chocolate Cake	1 Slice
	Coffee (Milk & Sugar)	1 Cup

Habits: Does not touch alcohol, cigarettes. No over-the-counter drugs except aspirin (see PI).

Geographic: Has lived on Long Island all her life. Travelled to Europe once with husband in 1969. Didn't like it.

Marit/Sexual: Preferred not to discuss since she sees gynecologist regularly.

Interpersonal Relationships: Lives with husband (postal worker). Married 22 years - unwilling to discuss relationship. Would like to open her own business but husband doesn't support the idea. Has friends at work. Socializes only occasionally.

Intrapersonal Functioning: Says she is satisfied with limited social and recreational activity as she works hard and needs rest. Yet has indicated wish for own business in real estate "where I can prove myself." Recognizes that she is rigid and highly self-controlled.

PATIENT PROFILE: This is a pleasant but highly rigid, self-controlled woman who seems unhappy but denies problems, who has no apparent financial or social difficulties. Lives with her husband.

PHYSICAL EXAMINATION

Vital Signs and Measurements: Ht. 163 cm. (5'4") Wt. 61.4 kg. (135 lbs) Temp. 37° C. (98.6°F.) oral; Pulse 80 reg.; Resp. 16 reg.; BP RA 135/80, LA 130/80 supine, LA 130/80 upright.

General: Mrs. A. is an alert, well-developed, moderately obese, 47-year-old white woman appearing about stated age in no acute distress. No speech defects.

Skin: Pink in color, good turgor, warm to touch, no excoriations or lesions.

Hair: Normal distribution and consistency.

Nails: No deformities, nail beds pink, no clubbing.

Head: Symmetrical, normocephalic. Normal hair distribution.

Face: No muscle weakness. Appropriate facial expression. Light touch intact.

Eyes: Lashes and brows present. No stare or ptosis. Normal ocular tension. Conjunctivae clear. Sclerae white. No defects of cornea or iris. Pupils equal, round, react to light and accommodation (PERRLA). Snellen 20/20 OD, 20/20 OS. Color intact for red-green. Fields normal by confrontation. Extraocular movements (EOM) normal, no nystagmus or strabismus.

Fundi: Red reflex: clear;
Discs: flat with sharp margins. Cup normal;
Vessels: arterioles and venules normal. No A-V nicking;
Retina: no hemorrhages or exudates. Macula normal, fo-
veal reflex present.

Ears: No masses, lesions of auricles or canals. No discharge. Both TM pearly-gray, no perforations, light reflex present. Watch ticking heard bilaterally. Weber test - normal.

Nose: Patent bilaterally. No septal deviation or perforation. Mucosa pink. Can identify alcohol.

Mouth: Can clench teeth. Mucosa and gingivae pink, no lesions or masses. Teeth in good repair. Tongue protrudes in mid-line. No tremor.

Pharynx: Mucosa pink, no lesions. Tonsils absent. Uvula rises in mid-line on phonation. Gag reflex present, bilaterally.

Neck: Full ROM. Veins not distended. Carotid pulsations equal and of good quality. Thyroid not palpable. Trachea in mid-line. No lymphadenopathy.

Thorax: Insp: Symmetrical, full expansion equal bilaterally.
AP diameter not increased.
Palp: No tenderness. No axillary adenopathy.

Lungs: Palp: Fremitus equal bilaterally.
      Perc: Lung fields resonant throughout.
      Ausc: Breath sounds normal. Vocal sounds normal. No
            rales, rhonchi, rubs.

Breasts: Symmetrical. Contour and consistency appropriate for
age and parity. No retraction or nipple discharge. No masses or
tenderness.

Heart: Insp: No heave. Apical impulse in 5th LICS medial to MCL.
      Palp: No heave, thrill or rib retraction.
      Perc: LBCD at MCL in 5th ICS.
      Ausc: Rate 80/min. regular. Sounds normal. S_2 (Aort) $>$
            S_2 (Pulm). S_2 split on inspiration. No murmurs,
            gallop, rubs.

Abdomen: Insp: Abdomen flat, no skin lesions, no hernia, no
            pulsations.
        Ausc: Normal bowel sounds q. ten seconds. No bruits.
        Palp: No tenderness or masses; spleen, kidneys not pal-
            pated, liver edge at costal margin, non-tender.
        Perc: Normal abdominal tympany. Liver 12 cm. long.

Back: Normal curvature, no spinal tenderness, no CVA tenderness.

Extremities: No skin, hair or nail abnormalities. Full range of
motion (ROM). Normal gait. Romberg negative. Muscle strength
intact. No venous dilation. Radial, femoral, dorsalis pedis and
post tibial pulses all palpable and equal. No lymphadenopathy. Biceps, triceps, patellar, and Achilles reflexes all 2+. Plantar reflex normal.

Genitalia: External: Normal pubic hair, no labial swellings or le-
                   sions. Normal clitoris. Introitus admits 2
                   fingers. No urethral redness, swelling or dis-
                   charge. Skene's and Bartholin's not inflamed.
                   Perineum intact, no scars.

          Internal: Vagina: No bulging or masses, mucosa intact
                        and pink.
                  Uterus: Anterior, average size, regular shape,
                        mobile, normal consistency.
                  Cervix: Compatible with nullipara, posterior
                        position, 0.5 cm. erosion 3 o'clock.
                  Adnexa: Tubes not palpated, ovaries not en-
                        larged, slight tenderness.
                  Cul-de-sac: No bulging, tenderness or masses.
                  Discharge: Clear, mucoid, 1+, no odor.
                  Pap: To lab.

Rectal: No external or internal hemorrhoids, no fissures or fistulae. Sphincter tone good. No masses or tenderness. No stool or visible blood on glove.

Neurological: Cerebral function: Alert and responsive, memory and orientation intact. Appropriate behavior and speech.

Cranial Nerves:
I - Identifies alcohol.
II - Vision 20/20 both eyes. Color intact. Visual fields by gross confrontation normal.
III, IV, VI - EOM intact. No ptosis. No nystagmus. PERRLA.
V - Sensory intact, jaw closure normal.
VII - Facial muscles symmetrical, no weakness.
VIII - Hearing intact. Weber no lateralization.
IX-X - Swallowing and gag reflex intact. Uvula in mid-line.
XI - Head movement and shrug of shoulders normal.
XII - Tongue protrudes in mid-line, no tremor.

Cerebellar function: Finger to nose, heel to shin co-ordination intact. Gait normal. Romberg negative.

Motor system: No atrophy, weakness, or tremors.

Sensory system: Intact to light touch, vibration. Pin-prick, hot-cold, deep pain not tested.

REFLEXES

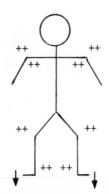

Problems
----
1. Headache - probably migraine
2. Sterility - patient or husband
3. Penicillin allergy
4. Inactive duodenal ulcer
5. Moderate obesity

Signature

Initial Note

Problem: Headache

S: Headache for 20 years. Began at about age 25 (2 years after marriage). Characteristically begins as pain in right temple, spreads within minutes to right side of head and neck, lasting 2-3 hours. Pain is boring and seems to penetrate skull. Occasionally requires her to stop work and lie down. Had 4-5 per year but now almost daily. No known cause or relief. Always afternoon. No scotomata; has nausea with severe attacks. One brother (age 40) has migraine.

O: Head, face, neck, ears, mouth, eyes, neurological within normal limits.

A: The pain and attack features are characteristic of migraine. Pt. is tense, rigid, overly-neat, which fits the typical personality pattern. Migraine in brother is also typical.

P: Dx. Per protocol, therapeutic trial of ergotamine, then referral to physician.

Rx. 2.0 mg. ergotamine tartrate at start of attack, then repeat 2 mg. at 30 min. and again at 1 hr. if necessary. Pt. will phone results.

Pt. Ed. Schedule revisits to explain in more detail this syndrome and its relationships to behavior and interpersonal relationships. Pt. told that medication for longer term use (methysergide) may be useful, but that alteration of life patterns and behavior is required. Further counseling may be scheduled with psychologist or psychiatrist in future.

Signature

APPENDIX II
DENVER DEVELOPMENTAL SCREENING TEST

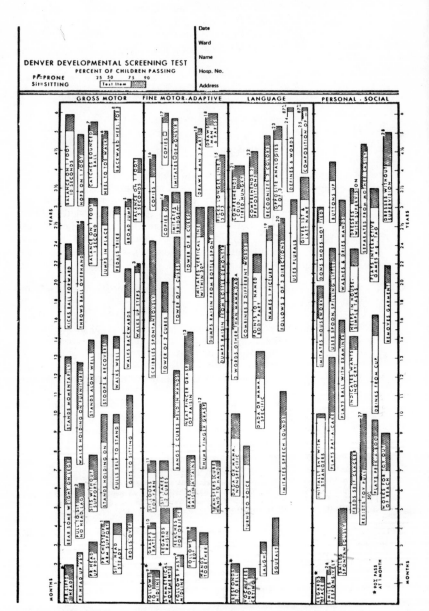

Reprinted with permission. © 1969, William K. Frankenburg, M. D.
and Josiah B. Dodds, Ph. D. , University of Colorado Medical Center.

1. Try to get child to smile by smiling, talking or waving to him. Do not touch him.
2. When child is playing with toy, pull it away from him. Pass if he resists.
3. Child does not have to be able to tie shoes or button in the back.
4. Move yarn slowly in an arc from one side to the other, about 6" above child's face. Pass if eyes follow 90° to midline. (Past midline; 180°)
5. Pass if child grasps rattle when it is touched to the backs or tips of fingers.
6. Pass if child continues to look where yarn disappeared or tries to see where it went. Yarn should be dropped quickly from sight from tester's hand without arm movement.
7. Pass if child picks up raisin with any part of thumb and a finger.
8. Pass if child picks up raisin with the ends of thumb and index finger using an overhand approach.

9. Pass any enclosed form. Fail continuous round motions	10. Which line is longer? (Not bigger.) Turn paper upside down and repeat. (3/3 or 5/6)	11. Pass any crossing lines.	12. Have child copy first. If failed, demonstrate

When giving items 9, 11 and 12, do not name the forms. Do not demonstrate 9 and 11.
13. When scoring, each pair (2 arms, 2 legs, etc.) counts as one part.
14. Point to picture and have child name it. (No credit is given for sounds only.)

15. Tell child to: Give block to Mommie; put block on table; put block on floor. Pass 2 of 3. (Do not help child by pointing, moving head or eyes.)
16. Ask child: What do you do when you are cold? .. hungry? .. tired? Pass 2 of 3.
17. Tell child to: Put block on table; under table; in front of chair; behind chair. Pass 3 of 4. (Do not help child by pointing, moving head or eyes.)
18. Ask child: If fire is hot, ice is ?; Mother is a woman, Dad is a ?; a horse is big, a mouse is ? Pass 2 of 3.
19. Ask child: What is a ball? .. lake? .. desk? .. house? .. banana? .. curtain? .. ceiling? .. hedge? .. pavement? Pass if defined in terms of use, shape, what it is made of or general category (such as banana is fruit, not just yellow). Pass 6 of 9.
20. Ask child: What is a spoon made of? .. a shoe made of? .. a door made of? (No other objects may be substituted.) Pass 3 of 3.
21. When placed on stomach, child lifts chest off table with support of forearms and/or hands.
22. When child is on back, grasp his hands and pull him to sitting. Pass if head does not hang back.
23. Child may use wall or rail only, not person. May not crawl.
24. Child must throw ball overhand 3 feet to within arm's reach of tester.
25. Child must perform standing broad jump over width of test sheet. (8-1/2 in.)

26. Tell child to walk forward, ∞∞∞∞➤ heel within 1 inch of toe. Tester may demonstrate. Child must walk 4 consecutive steps, 2 out of 3 trials.
27. Bounce ball to child who should stand 3 feet away from tester. Child must catch ball with hands, not arms, 2 out of 3 trials.

28. Tell child to walk backward, ◄∞∞∞∞ to within 1 inch of heel. Tester may demonstrate. Child must walk 4 consecutive steps, 2 out of 3 trials.
DATE AND BEHAVIORAL OBSERVATIONS (how child feels at time of test, relation to tester, attention span, verbal behavior, self-confidence, etc.):

To obtain original copies of the Anthropometric charts that appear on pps. 346 - 353, please write to MEDIFORM SYSTEMS, 32 Jameson Road, Newton, Massachusetts 02158.

PERCENTILE CHART FOR MEASUREMENTS OF INFANT BOYS

THIS CHART provides for infant boys standards of reference for body weight and recumbent length by month from birth to 28 months and for head circumference by week from birth to 28 weeks. It is based upon repeated measurements at selected ages of a group of more than 100 white infants of North European ancestry living under normal conditions of health and home life in Boston, Mass. The distribution of the measurements obtained from the infants at each age is expressed in percentiles, each percentile giving a value which represents a particular position in the normal range of occurrences. The number of the percentile refers to the position which a measurement of the given value would hold in any typical series of 100 infants. Thus, the 10th percentile gives the value for the tenth in any hundred; that is, 9 infants of the same sex and age would be expected to be smaller in the measurement under consideration while 90 would be expected to be larger than the figure given. Similarly the 90th percentile would indicate that 89 infants might be expected to be smaller than the figure given while 10 would be larger. The 50th percentile represents the median or midposition in the customary range. Here, the 10th and 90th percentiles are presented in heavy lines to show the limits within which most infants remain. The lighter lines in the graphs divide the distributions into segments for ready recognition and description of individual differences as well as of the "regularity" of progress. The 3rd and 97th percentiles represent unusual though not necessarily abnormal findings.

In line with common usage in the United States, the charts are ruled on a scale in pounds to represent weight. They are ruled, however, in centimeters to represent length and head circumference, because this scale facilitates accuracy in measuring and recording and centimeter rules and tapes are readily available. For the convenience of those preferring them, scales for kilograms and inches are placed outside of the principal scales and paralleling them. Therefore, if weights are taken in kilograms and lengths and head circumferences in inches, they may be plotted directly without conversion by placing a ruler at the appropriate points on the outer scales of the charts.

To determine the percentile position of any measurement at a given age, the vertical age line

is located and a dot is placed where this intersects the horizontal line representing the value obtained from the measurement. Vertical lines give age by one-month intervals for weight and length and one-week intervals for head circumference; horizontal lines give ½-pound, 1-cm. and 0.5-cm. intervals respectively. This permits by interpolation accurate placement for age to weeks, for weights to 2 ounces and for centimeters to 0.5 cm. Recognition of the position within or outside of the range held by an infant in respect to each measurement recorded calls attention to the relative size and build of the individual at the time. More importantly, comparisons of percentile positions held by these measurements at repeated periodic examinations indicate adherence to or possibly significant deviation from previous percentile positions. Under normal circumstances, one expects an infant to maintain a similar position from age to age — that is, on or near one percentile line or between the same two lines. Occasional sharp deviations or gradual but continuing shifts from one percentile position to another call for further investigation as to their causes. In all cases, readings of measurements should be checked and care should be taken to secure the same position of the infant at all examinations. The following procedures were used in obtaining these norms and therefore are recommended:

Body Weight — The infant is weighed without clothing, preferably on special infant scales.

Recumbent Length — The infant lies relaxed on a firm surface parallel to a centimeter rule or on a special infant measuring board which permits the following procedure. The soles of the feet are held firmly against a fixed upright at the zero mark on the rule, and a movable square is brought firmly against the vertex. Care must be taken to secure extension at the knees, and the head should be held so that the eyes face the ceiling.

Head Circumference — This measurement is more satisfactory if taken with the infant lying on his back. The tape is passed around the head from above and placed anteriorly over the lower forehead just above the supraorbital ridges. With the position of the tape thus fixed anteriorly, the largest circumference is obtained by passing it posteriorly over the most prominent part of the occiput.

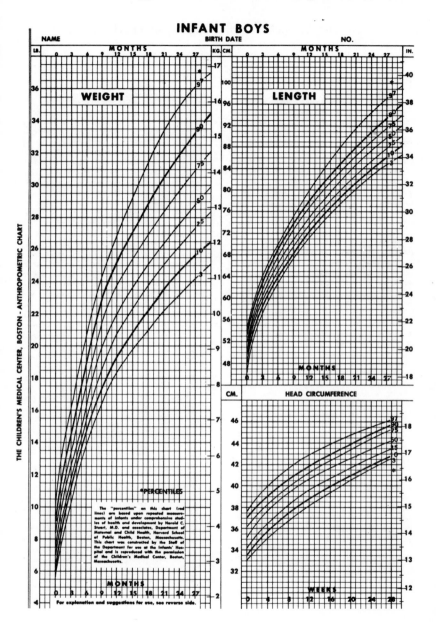

PERCENTILE CHART FOR MEASUREMENTS OF BOYS

THIS CHART provides for boys standards of reference for body weight and recumbent length at ages between 2 and 6 years and for weight and standing height from 6 to 13 years. It is based upon repeated measurements at selected ages of a group of more than 100 white boys of North European ancestry living under normal conditions of health and home life in Boston, Mass. The distribution of the measurements obtained from these children at each age is expressed in percentiles, each percentile giving a value which represents a particular position in the normal range of occurrences. The number of the percentile refers to the position which a measurement of the given value would hold in any typical series of 100 children. Thus, the 10th percentile gives the value for the tenth in any hundred; that is, 9 children of the same sex and age would be expected to be smaller in the measurement under consideration while 90 would be expected to be larger than the figure given. Similarly the 90th percentile would indicate that 89 children might be expected to be smaller than the figure given while 10 would be larger. The 50th percentile represents the median or midposition in the customary range. Here, the 10th and 90th percentiles are represented in heavy lines to show the limits within which most children remain. The lighter lines in the graphs divide the distribution into segments for ready recognition and description of individual differences as well as of the "regularity" of progress. The 3rd and 97th percentiles represent unusual though not necessarily abnormal findings.

In line with common usage in the United States, the charts are ruled on a scale in pounds to represent weight. They are ruled, however, in centimeters to represent length under 6 years and height thereafter, because this scale facilitates accuracy in measuring and recording and centimeter rules and tapes are readily available. For the convenience of those preferring them, scales for kilograms and inches are placed outside of the principal scales and paralleling them. Therefore, if weights are taken in kilograms and lengths and heights in inches, they may be plotted directly without conversion by placing a ruler at the appropriate points on the outer scales of the chart.

To determine the percentile position of any measurement at a given age, the vertical age line is located and a dot is placed where this intersects the horizontal line representing the value obtained from the measurement. Vertical lines give age by 2-month intervals and horizontal lines by 2-pound and 2-cm. intervals. This permits by interpolation accurate placement for age to ½ month and for measurements to ½ pound or 0.5 cm. Recognition of the position held by a child within or outside of the range in respect to each measurement recorded calls attention to the relative size and build of the individual at the time. More importantly, comparisons of percentile positions held by these measurements at repeated periodic examinations indicate adherence to or possibly significant deviation from previous percentile positions. Under normal circumstances, one expects a child to maintain a similar position from age to age — that is, on or near one percentile line or between the same two lines. Occasionally encountered sharp deviations or more gradual but continuing shifts from one percentile position to another call for further investigation as to their causes. In all cases, readings of measurements should be checked and care should be taken to secure the same position of the child accurately at all examinations. The following procedures were used in obtaining these norms and therefore are recommended:

Body Weight — The child is weighed without clothing except light undergarments.

Recumbent Length — The child lies relaxed on a firm surface parallel to a centimeter rule. The soles of the feet are held firmly against a fixed upright at the zero mark on the rule, and a movable square is brought firmly against the vertex. The head is held so that the eyes face the ceiling.

Height — The child's heels should be near together, and heels, buttocks and occiput should be against a firm vertical upright mounting the measuring stick. The eyes should be horizontal and approximately in the same plane as the external auditory canals. A right angle triangle or other movable device should be placed firmly on the head at right angles to the measuring stick and the measurement read after a satisfactory position has been adopted.

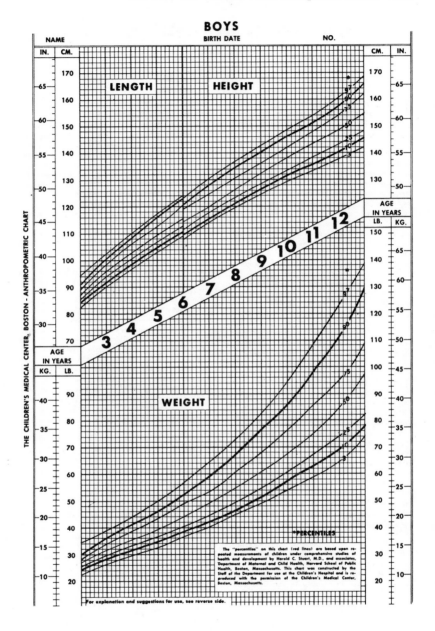

PERCENTILE CHART FOR MEASUREMENTS OF INFANT GIRLS

THIS CHART provides for infant girls· standards of reference for body weight and recumbent length by month from birth to 28 months and for head circumference by week from birth to 28 weeks. It is based upon repeated measurements at selected ages of a group of more than 100 white infants of North European ancestry living under normal conditions of health and home life in Boston, Mass. The distribution of the measurements obtained from the infants at each age is expressed in percentiles, each percentile giving a value which represents a particular position in the normal range of occurrences. The number of the percentile refers to the position which a measurement of the given value would hold in any typical series of 100 infants. Thus, the 10th percentile gives the value for the tenth in any hundred; that is, 9 infants of the same sex and age would be expected to be smaller in the measurement under consideration while 90 would be expected to be larger than the figure given. Similarly the 90th percentile would indicate that 89 infants might be expected to be smaller than the figure given while 10 would be larger. The 50th percentile represents the median or midposition in the customary range. Here, the 10th and 90th percentiles are presented in heavy lines to show the limits within which most infants remain. The lighter lines in the graphs divide the distributions into segments for ready recognition and description of individual differences as well as of the "regularity" of progress. The 3rd and 97th percentiles represent unusual though not necessarily abnormal findings.

In line with common usage in the United States, the charts are ruled on a scale in pounds to represent weight. They are ruled, however, in centimeters to represent length and head circumference, because this scale facilitates accuracy in measuring and recording and centimeter rules and tapes are readily available. For the convenience of those preferring them, scales for kilograms and inches are placed outside of the principal scales and paralleling them. Therefore, if weights are taken in kilograms and lengths and head circumferences in inches, they may be plotted directly without conversion by placing a ruler at the appropriate points on the outer scales of the charts.

To determine the percentile position of any measurement at a given age, the vertical age line is located and a dot is placed where this intersects the horizontal line representing the value obtained from the measurement. Vertical lines give age by one-month intervals for weight and length and one-week intervals for head circumference; horizontal lines give ½-pound, 1-cm. and 0.5-cm. intervals respectively. This permits by interpolation accurate placement for age to weeks, for weights to 2 ounces and for centimeters to 0.5 cm. Recognition of the position within or outside of the range held by an infant in respect to each measurement recorded calls attention to the relative size and build of the individual at the time. More importantly, comparisons of percentile positions held by these measurements at repeated periodic examinations indicate adherence to or possibly significant deviation from previous percentile positions. Under normal circumstances, one expects an infant to maintain a similar position from age to age — that is, on or near one percentile line or between the same two lines. Occasional sharp deviations or gradual but continuing shifts from one percentile position to another call for further investigation as to their causes. In all cases, readings of measurements should be checked and care should be· taken to secure the same position of the infant at all examinations. The following procedures were used in obtaining these norms and therefore are recommended:

Body Weight — The infant is weighed without clothing, preferably on special infant scales.

Recumbent Length — The infant lies relaxed on a firm surface parallel to a centimeter rule or on a special infant measuring board which permits the following procedure. The soles of the feet are held firmly against a fixed upright at the zero mark on the rule, and a movable square is brought firmly against the vertex. Care must be taken to secure extension at the knees, and the head should be held so that the eyes face the ceiling.

Head Circumference — This measurement is more satisfactory if taken with the infant lying on his back. The tape is passed around the head from above and placed anteriorly over the lower forehead just above the supraorbital ridges. With the position of the tape thus fixed anteriorly, the largest circumference is obtained by passing it posteriorly over the most prominent part of the occiput.

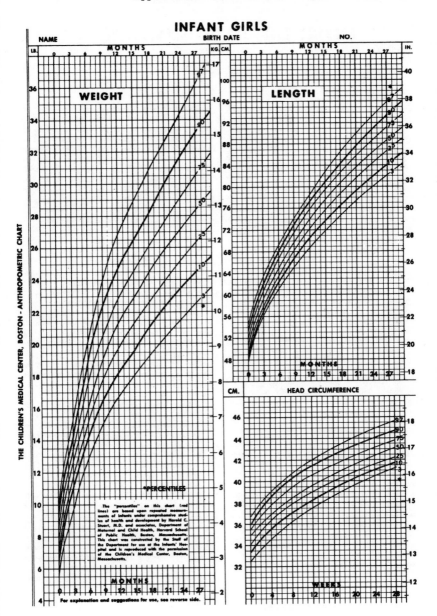

INFANT GIRLS

PERCENTILE CHART FOR MEASUREMENTS OF GIRLS

THIS CHART provides for girls standards of reference for body weight and recumbent length at ages between 2 and 6 years and for weight and standing height from 6 to 13 years. It is based upon repeated measurements at selected ages of a group of more than 100 white girls of North European ancestry living under normal conditions of health and home life in Boston, Mass. The distribution of the measurements obtained from these children at each age is expressed in percentiles, each percentile giving a value which represents a particular position in the normal range of occurrences. The number of the percentile refers to the position which a measurement of the given value would hold in any typical series of 100 children. Thus, the 10th percentile gives the value for the tenth in any hundred; that is, 9 children of the same sex and age would be expected to be smaller in the measurement under consideration while 90 would be expected to be larger than the figure given. Similarly the 90th percentile would indicate that 89 children might be expected to be smaller than the figure given while 10 would be larger. The 50th percentile represents the median or midposition in the customary range. Here, the 10th and 90th percentiles are represented in heavy lines to show the limits within which most children remain. The lighter lines in the graphs divide the distribution into segments for ready recognition and description of individual differences as well as of the "regularity" of progress. The 3rd and 97th percentiles represent unusual though not necessarily abnormal findings.

In line with common usage in the United States, the charts are ruled on a scale in pounds to represent weight. They are ruled, however, in centimeters to represent length under 6 years and height thereafter, because this scale facilitates accuracy in measuring and recording and centimeter rules and tapes are readily available. For the convenience of those preferring them, scales for kilograms and inches are placed outside of the principal scales and paralleling them. Therefore, if weights are taken in kilograms and lengths and heights in inches, they may be plotted directly without conversion by placing a ruler at the appropriate points on the outer scales of the chart.

To determine the percentile position of any measurement at a given age, the vertical age line is located and a dot is placed where this intersects the horizontal line representing the value obtained from the measurement. Vertical lines give age by 2-month intervals and horizontal lines by 2-pound and 2-cm. intervals. This permits by interpolation accurate placement for age to ½ month and for measurements to ½ pound or 0.5 cm. Recognition of the position held by a child within or outside of the range in respect to each measurement recorded calls attention to the relative size and build of the individual at the time. More importantly, comparisons of percentile positions held by these measurements at repeated periodic examinations indicate adherence to or possibly significant deviation from previous percentile positions. Under normal circumstances, one expects a child to maintain a similar position from age to age — that is, on or near one percentile line or between the same two lines. Occasionally encountered sharp deviations or more gradual but continuing shifts from one percentile position to another call for further investigation as to their causes. In all cases, readings of measurements should be checked and care should be taken to secure the same position of the child accurately at all examinations. The following procedures were used in obtaining these norms and therefore are recommended:

Body Weight — The child is weighed without clothing except light undergarments.

Recumbent Length — The child lies relaxed on a firm surface parallel to a centimeter rule. The soles of the feet are held firmly against a fixed upright at the zero mark on the rule, and a movable square is brought firmly against the vertex. The head is held so that the eyes face the ceiling.

Height — The child's heels should be near together, and heels, buttocks and occiput should be against a firm vertical upright mounting the measuring stick. The eyes should be horizontal and approximately in the same plane as the external auditory canals. A right angle triangle or other movable device should be placed firmly on the head at right angles to the measuring stick and the measurement read after a satisfactory position has been adopted.

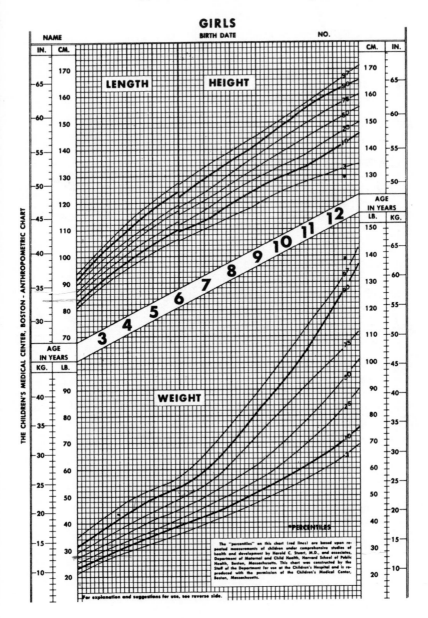

CREDITS FOR ILLUSTRATIONS

DR. CLARENCE BERGER, Brooklyn, N.Y.:
Original photograph for Fig. 8.5

MS. WANDA DePAUL, Brooklyn, N.Y.:
Drawings for Figs. 12.1, 12.2

DR. ARTHUR FRIEDLANDER, VA Hospital, Northport, N.Y.:
Original photographs for Figs. 10.6, 10.7, 10.8, 10.9, 10.10, 10.11, 10.12

MS. KATHY GEBHARDT, SUNY at Stony Brook:
Drawings for Figs. 4.1, 8.8, 12.10, 12.11, 12.12, 12.13, 12.14, 12.15

MR. ANTOL HERSKOVITZ and MR. LEE RICHMOND, Health Sciences Media Services, SUNY at Stony Brook:
Figs. 12.3, 12.4, 12.5, 12.6, 12.7, 12.8, 12.9, 17.3, 17.4, 17.5, 17.6, 17.7, 17.8

DR. INDERJIT KATYAL, VA Hospital, Northport, N.Y.:
Phonocardiograms for Figs. 13.6, 13.10

DR. BERNARD POTTER, Dix Hills, N.Y.:
Original photographs for Figs. 7.4, 7.6

MR. ROBERT SCHWARTZ, The Coney Island Hospital, Brooklyn, N.Y.:
Original photographs for Figs. 6.1, 9.3, 9.4, 9.7, 11.8, 14.5, 15.4

MRS. BARBARA-JANE SINNI, Bellport, N.Y.:
Drawings for Figs. 7.5, 17.9

WALTER REED ARMY MEDICAL CENTER, Washington, D.C.:
Original photographs for Figs. 7.1, 8.2, 9.5

MR. ROBERT VOLLMER, VA Hospital, Northport, N.Y.:
Front and back cover designs

MR. ALFRED YOUNG, VA Hospital, Northport, N.Y.:
Drawings for Figs. 8.1, 9.1, 9.18, 9.20, 9.21, 9.22, 10.2, 11.4, 11.5, 11.10, 13.1, 13.2, 13.7, 13.8, 13.9, 13.11, 14.2, 14.3, 15.2, 16.2, 17.1, 17.2

MR. THEODORE WILLERS: VA Hospital, Northport, N.Y., served as general advisor and consultant for the design and layout of all illustrations. In addition, he photographed drawings, copied photographs from other credited sources above, and did original photography for all other illustrations in this textbook.

CHAPTERS 21 AND 22: Produced by the SPAN Project, School of Nursing, SUNY at Stony Brook, in conjunction with the Division of Media Services, Health Sciences Center. Supported in part by PHS Special Training Grant No. 02D-000-008-01/2.

GENERAL REFERENCES

Bates, B.: A Guide to Physical Examination, J.P. Lippincott Co., Philadelphia, 1974.

Buckingham, W.B., Sparberg, M., and Brondfonbrener, M.: A Primer of Clinical Diagnosis, Harper and Row, New York, 1971.

Burnside, J.W.: Adam's Physical Diagnosis, 15th Edition, Williams and Wilkins Co., Baltimore, 1974.

DeGowin, E.L. and DeGowin, R.L.: Bedside Diagnostic Examination, 3rd Edition, The Macmillan Co., London, 1976.

Delp, M.H. and Manning, R.T.: Major's Physical Diagnosis, 8th Edition, W.B. Saunders Co., Philadelphia, 1975.

Hochstein, E. and Rubin, A.L.: Physical Diagnosis, McGraw-Hill, New York, 1964.

Morgan, W.L., Jr. and Engel, G.L.: The Clinical Approach to the Patient, W.B. Saunders Co., Philadelphia, 1969.

Prior, J.A. and Silberstein, J.S.: Physical Diagnosis, 5th Edition, The C.V. Mosby Co., St. Louis, 1977.

Sana, J.M. and Judge, R.D.: Physical Appraisal Methods in Nursing Practice, Little, Brown and Co., Boston, 1975.

Stern, T.N.: Clinical Examination, Year Book Medical Publishers, Chicago, 1964.

INDEX

Other Books of Interest

Volume ☐1☐ **MEDICAL-SURGICAL NURSING**

A review consisting of 1500 multiple choice questions and answers referenced to textbooks.

Edited by Marguerite C. Holmes, R.N., M.A., Ed.D. and Harriet Levine, R.N., M.A.

Volume ☐2☐ **PSYCHIATRIC-MENTAL HEALTH NURSING**

A review consisting of 1500 multiple choice questions and answers referenced to textbooks.

Edited by Francis B. Arje, R.N., M.A., Charlotte H. Martin, R.N., M.A., and Irene L. Sell, R.N., M.A.

Volume ☐3☐ **MATERNAL AND CHILD HEALTH NURSING**

A review consisting of 1500 multiple choice questions and answers referenced to textbooks.

Edited by Joanne K. Griffen, R.N., M.A., Agnes V. Murray, R.N., M.A., Estelle B. Resnick, R.N., B.S., M.A., and Jean W. Tease, R.N., M.S., C.N.M.

Volume ☐4☐ **BASIC SCIENCES**

A review consisting of 1800 multiple choice questions and answers referenced to textbooks.

Edited by Marguerite C. Holmes, R.N., M.A., Ed.D., Harriet Levine, R.N., M.A., Daniel B. Murphy, Ph.D., James J. Murphy, M.S., and Victor A. Stanionis, M.S.

Volume ☐5☐ **ANATOMY AND PHYSIOLOGY**

A review consisting of 1500 multiple choice questions and answers referenced to textbooks.

Edited by Marvin I. Gottlieb, M.D., Ph.D. and Marguerite C. Holmes, R.N., M.A., Ed.D.

Volume `6` **PHARMACOLOGY**

A review consisting of 1500 multiple choice questions and answers referenced to textbooks.

Edited by Maurice B. Feinstein, Ph.D. and Harriet Levine, R.N., B.S., M.A.

Volume `7` **MICROBIOLOGY**

A review consisting of 1500 multiple choice questions and answers referenced to textbooks.

Edited by Daniel Kaminsky, M.S., Arlene Levey, R.N., M.A., and Alice Ehrhart, R.N., M.A.

Volume `8` **NUTRITION AND DIET THERAPY**

A review consisting of 1500 multiple choice questions and answers referenced to textbooks.

Edited by Rose Mirenda, Ed.D., Antoinette V. Grundy, B.S., M.A., and Esther K. Plotner, B.S.

Volume `9` **COMMUNITY HEALTH NURSING**

A review consisting of 1600 multiple choice questions and answers referenced to textbooks.

Edited by Martha M. Borlick, R.N., Ed.D., F.A.P.H.A., Beverly Henry Bowns, R.N., Dr. P.H., F.A.P.H.A., Velena Boyd, R.N., M.P.H., F.A.P.H.A., and Carolyn Feher Waltz, R.N., M.S.N.

Volume `10` **HISTORY AND LAW OF NURSING**

A review consisting of 1500 multiple choice questions and answers referenced to textbooks.

Edited by Harriet Levine, R.N., M.A. and Francis P. F. Minno, Esq.

Volume `11` **FUNDAMENTALS OF NURSING**

A review consisting of 1500 multiple choice questions and answers referenced to textbooks.

Edited by Margaret Magnus, Ph.D., R.N.

NURSING EXAMINATION REVIEW BOOKS @ $5.00 *each*

____ Vol. 1 — (#501) Medical-Surgical Nursing
____ Vol. 2 — (#502) Psych/Mental Health Nursing
____ Vol. 3 — (#503) Maternal & Child Health Nurs
____ Vol. 4 — (#504) Basic Sciences
____ Vol. 5 — (#505) Anatomy and Physiology
____ Vol. 6 — (#506) Pharmacology
____ Vol. 7 — (#507) Microbiology
____ Vol. 8 — (#508) Nutrition and Diet Therapy
____ Vol. 9 — (#509) Community Health Nursing
____ Vol. 10 — (#510) History and Law of Nursing
____ Vol. 11 — (#511) Fundamentals of Nursing
____ (#711) Practical Nursing Exam Review — Vol. 1

Available September 1, 1978

GYNECOLOGIC NURSING

NURSING OUTLINE SERIES
by
GLORIA C. ESSOKA, R.N., B.S., M.S.
RUTH L. HARRISON, R.N., B.S., M.A.
CHRISTINE W. MILLER, R.N., B.S., M.A.
JEANNE L. PALETTA, R.N., B.S., M.A.
JAVU S. PARIKH, R.N., C.N.M., B.S., M.S.
FRANCES W. QUINLESS, R.N., B.S., M.A.
PHYLLIS J. SHANLEY, R.N., B.S.

About 185 pages   ●   1978   ●   About $7.00

This volume was conceived to meet the long-felt need for a text devoted to gynecologic nursing. Specifically geared to nursing students and practicing nurses caring for patients with gynecologic problems, this book presents pertinent information in convenient outline form for ease of study and review. The first two chapters serve to reacquaint the reader with fundamentals of the discipline — reproductive biology and patient assessment. The remaining chapters are organized by developmental stages, and include representative nursing situations with problem identification and goal-oriented questions. The problems are designed as guides to the application of nursing process to gynecologic nursing care.

Table of Contents: Biology Related to Reproductive Functioning / Assessment of Individuals and Families Experiencing Gynecologic Problems / The Pre-pubertal Years / The Adolescent Years / The Young Adult / The Middle Years / The Mature Years.   **(#388)**

Maternity Nursing

Nursing Outline Series
Second Edition
by ARLYNE FRIESNER, Ed.D., R.N.
Consultant in Nursing Education
Department of Baccalaureate and
Higher Degree Programs — National League for Nursing
BEVERLY RAFF, Ph.D., R.N.
Associate Professor, School of Nursing
Adelphi University, Garden City, New York

219 pages   ●   1977   ● $6.00

Formerly entitled *Obstetric Nursing — Nursing Outline Series*, this latest edition is designed to meet the needs of students and graduate nurses for a concise but thorough review of maternity nursing. It will also serve as a useful reference manual for the maternity nurse directly involved in nursing care. It clearly delineates the important physiological and psychological changes occurring during the maternity cycle, and the related nursing implications. Emphasizing the nurse's involvement in *all* levels of health care — preventative, curative, and rehabilitative — this text is categorized into the following major sections: Trends in Maternal Care, The Prenatal Period, The Intrapartal Period, The Postnatal Period, and Newborn. Questions and bibliographies of current literature appear at the end of each section.   **(#377)**

Other Books Available

Prices subject to change.

P

Other Books Available

Prices subject to change.   MF

Other Books Available

Prices subject to change.

MB